Second Edition

MEDICAL ASSISTING
ENDOCRINOLOGY & REPRODUCTION—MODULE F

Material Selected from:

Medical Terminology with Human Anatomy, Fourth Edition
by Jane Rice

Structure & Function of the Human Body
by Frederic H. Martini and Edwin F. Bartholomew

Pediatric Nursing: Caring for Children, Second Edition
by Jane Ball and Ruth Bindler

Essentials of Medical Assisting: Administrative and Clinical Competencies
by Bonnie F. Fremgen

Quick Reference to Pediatric Clinical Skills
by Ruth Bindler and Jane Ball
for *Pediatric Nursing: Caring for Children*, Second Edition
by Jane Ball and Ruth Bindler

Workbook
by Bonnie F. Fremgen and Kathleen Wallington
for *Essentials of Medical Assisting: Administrative and Clinical Competencies*
by Bonnie F. Fremgen

Medical Assistant Test Review Programmed Learner
by Bonnie F. Fremgen, Kathleen Wallington, and Mary King

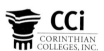

CCi
CORINTHIAN
COLLEGES, INC.

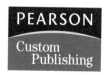

PEARSON

Custom
Publishing

Cover photograph courtesy of Index Stock Imagery.

Excerpts taken from:

Medical Terminology with Human Anatomy, Fourth
Edition by Jane Rice
Copyright © 1999, 1995, 1991
by Appleton & Lange
Published by Prentice-Hall, Inc.
A Pearson Education Company
Upper Saddle River, New Jersey 07458

Structure & Function of the Human Body by
Frederic H. Martini and Edwin F. Bartholomew
Copyright © 1999 by Frederic H. Martini, Inc.
Published by Prentice-Hall, Inc.

Pediatric Nursing: Caring for Children, Second
Edition by Jane Ball and Ruth Bindler
Copyright © 1999, 1995 by Appleton & Lange
Published by Prentice-Hall, Inc.

*Essentials of Medical Assisting: Administrative and
Clinical Competencies* by Bonnie F. Fremgen
Copyright © 1998 by Prentice-Hall, Inc.

Quick Reference to Pediatric Clinical Skills
by Ruth Bindler and Jane Ball for *Pediatric
Nursing: Caring for Children*, Second Edition
by Jane Ball and Ruth Bindler
Copyright © 1999, 1995 by Appleton & Lange
Published by Prentice-Hall, Inc.

Workbook by Bonnie F. Fremgen and Kathleen
Wallington for *Essentials of Medical Assisting:
Administrative and Clinical Competencies*
by Bonnie F. Fremgen
Copyright © 1998 by Prentice-Hall, Inc.

Medical Assistant Test Review Programmed Learner
by Bonnie F. Fremgen, Kathleen Wallington,
and Mary King
Copyright © 1999 Prentice-Hall, Inc.

This special edition published in cooperation with Pearson Custom Publishing.

Printed in the United States of America

10 9 8 7 6 5 4 3 2 1

ISBN 0-536-84474-7

2004520027

EH/LD

Please visit our web site at *www.pearsoncustom.com*

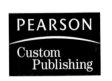

PEARSON CUSTOM PUBLISHING
75 Arlington Street, Suite 300, Boston, MA 02116
A Pearson Education Company

Credits and Acknowledgments

CCi Medical Assisting Program Series (Modules A-G)

Publisher

Pearson Custom Publishing in cooperation with Corinthian Colleges, Inc.

Editors and Project Managers

Alicia Mata, BSBM, CMA, Allied Health Program Manager, CCi

Kathy Case, MSN, RN, Program Manager Health Sciences

Donna Patterson, AA, CMA, Program Coordinator

Authors

Cheryl Niblett, CMA, BSC, Medical Assistant Program Chair

Kellie Stock, CMA, Medical Assistant Program Chair

Ted Volkmann, BS, Mathematics

Shaun Holland, CMA, Lead Medical Assistant Instructor

Tanya Mercer, Medical Assistant Instructor

Irma Blanco, BS, Director of Education

Blanca Zepeda, AA, CMA, Medical Assistant Program Chair

Vince Dick, Medical Assistant Instructor

Claudia Chaparro, AA, CMA, Medical Assistant Instructor

Sally Stegmeier, CMA, Medical Assistant Instructor

Berta Williams, NRCMA, Director of Education

Brad Johnson, Medical Assistant Program Chair

Jennifer Montoya, Medical Assistant Instructor

Steve Dovalina, CMA, Medical Assistant Instructor

Gwen Schrader, Medical Assistant Program Chair

Christine Cusano, AA, CMA, Medical Assistant & Medical Administrative Assistant Instructor

Maria Leal, Allied Health Instructor

Rachael Washington, Placement Representative

Amanda Gaugler, BS, Director of Education

Niki Good, BA Education, School President

Jacqueline Ferguson, BA, Academic Dean

Joan Jeong, BA, AA, CMA, Medical Program Director

John Etheridge, Medical Assistant Program Chair

Judith Enlow, CMA, Medical Assistant Instructor and Program Chair

Marchelle (Mickey) Weaver, BSBA, Director of Education

Kathryn Cremeans, Medical Assistant Program Chair

Sandra Shepherd, Medical Assistant Instructor

Dorit Soltanovich, MD, Medical Program Director

Dottie Fields, RMA, Education Chair, Medical Assistant and Medical Administrative Assistant Programs

CONTENTS

4. ANATOMY AND PHYSIOLOGY OF THE SKELETAL SYSTEM 91

Material selected from: *Structure & Function of the Human Body*
by Frederic H. Martini and Edwin F. Bartholomew

5. MEDICAL TERMINOLOGY OF THE MALE REPRODUCTIVE SYSTEM 127

Material selected from: *Medical Terminology with Human Anatomy*, Fourth Edition
by Jane Rice

12.   PEDIATRICS 317

Material selected from: *Essentials of Medical Assisting: Administrative and Clinical Competencies*
by Bonnie F. Fremgen
And *Quick References to Pediatric Clinical Skills*
by Bindler & Ball

SECTION THREE: CERTIFICATION EXAM PREPARATION 367

13.   CERTIFICATION EXAM PREPARATION 369

APPENDICES 375

Content provided by Corinthian Colleges, Inc.

Content provided by Corinthian Colleges, Inc.

Section One
MEDICAL TERMINOLOGY AND ANATOMY AND PHYSIOLOGY

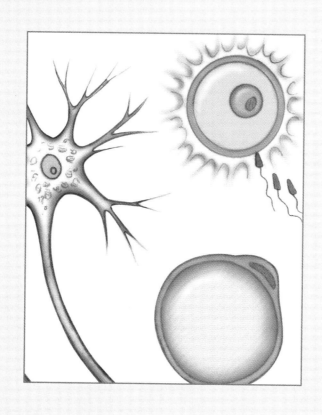

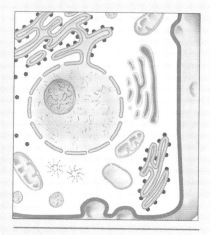

- Anatomy and Physiology Overview
- The Human Body: Levels of Organization
- Anatomical Locations and Positions
- Terminology With Surgical Procedures & Pathology
- Vocabulary Words
- Abbreviations
- Drug Highlights
- Communication Enrichment
- Patient Information Form (Información de Paciente)
- Chapter Review Section

    Learning Exercises

    Word Parts Study Sheet

    Review Questions

MEDICAL TERMINOLOGY: THE ORGANIZATION OF THE BODY

OBJECTIVES _____

On completion of this chapter, you should be able to:

- Define terms that describe the body and its structural units.

- List the systems of the body and give the organs in each system.

- Define terms that are used to describe direction, planes, and cavities of the body.

- Analyze, build, spell, and pronounce medical words that relate to surgical procedures and pathology.

- Identify and give the meaning of selected vocabulary words.

- Identify and define selected abbreviations.

- Review Drug Highlights presented in this chapter.

- Understand word analysis as it relates to Head-to-Toe Assessment.

- Successfully complete the study and review section.

▶ ANATOMY AND PHYSIOLOGY OVERVIEW

This chapter introduces you to terms describing the body and its structural units. To aid you, these terms have been grouped into two major sections: the first offering an overview of the units that make up the human body, and the second covering terms used to describe anatomical positions and locations. The human body is made up of atoms, molecules, organelles, cells, tissues, organs, and systems. See Figure 1–1. All of these parts normally function together in a unified and complex process. During *homeostasis* these processes allow the body to perform at its maximum potential.

▶ THE HUMAN BODY: LEVELS OF ORGANIZATION

ATOMS

An *atom* is the smallest chemical unit of matter. It consists of a nucleus that contains protons and neutrons and is surrounded by electrons. The *nucleus* is at the center of the atom and a *proton* is a positively charged particle, while a *neutron* is without an electrical charge. The *electron* is a negatively charged particle that revolves about the nucleus of an atom.

Chemical elements are made up of atoms. In chemistry, an *element* is a substance that cannot be separated into substances different from itself by ordinary chemical means. It is the basic component of which all matter is composed. There are at least 105 different chemical elements that have been identified.

Elements found in the human body include aluminum, carbon, calcium, chlorine, cobalt, copper, fluorine, hydrogen, iodine, iron, maganese, magnesium, nitrogen, oxygen, phosphorus, potassium, sodium, sulfur, and zinc.

ELEMENTS FOUND IN THE HUMAN BODY

Symbol	Element	Atomic Weight
Al	aluminum	13
C	carbon	6
Ca	calcium	20
Cl	chlorine	17
Co	cobalt	27
Cu	copper	29
F	fluorine	9
H	hydrogen	1
I	iodine	53
Fe	iron	26
Mn	manganese	25
Mg	magnesium	12
N	nitrogen	7
O	oxygen	8
P	phosphorus	15
K	potassium	19
Na	sodium	11
S	sulfur	16
Zn	zinc	30

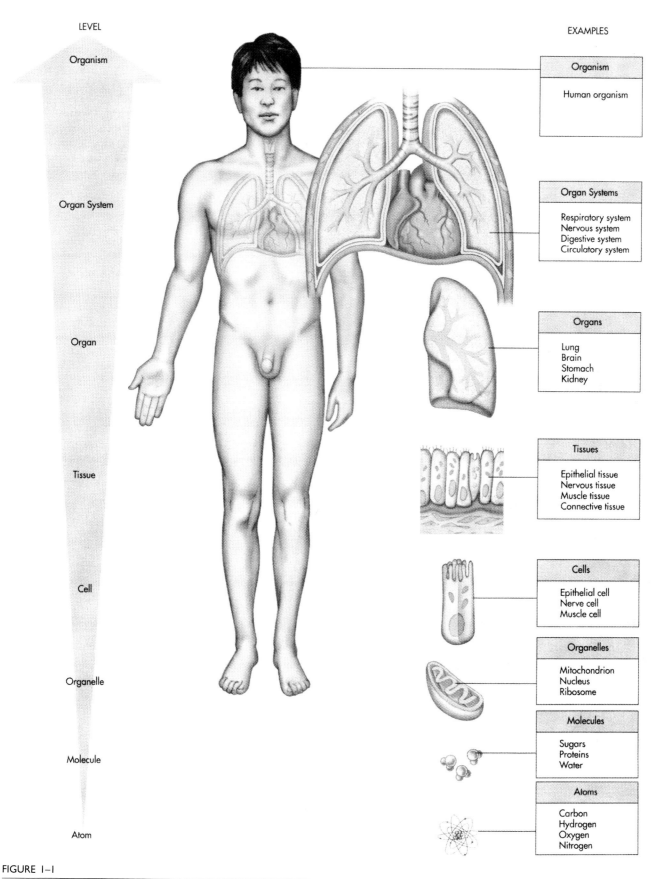

LEVEL

Organism

Organ System

Organ

Tissue

Cell

Organelle

Molecule

Atom

EXAMPLES

Organism

Human organism

Organ Systems

Respiratory system
Nervous system
Digestive system
Circulatory system

Organs

Lung
Brain
Stomach
Kidney

Tissues

Epithelial tissue
Nervous tissue
Muscle tissue
Connective tissue

Cells

Epithelial cell
Nerve cell
Muscle cell

Organelles

Mitochondrion
Nucleus
Ribosome

Molecules

Sugars
Proteins
Water

Atoms

Carbon
Hydrogen
Oxygen
Nitrogen

FIGURE 1–1

The human body: levels of organization.

MOLECULES

A *molecule* is a chemical combination of two or more atoms that form a specific chemical compound. In a water molecule (H_2O), oxygen forms polar covalent bonds with two hydrogen atoms. *Water* is a tasteless, clear, odorless liquid that makes up 65% of a male's body weight and 55% of a female's body weight. Water is the most important constituent of all body fluids, secretions, and excretions. It is an ideal transportation medium for inorganic and organic compounds.

CELLS

The body consists of millions of cells working individually and with each other to sustain life. For the purposes of this book, *cells* are considered the basic building blocks for the various structures that together make up the human being. There are several types of cells, each specialized to perform specific functions. The size and shape of a cell are generally related directly to its function. See Figure 1–3. For example, cells forming the skin overlap each other to form a protective barrier, whereas nerve cells are usually elongated with branches connecting to other cells for the transmission of sensory impulses. Despite these differences, however, cells can generally be said to have a number of common components. The common parts of the cell are the *cell membrane* and the *protoplasm.*

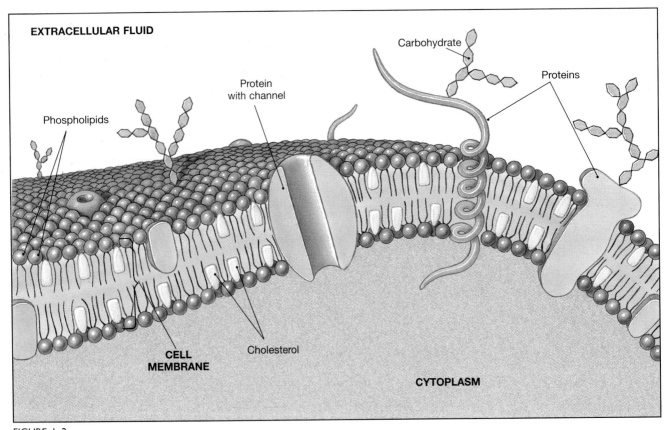

FIGURE 1–2

The Cell Membrane.

The Cell Membrane

The outer covering of the cell is called the *cell membrane.* Cell membranes have the capability of allowing some substances to pass into and out of the cell while denying passage to other substances. This selectivity allows cells to receive nutrition and dispose of waste just as the human being eats food and disposes of waste.

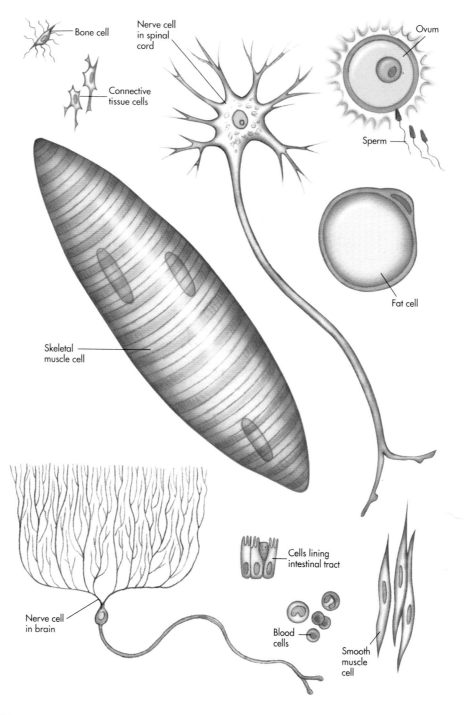

FIGURE 1–3

Cells may be described as the basic building blocks of the human body. They have many different shapes and vary in size and function. These examples show the range of forms and sizes with the dimensions they would have if magnified approximately 500 times.

TABLE 1–1 Functions of Generalized Cell

Appearance	Structure	Function
	Cell Membrane	Separates cell contents from external environment, provides sensitivity to environment, regulates the movement of substances in and out of
cell	**Cytoplasm**	Establishes internal environment of cell, contains intracellular fluid, organelles, and raw materials for their use
	NONMEMBRANOUS ORGANELLES	
	Microvilli	Increase surface area for efficient absorption of materials
	Cilia	Produce movement of materials over cell surface
	Centrioles	Aid movement of chromosomes during cell division
	Ribosomes	Site of protein assembly
	MEMBRANOUS ORGANELLES	
	Endoplasmic Reticulum (ER)	Production of cellular materials; intracellular storage and transport
	Rough ER	Protein synthesis
	Smooth ER	Lipid and carbohydrate synthesis
	Golgi apparatus	Storage and packaging center of cellular materials into vesicles for export out of the cell or use in the cell
	Lysosomes	Remove damaged organelles or cells; "suicide bags"
	Mitochondria	Produce most of the ATP energy for the cell
	Nucleus	Control center of cell; stores hereditary information in chromosomes; controls protein synthesis
	Nucleolus	Site of ribosome production

Protoplasm

The substance within the cell membrane is called *protoplasm*. Protoplasm is composed of cytoplasm and karyoplasm. These substances and their functions are described below.

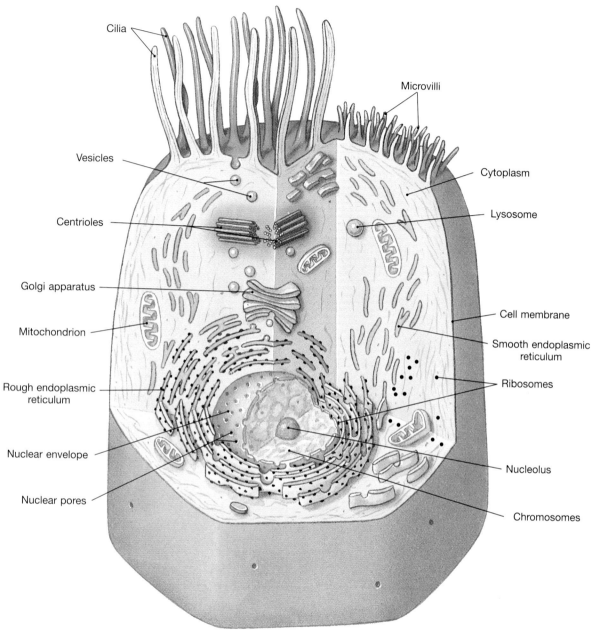

FIGURE 1–4

A Generalized Cell of the Human Body.

Karyoplasm.   Enclosed by its own membrane, *karyoplasm* is the substance of the cell's nucleus and contains the genetic matter necessary for cell reproduction as well as control over activity within the cell's cytoplasm.

Cytoplasm.   All protoplasm outside the nucleus is called *cytoplasm.* The cytoplasm provides storage and work areas for the cell. The work and storage elements of the cell, called organelles, are the endoplasmic reticulum, ribosomes, Golgi apparatus, mitochondria, lysosomes, and centrioles. See Figure 1–4 and Table 1–2.

TABLE 1–2   Major Cell Structures and Primary Functions

Cell Structures	Primary Functions
Cell membrane	Protects the cell; provides for communication via receptor proteins; surface proteins serve as positive identification tags; allow some substances to pass into and out of the cell while denying passage to other substances; this selectivity allows cells to receive nutrition and dispose of waste
Protoplasm	Composed of cytoplasm and karyoplasm
Karyoplasm	Substance of the cell's nucleus; contains the genetic matter necessary for cell reproduction as well as control over activity within the cell's cytoplasm
Cytoplasm	All protoplasm outside the nucleus. The cytoplasm provides storage and work areas for the cell:
Ribosomes	Make enzymes and other proteins; nicknamed "protein factories"
Endoplasmic reticulum (ER)	Carries proteins and other substances through the cytoplasm
Golgi apparatus	Chemically processes the molecules from the endoplasmic reticulum, then packages them into vesicles; nicknamed "chemical processing and packaging center"
Mitochondria	Complex, energy-releasing chemical reactions occur continuously; nicknamed "power plants"
Lysosomes	Contain enzymes that can digest food compounds; nicknamed "digestive bags"
Centrioles	Play an important role in cell reproduction
Cilia	Hair-like processes that project from epithelial cells; help propel mucus, dust particles, and other foreign substances from the respiratory tract
Flagellum	"Tail" of the sperm that makes it possible for the sperm to "swim" or move toward the ovum
Nucleus	Controls every organelle (little organ) in the cytoplasm; contains the genetic matter necessary for cell reproduction as well as control over activity within the cell's cytoplasm

TISSUES

A *tissue* is a grouping of similar cells that together perform specialized functions. There are four basic types of tissue in the body: *epithelial, connective, muscle,* and *nerve.* Each of the four basic tissues has several subtypes named for their shape, appearance, arrangement, or function. The four basic types of tissue are described for you.

Epithelial Tissue
Epithelial tissue appears as sheet-like arrangements of cells, sometimes several layers thick, that form the outer layer of the skin, cover the surfaces of organs, line the walls of cavities, and form tubes, ducts, and portions of certain glands. The functions of epithelial tissues are protection, absorption, secretion, and excretion.

Connective Tissue
The most widespread and abundant of the body tissues, *connective tissue* forms the supporting network for the organs of the body, sheaths the muscles, and connects muscles to bones and bones to joints. Bone is a dense form of connective tissue.

Muscle Tissue

There are three types of *muscle tissue:* voluntary or striated, cardiac, and involuntary or smooth. Striated and smooth muscles are so described because of their appearance. Cardiac muscle is a specialized form of striated tissue under the control of the autonomic nervous system. Involuntary or smooth muscles are also controlled by this system. The striated or voluntary muscles are controlled by the person's will.

Nerve Tissue

Nerve tissue consists of nerve cells (neurons) and interstitial tissue. It has the properties of excitability and conductivity, and functions to control and coordinate the activities of the body.

ORGANS

Tissues serving a common purpose or function make up structures called *organs.* Organs are specialized components of the body such as the brain, skin, or heart.

SYSTEMS

A group of organs functioning together for a common purpose is called a *system.* The various body systems function in support of the body as a whole. Listed in Figure 1–5 are the organ systems of the body.

▶ ANATOMICAL LOCATIONS AND POSITIONS

Four primary reference systems have been adopted to provide uniformity to the anatomical description of the body. These reference systems are *direction, planes, cavities,* and *structural unit.* The standard anatomical position for the body is erect, head facing forward, arms by the sides with palms to the front. Left and right are from the subject's point of view, not the examiner's.

DIRECTION

The following terms are used to describe direction:

- **Superior.** Above, in an upward direction
- **Anterior.** In front of or before
- **Posterior.** Toward the back
- **Cephalad.** Toward the head
- **Medial.** Nearest the midline
- **Lateral.** To the side
- **Proximal.** Nearest the point of attachment
- **Distal.** Away from the point of attachment
- **Ventral.** The same as anterior, the front side
- **Dorsal.** The same as posterior, the back side

PLANES

The terms defined below are used to describe the imaginary planes that are depicted in Figure 1–6 as passing through the body and dividing it into various sections.

Intraderma
Brachioradialis

Know this

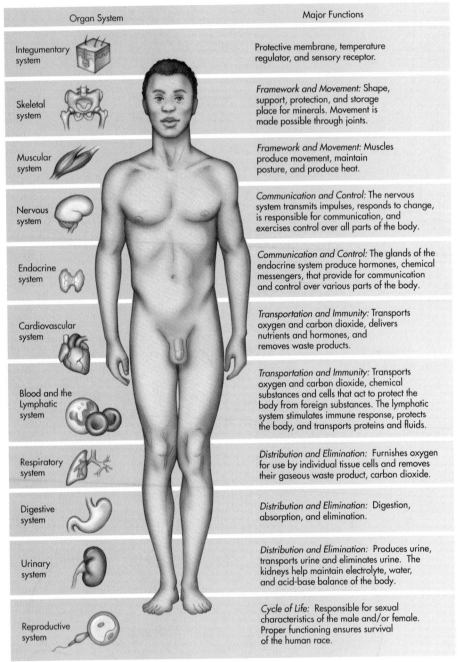

Organ System	Major Functions
Integumentary system	Protective membrane, temperature regulator, and sensory receptor.
Skeletal system	*Framework and Movement:* Shape, support, protection, and storage place for minerals. Movement is made possible through joints.
Muscular system	*Framework and Movement:* Muscles produce movement, maintain posture, and produce heat.
Nervous system	*Communication and Control:* The nervous system transmits impulses, responds to change, is responsible for communication, and exercises control over all parts of the body.
Endocrine system	*Communication and Control:* The glands of the endocrine system produce hormones, chemical messengers, that provide for communication and control over various parts of the body.
Cardiovascular system	*Transportation and Immunity:* Transports oxygen and carbon dioxide, delivers nutrients and hormones, and removes waste products.
Blood and the Lymphatic system	*Transportation and Immunity:* Transports oxygen and carbon dioxide, chemical substances and cells that act to protect the body from foreign substances. The lymphatic system stimulates immune response, protects the body, and transports proteins and fluids.
Respiratory system	*Distribution and Elimination:* Furnishes oxygen for use by individual tissue cells and removes their gaseous waste product, carbon dioxide.
Digestive system	*Distribution and Elimination:* Digestion, absorption, and elimination.
Urinary system	*Distribution and Elimination:* Produces urine, transports urine and eliminates urine. The kidneys help maintain electrolyte, water, and acid-base balance of the body.
Reproductive system	*Cycle of Life:* Responsible for sexual characteristics of the male and/or female. Proper functioning ensures survival of the human race.

FIGURE 1–5

Organ systems of the body with major functions.

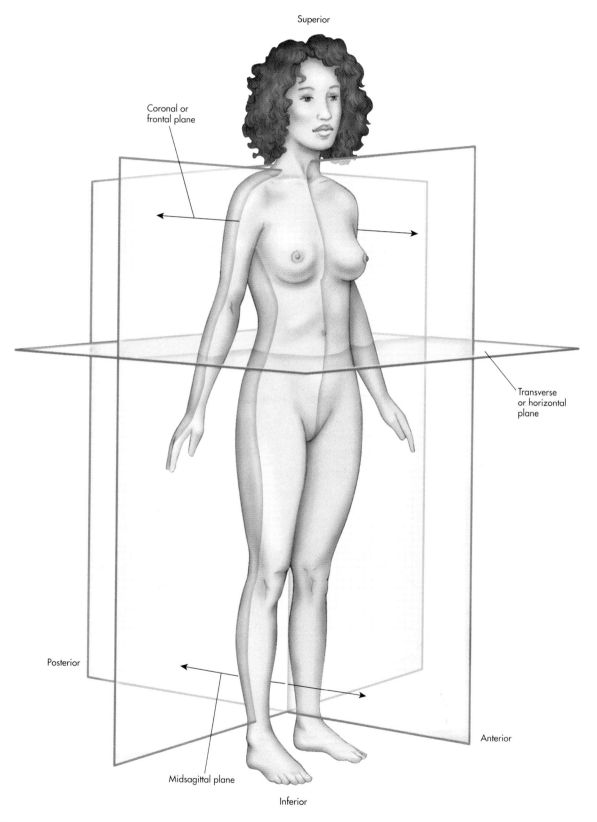

FIGURE 1–6

Planes of the body: coronal or frontal, transverse, and midsagittal.

Midsagittal Plane

The *midsagittal plane* vertically divides the body as it passes through the midline to form a *right* and *left half.*

Transverse or Horizontal Plane

A *transverse* or *horizontal plane* is any plane that divides the body into *superior* and *inferior* portions.

Coronal or Frontal Plane

A *coronal* or *frontal plane* is any plane that divides the body at right angles to the midsagittal plane. The coronal plane divides the body into *anterior* (ventral) and *posterior* (dorsal) portions.

CAVITIES

A *cavity* is a hollow space containing body organs. Body cavities are classified into two groups according to their location. On the front are the *ventral* or *anterior cavities* and on the back are the *dorsal* or *posterior cavities.* The various cavities found in the human body are depicted in Figure 1–7.

The Ventral Cavity

The *ventral cavity* is the hollow portion of the human torso extending from the neck to the pelvis and containing the heart and the organs of respiration, digestion, reproduction, and elimination. The ventral cavity can be subdivided into three distinct areas: thoracic, abdominal, and pelvic.

The Thoracic Cavity.   The *thoracic cavity* is the area of the chest containing the heart and the lungs. Within this cavity, the space containing the *heart* is called the *pericardial* cavity and the spaces surrounding each *lung* are known as the *pleural* cavities. Other organs located in the thoracic cavity are the esophagus, trachea, thymus, and certain large blood and lymph vessels.

The Abdominal Cavity.   The *abdominal cavity* is the space below the diaphragm, commonly referred to as the belly. It contains the kidneys, stomach, intestines, and other organs of digestion.

The Pelvic Cavity.   The *pelvic cavity* is the space formed by the bones of the pelvic area and contains the organs of reproduction and elimination.

The Dorsal Cavity

Containing the structures of the nervous system, the *dorsal cavity* is subdivided into the cranial cavity and the spinal cavity.

The Cranial Cavity.   The *cranial cavity* is the space in the skull containing the brain.

The Spinal Cavity.   The *spinal cavity* is the space within the bony spinal column that contains the spinal cord and spinal fluid.

The Abdominopelvic Cavity

The *abdominopelvic cavity* is the combination of the abdominal and pelvic cavities. It is divided into nine regions.

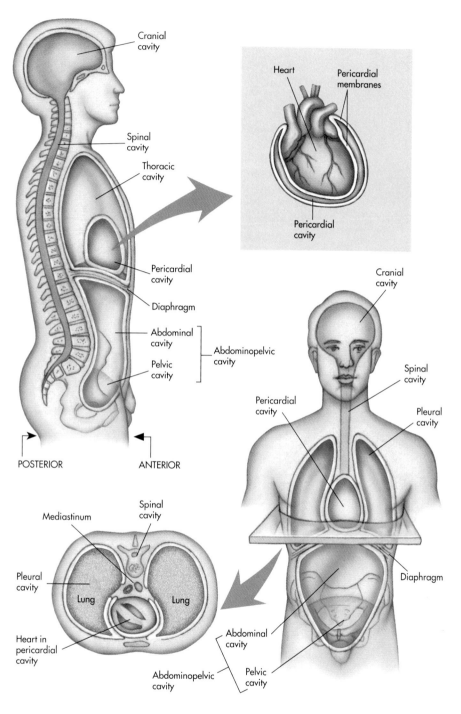

FIGURE 1–7

Body cavities.

NINE REGIONS OF THE ABDOMINOPELVIC CAVITY

As a ready reference for locating visceral organs, anatomists divided the abdominopelvic cavity into nine regions. A tic-tac-toe pattern drawn across the abdominopelvic cavity (Fig. 1–8A) delineates these regions:

- **Right hypochondriac**—upper right region at the level of the ninth rib cartilage
- **Left hypochondriac**—upper left region at the level of the ninth rib cartilage
- **Epigastric**—region over the stomach
- **Right lumbar**—right middle lateral region
- **Left lumbar**—left middle lateral region
- **Umbilical**—in the center, between the right and left lumbar region; at the navel
- **Right iliac (inguinal)**—right lower lateral region
- **Left iliac (inguinal)**—left lower lateral region
- **Hypogastric**—lower middle region below the navel

ABDOMEN DIVIDED INTO QUADRANTS

The *abdomen* is divided into four corresponding regions that are used for descriptive and diagnostic purposes. By using these regions one may describe the exact location of pain, a skin lesion, surgical incision, and/or abdominal tumor. The four *quadrants* are (Fig. 1–8B):

- Right upper (RUQ)
- Left upper (LUQ)
- Right lower (RLQ)
- Left lower (LLQ)

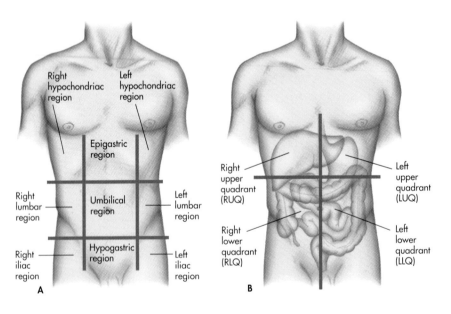

FIGURE 1–8

(A) The nine regions of the abdominopelvic cavity. **(B)** The four regions of the abdomen that are referred to as quadrants.

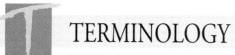

TERMINOLOGY

WITH SURGICAL PROCEDURES & PATHOLOGY

TERM	WORD PARTS			DEFINITION
adipose (ăd″ ĭ-pōs)	adip ose	R S	fat like	Fatty tissue throughout the body
ambilateral (ăm″ bĭ-lăt′ ĕr-ăl)	ambi later al	P R S	both side pertaining to	Pertaining to both sides
anatomy (ăn-ăt′ ō-mē)	ana tomy	P S	up incision	Literally means to cut up; the study of the structure of an organism such as humans
android (ăn′ droyd)	andr oid	R S	man resemble	To resemble man
bilateral (bī-lăt′ ĕr-ăl)	bi later al	P R S	two side pertaining to	Pertaining to two sides
biology (bi-ŏl′ ō-jē)	bio logy	CF S	life study of	The study of life
caudal (kŏd′ ăl)	caud al	R S	tail pertaining to	Pertaining to the tail
chromosome (krō-mō-sōm)	chromo some	P S	color body	Microscopic bodies that carry the genes that determine hereditary characteristics
cytology (sī-tŏl′ ō-jē)	cyto logy	CF S	cell study of	The study of cells
dehydrate (dē-hī′ drāt)	de hydr ate	P R S	down, away from water use, action	To remove water away from the body
diffusion (di-fū′ zhŭn)	dif fus ion	P R S	apart to pour process	A process in which parts of a substance move from areas of high concentration to areas of lower concentration
ectogenous (ĕk-tŏj′ ĕ-nŭs)	ecto gen ous	P R S	outside formation, produce pertaining to	Pertaining to formation outside the organism or body

Terminology - continued

TERM	WORD PARTS			DEFINITION
ectomorph (ĕk′ tō-morf)	ecto morph	P S	outside form, shape	A slender physical body form
endomorph (ĕn″ dō-morf)	endo morph	P S	within form, shape	A round physical body form
histology (hĭs-tŏl′ ō-jē)	histo logy	CF S	tissue study of	The study of tissue
homeostasis (hō″ mē-ō-stā′ sĭs)	homeo stasis	P S	similar, same control, stopping	The state of equilibrium maintained in the body's internal environment

 TERMINOLOGY SPOTLIGHT

To maintain **homeostasis** it is essential that the body be supplied with adequate fluids. Water is the most important constituent of the human body and is essential to every body process. Bones depend on water intake to provide adequate blood for delivery and removal of calcium. The intestines and kidneys use water to remove waste. Muscles need water to remove acids that would otherwise build up, causing cramps and diminishing muscle action. Nerve function depends on the presence of certain minerals, which are kept in balance by water levels in the body. The immune system depends on sufficient water to ensure blood flow for delivery of immune cells and removal of diseased cells. Water in saliva and the stomach aids digestion and absorption of nutrients.

It is recommended that the average healthy adult drink eight 8-ounce glasses of water per day. One may need more than eight glasses of water per day before, during, and after exercise, in warm weather, during and after drinking alcohol or caffeine, when breast-feeding, during illness, with certain medications, after surgery, and/or with severe burns or bleeding.

karyogenesis (kăr″ i-ō-jĕn′ ĕ-sĭs)	karyo genesis	CF S	cell's nucleus formation, produce	Formation of a cell's nucleus
mesomorph (mĕs′ ō-morf)	meso morph	P S	middle form, shape	A well-proportioned body form
pathology (pă-thŏl′ ō-jē)	patho logy	CF S	disease study of	The study of disease
perfusion (pur-fū′ zhŭn)	per fus ion	P R S	through to pour process	The process of pouring through
physiology (fiz″ i-ŏl′ ō-jē)	physio logy	CF S	nature study of	The study of the nature of living organisms

continued

Terminology - continued

TERM	WORD PARTS			DEFINITION
pinocytosis (pī″ nō-si-tō′ sis)	pino cyt osis	CF R S	to drink cell condition of	The condition whereby a cell absorbs or ingests nutrients and fluids
protoplasm (prō-tō-plăzm)	proto plasm	P S	first a thing formed, plasma	The essential matter of a living cell
somatotrophic (sō″ mă-tō-trŏf′ ĭk)	somato troph ic	CF R S	body a turning pertaining to	Pertaining to stimulation of body growth
topical (tŏp′ ĭ-kăl)	topic al	R S	place pertaining to	Pertaining to a place, definite locale
unilateral (ū″ nĭ-lăt′ ĕr-ăl)	uni later al	P R S	one side pertaining to	Pertaining to one side
visceral (vĭs′ ĕr-ăl)	viscer al	R S	body organs pertaining to	Pertaining to body organs enclosed within a cavity, especially abdominal organs

VOCABULARY WORDS

Vocabulary words are terms that have not been divided into component parts. They are common words or specialized terms associated with the subject of this chapter. These words are provided to enhance your medical vocabulary.

WORD	DEFINITION
anterior (an-tĕr′ ē-ōr)	In front of, before
anthropometry (ăn-thrō-pŏm′ ĕt-rē)	The measurement of the human body; includes measurement of the skull, bones, height, weight, and skin fold evaluation for subcutaneous fat estimation
apex (ā′ pĕks)	The pointed end of a cone-shaped structure

Vocabulary - continued

WORD	DEFINITION
base (bās)	The lower part or foundation of a structure
center (sĕn′ tĕr)	The midpoint of a body or activity
cephalad (sĕf′ ă-lăd)	Toward the head
cilia (sĭl′ ē-ă)	Hair-like processes that project from epithelial cells; they help propel mucus, dust particles, and other foreign substances from the respiratory tract
deep (dēp)	Far down from the surface
distal (dĭs′ tăl)	Farthest from the center or point of origin
dorsal (dōr′ săl)	Pertaining to the back side of the body
filtration (fĭl-trā′ shŭn)	The process of filtering or straining particles from a solution
gene (jēn)	The hereditary unit that transmits and determines one's characteristics or hereditary traits
horizontal (hŏr′ă-zŏn′ tăl)	Pertaining to the horizon, of or near the horizon, lying flat, even, level
human genome (hū′ măn jē′ nōm)	The complete set of genes and chromosomes tucked inside each of the body's trillions of cells
inferior (ĭn-fē′ rē-or)	Located below or in a downward direction
inguinal (ĭng′ gwĭ-năl)	Pertaining to the groin, of or near the groin
internal (ĭn-tĕr′ nal)	Pertaining to within or the inside
lateral (lăt′ ĕr-ăl)	Pertaining to the side

continued

Vocabulary - continued

WORD	DEFINITION
medial (mē′ dē al)	Pertaining to the middle or midline
organic (or-găn′ĭk)	Pertaining to an organ
phenotype (fē′ nō-tīp)	The physical appearance or type of makeup of an individual
posterior (pŏs-tē′ rĭ-ōr)	Toward the back
prions (prē′ ons)	An entirely new genre of disease-causing agents that are made of proteins and do not contain any genes or genetic material. This detail distinguishes them from all other kinds of infectious agents such as viruses, bacteria, fungi, and parasites. In 1997, Doctor Stanley B. Prusiner, an American scientist, was awarded the Nobel Prize in Medicine for his discovery of prions. His work has proved invaluable in the study of mad cow disease and the human brain disease "new variant" Creutzfeldt-Jakob disease, believed to be caused by eating beef from affected cattle. Prusiner's discovery may lead to a better understanding of Alzheimer's disease and other neurodegenerative syndromes.
proximal (prŏk′ sĭm-ăl)	Nearest the center or point of origin; nearest the point of attachment
superficial (sū″ pĕr-fĭsh′ ăl)	Pertaining to the surface, on or near the surface
superior (sū-pēr′ rĭ-ōr)	Located above or in an upward direction
systemic (sis-tĕm′ ĭk)	Pertaining to the body as a whole
ventral (vĕn′ trăl)	Pertaining to the front side of the body, abdomen, belly surface
vertex (vĕr′ tĕks)	The top or highest point; the top or crown of the head

ABBREVIATIONS

abd	abdomen, abdominal		**lat**	lateral
A&P	anatomy and physiology		**LLQ**	left lower quadrant
AP	anterior–posterior		**LUQ**	left upper quadrant
CNS	central nervous system		**PA**	posterior–anterior
CV	cardiovascular		**resp**	respiratory
ER	endoplasmic reticulum		**RLQ**	right lower quadrant
GI	gastrointestinal		**RUQ**	right upper quadrant

DRUG HIGHLIGHTS

A drug is a medicinal substance that may alter or modify the functions of a living organism. There are thousands of drugs that are available as over-the-counter (OTC) medicines and do not need a prescription. A prescription is a written legal document that gives directions for compounding, dispensing, and administering a medication to a patient.

In general, there are five medical uses for drugs and these are: therapeutic, diagnostic, curative, replacement, and preventive or prophylactic.

- **Therapeutic Use.** Used in the treatment of a disease or condition, such as an allergy, to relieve the symptoms or to sustain the patient until other measures are instituted.
- **Diagnostic Use.** Certain drugs are used in conjunction with radiology to allow the physician to pinpoint the location of a disease process.
- **Curative Use.** Certain drugs, such as antibiotics, kill or remove the causative agent of a disease.
- **Replacement Use.** Certain drugs, such as hormones and vitamins, are used to replace substances normally found in the body.
- **Preventive or Prophylactic Use.** Certain drugs, such as immunizing agents, are used to ward off or lessen the severity of a disease.

Drug Names   Most drugs may be cited by their chemical, generic, and trade or brand (proprietary) name. The chemical name is usually the formula that denotes the composition of the drug. It is made up of letters and numbers that represent the drug's molecular structure. The generic name is the drug's official name and is descriptive of its chemical structure. The generic name is written in lowercase letters. A generic drug can be manufactured by more than one pharmaceutical company. When this is the case, each company markets the drug under its own unique trade or brand name. A trade or brand name is registered by the US Patent Office as well as approved by the US Food and Drug Administration (FDA). A trade or brand name is written with a capital.

Undesirable Actions of Drugs   Most drugs have the potential for causing an action other than their intended action. For example, antibiotics that are administered orally may disrupt the normal bacterial flora of the gastrointestinal tract and cause gastric discomfort. This type of reaction is known as a side effect. An adverse reaction is an unfavorable or harmful unintended action of a drug. For example, the adverse reaction of Demerol may be lightheadedness, dizziness, sedation, nausea, and sweating. A drug interaction may occur when one drug potentiates or diminishes the action of another drug. These actions may be desirable or undesirable. Drugs may also interact with foods, alcohol, tobacco, and other substances.

Medication Order and Dosage

The medication order is given for a specific patient and denotes the name of the drug, the dosage, the form of the drug, the time for or frequency of administration, and the route by which the drug is to be given.

The dosage is the amount of medicine that is prescribed for administration. The form of the drug may be liquid, solid, semisolid, tablet, capsule, transdermal therapeutic patch, etc. The route of administration may be by mouth, by injection, into the eye(s), ear(s), nostril(s), rectum, vagina, etc.

It is important for the patient to know when and how to take a medication. The following are some hows, whens, and directions for taking medications. To assist you in communicating this information to a patient, both English and Spanish are provided for you to use.

English	Spanish	English	Spanish
When	*Cuándo*	*When*	*Cuándo*
every hour	cada hora (că-dă ŏ-ră)	after meals	después de comer (dĕs-pū-ĕs dĕ cō-mĕr)
every two hours	cada dos horas (că-dă dōs ō-răs)	before breakfast	antes de desayunar (ăn-tĕs dĕ dĕ-să-jū-năr)
every three hours	cada tres horas (că-dă trĕs ō-ră s)	after breakfast	después de desayunar (dĕs-pū-ĕs dĕ dĕ-să-jū-năr)
every four hours	cada cuatro horas (că-dă kū-ă-trō ō-răs)	before lunch	antes de merendar (ăn-tĕs dĕ mĕ-rĕn-dăr)
every six hours	cada seis horas (că-dă sĕ-ĭs ō-răs)	after dinner	después de cenar (dĕs-pū-ĕs dĕ sĕ-năr)
every eight hours	cada ocho horas (că-dă ō-chō ō-răs)	at night	por la noche (pōr lă nō-chĕ)
every twelve hours	cada doce horas (că-dă dō-sĕ ō-răs)	in the morning	por la mañana (pōr lă mă-nyă-nă)
before meals	antes de comer (ăn-tĕs dĕ cō-mĕr)	at bedtime	al acostarse (ăl ă-cōs-tăr-sĕ)
How	*Cómo*	*How*	*Cómo*
with meals	con la comida (kōn lă kō-mĭ-dă)	in the right eye	en el ojo derecho (ĕn ĕl ō-hō dĕ-rĕ-chō)
with milk	con leche (kōn lĕ-chĕ)	in the left eye	en el ojo izquierdo (ĕn ĕl ō-hō ĭs-kĭ-ĕr-dō)
with food	con alimento (kōn ă-lĭ-mĕn-tō)	in both eyes	en los dos ojos (ĕn lōs dōs ō-hōs)
with antacid	con anti-acido (kōn ăn-tĭ ă-cĭ-dō)	in the right ear	en el oido derecho (ĕn ĕl ō-ĭ-dō dĕ-rĕ-chō)

How	*Cómo*	*How*	*Cómo*
in the left ear	en el oido izquierdo (ĕn ĕl ō-ĭ-dō ĭs-kĭ-*ĕr*-dō)	into the rectum	en el recto (ĕn ĕl *rĕc*-tō)
in both ears	en los dos oidos (ĕn lōs dōs ō-ĭ-dōs)	into the vagina	en la vagina (ĕn lă vă-*hĭ*-nă)
into the nostrils	en la nariz (ĕn lă nă-*rĭz*)		

Directions	*Dirección*	*Directions*	*Dirección*
chew	mascar (măs-*kăr*)	shake well	agitar bien (ă-hĭ-tăr bĭ-ĕn)
do not chew	no mascar (nō măs-*kăr*)	for external use	para uso externo (pă-ră *ū*-sō ĕx-*tĕr*-nō)
avoid sunlight	evitar sol (ĕ-vĭ-tăr sōl)	keep refrigerated	mantener en el refrigerador (măn-tĕ-*nĕr* ĕn ĕl rĕ-frĭ-hĕ-ră-*dōr*)
avoid alcohol	evitar alcohol (ĕ-vĭ-tăr ăl-kō ōhl)		

COMMUNICATION ENRICHMENT

This segment is provided for those who wish to enhance their ability to communicate in either English or Spanish.

▶ Head-to-Toe Assessment

Body Area	Spanish	Component Part/Terminology
abdomen (belly)	vientre (vĭ-*ĕn*-trĕ)	abdomino (ăb-*dō*-mĭ-nō)
ankle	tobillo (tō-bĭ-yō)	ankylo (ăn-*kĭ*-lō)
arm	brazo (*bră*-zō)	brachi (*bnĭ*-chĭ)
back	espalda (ĕs-*pāl*-dă)	posterior (pōs-tĕ-rĭ-ōr)
bones	huesos (*wĕ*-sos)	osteo (ōs-tĕ-ō)

Body Area	Spanish	Component Part/Terminology
breast	ceno (*sĕ*-nō)	mast/mammo/mammary (măst; *măm*-ō; *măm*-ă-rē)
cheek	mejilla (*mĕ*-jĭ-yă)	bucco/buccal (*bŭk*-kō; *bŭk*-ăl)
chest	pecho (*pĕ*-chō)	thoraco (thō-*nă*-kō)
ear	oido (ō-*ē*-dō)	oto (ō-tō)
elbow	codo (*kō*-dō)	cubital (cū-bĭ-*tăl*)
eye	ojo (*ō*-hō)	ophthalmo; oculo; opto (ōp-*thăl*-mō; ō-kū-lō; *ōp*-tō)
finger	dedo (*dĕ*-dow)	dactylo/digit/phalanx (*dăk*-tĭ-lō; *dĭj*-ĭt; *făl*-ănks)
foot	pie (pĭĕ)	illus (il-lus-)
gums	encías (ĕn-*sĭ*-ăs)	gingiv (gĭn-gĭv-)
hand	mano (*mă*-nō)	manus (mă-nūs)
head	cabeza (*aĭ*-bē-ză)	cephalo (sĕ-fă-lō)
heart	corazón (kō-ră-*zōn*)	cardio (kăr-dĭ-ō)
hip	cadera (kă-*dĕ*-ră)	coxa (*kŏk*-să)
leg	pierna (pī-*ĕr*-nă)	crural; femoral (crū-răl; fĕ-mō-răl)
liver	higado (hĭ-gă-dō)	hepato (hĕ-pă-tō)
lungs	pulmones (pūl-*mō*-nĕs)	pulmo (pūl-mō)
mouth	boca (*bō*-kă)	oro (ō-rō)

Body Area	Spanish	Component Part/Terminology
muscles	músculos (*mūs*-kū-lōs)	musculo (mūs-cū-lō)
navel	ombligo (*om*-blĭ-gō)	umbilic/umbilicus (ŭm-bĭ-*lĭ*-k; ŭm-bĭ-*lĭ*-kŭs)
neck	cuello (*kŭe*-jō)	cervico (*sĕr*-vĭ-cō)
nerves	nervios (*ner*-vĭ-ōs)	neuro (*nū*-rō)
nose	nariz (*nă*-rĭz)	rhino; naso (*rĭ*-nō; *nă*-sō)
ribs	costillas (cōs-*tĭ*-yăs)	costo (*cōs*-tō)
side	costado (cōs-*tă*-dō)	lateral (lă-tĕ-*răl*)
skin	piel (pē-ĕl)	derma (*dĕr*-mă)
skull	cráneo (*krā*-nĕ-ō)	cranio; cranial (*kră*-nĭ-ō; *knă*-nē-ăl)
stomach	estómago (ĕs-tō-*mă*-gō)	gastro (*găs*-trō)
teeth	dientes (*dĭĕn*-tĕs)	denti (*dĕn*-tĭ)
temples	templo (*ti*-ĕm-plō)	tempora (tĕm-*pō*-ră)
thigh	muslo (*mŭs*-lō)	femoral; crural (fĕ-mō-răl; crŭ-răl)
throat	garganta (găr-*găn*-tă)	pharyngo (fă-*rĭn*-hō)
thumb	dedo pulgar (*dĕ*-dow *pŭl*-găr)	pollex (*pōl*-lĕx)
tongue	lengua (*lĕn*-gŭ-ă)	linguo; glosso (lĭn-gū-ō; glōs-sō)
wrist	muñeca (*mŭ*-ñĕ-kă)	carpo (*căr*-pō)

► PATIENT INFORMATION FORM (INFORMACIÓN DE PACIENTE)

The patient information form is an essential part of the patient's record. This form is filled out by the patient on the first visit to the physician's office and then updated as necessary. It provides data that relate directly to the patient including last name, first name, sex, date of birth, marital status, street address, city, state, zip code, telephone number, social security number, employment status, address of employer, telephone number at employment agency, and vital information concerning who should be contacted in case of an emergency. Also included is information about who is responsible for the patient's bill.

The following is an example of a patient information form. *Note that it is in **Spanish** with English subtitles.*

INFORMACIÓN DE PACIENTE
(Patient Information)

Apellido _____   **Nombre** _____   **Sexo** _____
(Last Name)   (First Name)   (Sex)

Fecha de Nacamiento _____   **Estado Civil:** C_____ S_____ V_____ D_____
(Date of Birth)   (Marital Status: M, S, W, D)

Dirección _____   **Ciudad** _____   **Estado** _____
(Street Address)   (City)   (State)

Código Postal _____   **Teléfono** (____)_____   **# Seg. Social** _____
(Zip Code)   (Telephone)   (Social Security #)

Empleo _____   **Dirección de Empleo** _____
(Employment)   (Address of Employment)

Teléfono de Empleo (____)_____
(Work Telephone)

Contacto Emergencia (Alguien Qué No Vive En Su Casa)
(Who to Contact in Case of an Emergency)

Nombre _____   **Relación** _____
(Name)   (Relationship)

Dirección _____   **Ciudad** _____   **Estado** _____
(Street Address)   (City)   (State)

Código Postal _____   **Teléfono** (____)_____
(Zip Code)   (Telephone)

Quién Es Resposable de la Cuenta de Paciente
(Who is responsible for the patient's bill?)

Apellido _____   **Nombre** _____   **Sexo** _____
(Last Name)   (First Name)   (Sex)

Fecha de Nacamiento _____   **Teléfono** (____)_____   **# Seg. Social** _____
(Date of Birth)   (Telephone)   (Social Security #)

Dirección _____   **Ciudad** _____   **Estado** _____
(Street Address)   (City)   (State)

CHAPTER REVIEW SECTION

LEARNING EXERCISES

▶ **Anatomy and Physiology**

Write your answers to the following questions. Do not refer back to the text.

1. The _____ consist of millions of _____ working individually and

   with each other to _____ life.

2. The outer covering of the cell is known as the _____ which has the
   capability of allowing some substances to pass into and out of the cell.

3. The substance within the cell is known as _____ and is composed of

   _____ and _____.

4. The cell's nucleus is composed of _____, which contains its genetic material.

5. The two primary functions of the cell's nucleus are _____

   and _____.

6. List the four functions of epithelial tissue.

   a. _____   b. _____

   c. _____   d. _____

7. _____ tissue is the most widespread and abundant of the four body tissues.

8. Name the three types of muscle tissue.

   a. _____   b. _____   c. _____

9. Two properties of nerve tissue are _____ and _____.

10. Define organ. _____.

11. Define body system. _____.

12. Name the organ systems listed in this text.

    a. _____   b. _____

    c. _____   d. _____

    e. _____   f. _____

    g. _____   h. _____

    i. _____   j. _____

    k. _____

13. Define the following directional terms:

a. Superior _____   b. Anterior _____

c. Posterior _____   d. Cephalad _____

e. Medial _____   f. Lateral _____

g. Proximal _____   h. Distal _____

i. Ventral _____   j. Dorsal _____

14. The _____ _____ vertically divides the body. It passes through the midline to form a right and left half.

15. The _____ plane is any plane that divides the body into superior and inferior portions.

16. The _____ plane is any plane that divides the body at right angles to the plane described in question 14.

17. List the three distinct cavities that are located in the ventral cavity.

a. _____   b. _____   c. _____

18. Name the two distinct cavities located in the dorsal cavity.

a. _____   b. _____

▶ Word Parts

1. In the spaces provided, write the definition of these prefixes, roots, combining forms, and suffixes. Do not refer to the listings of terminology words. Leave blank those terms you cannot define.

2. After completing as many as you can, refer back to the terminology word listings to check your work. For each word missed or left blank, write the term and its definition several times on the margins of these pages or on a separate sheet of paper.

3. To maximize the learning process, it is to your advantage to do the following exercises as directed. To refer to the terminology listings before completing these exercises invalidates the learning process.

Prefixes

Give the definitions of the following prefixes:

1. ambi- _Both_

2. ana- _Up_

3. bi- _Two_

4. chromo- _Color_

5. de- _Down_

6. dif- _apart_

7. ecto- _Outside_   8. endo- _Within_

9. homeo- _Similar_   10. meso- _Middle_

11. per- _through_   12. proto- _disease_

13. uni- _One_

Roots and Combining Forms

Give the definitions of the following roots and combining forms:

1. adip _Fat_   2. andr _Man_

3. bio _life_   4. caud _tail_

5. cyt _cell_   6. cyto _Cell_

7. fus _to pour_   8. gen _Formation_

9. histo _tissue_   10. hydr _water_

11. karyo _Cells nucles_   12. later _Side_

13. patho _diseas_   14. physio _nature_

15. pino _drink_   16. somato _body_

17. topic _place_   18. troph _turning_

19. viscer _body organs_

Suffixes

Give the definitions for the following suffixes:

1. -al _pretinding_   2. -ate _____

3. -genesis _____   4. -ic _____

5. -ion _____   6. -logy _____

7. -morph _____   8. -oid _____

9. -ose _____   10. -osis _____

11. -ous _____   12. -plasm _____

13. -some _____   14. -stasis _____

15. -tomy _____

Identifying Medical Terms

In the spaces provided, write the medical terms for the following meanings:

1. _____ To resemble man

2. _____ Pertaining to two sides

3. _____ The study of cells

4. _____ A slender physical body form

5. _____ Formation of a cell's nucleus

6. _____ Pertaining to the stimulation of body growth

7. _____ Pertaining to one side

Spelling

In the spaces provided, write the correct spelling of these misspelled terms:

1. adpose _____ 2. caual _____

3. cytlogy _____ 4. difusion _____

5. histlogy _____ 6. mesmorph _____

7. prefusion _____ 8. pincytosis _____

9. somattrophic _____ 10. unlateral _____

WORD PARTS STUDY SHEET

Word Parts	Give the Meaning
Head-to-Toe-Assessment	
abdomino-	_____
ankylo-	_____
brachi-	_____
posterior-	_____
osteo-	_____
bucco-	_____
mast-, mammo-	_____
thoraco-	_____

oto-   _____

cubital-   _____

ophthalmo-, oculo-, opto-   _____

dactylo-   _____

illus-   _____

gingiv-   _____

manus-   _____

cephalo-   _____

cardio-   _____

coxa-   _____

crural-, femoral-   _____

hepato-   _____

pulmo-   _____

oro-   _____

musculo-   _____

umbilic-   _____

cervico-   _____

neuro-   _____

rhino-, naso-   _____

costo-   _____

lateral-   _____

derma-   _____

cranio-   _____

gastro-   _____

denti-   _____

tempora-   _____

pharyngo-   _____

linguo-, glosso-   _____

carpo-   _____

REVIEW QUESTIONS

▶ **Matching**

Select the appropriate lettered meaning for each numbered line.

K   1. ambilateral
J   2. anatomy
G   3. anthropometry
C   4. chromosome
B   5. cilia
A   6. homeostasis
H   7. human genome
D   8. phenotype
I   9. physiology
E   10. vertex

a. Hair-like processes that project from epithelial cells
b. The top or highest point
c. Pertaining to both sides
d. The study of the structure of an organism such as humans
e. The measurement of the human body
f. Microscopic bodies that carry the genes that determine hereditary characteristics
g. The complete set of genes and chromosomes
h. The physical appearance or type of makeup of an individual
i. The state of equilibrium maintained in the body's internal environment
j. The study of the nature of living organism
k. The study of disease

▶ **Abbreviations**

Place the correct word, phrase, or abbreviation in the space provided.

1. abdomen   Abd
2. A&P   anatomy & physiology
3. CNS   Central nervous system
4. cardiovascular   CV
5. gastrointestinal   GI
6. lat   leteral
7. resp   respiratory
8. ER   endoplasmic reticlum
9. AP   anterior - Posterior
10. PA   posterior - anterior

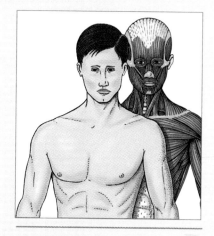

INTRODUCTION TO THE STRUCTURE AND FUNCTION OF THE HUMAN BODY

OBJECTIVES

- Define the terms *anatomy* and *physiology*.

- Identify the major levels of organization in humans and other living organisms.

- Explain the importance of homeostasis.

- Describe how positive and negative feedback are involved in homeostatic regulation.

- Use anatomical terms to describe body regions, body sections, and relative positions.

- Identify the major body cavities and their subdivisions.

- Distinguish between *visceral* and *parietal* portions of *serous membranes*.

The world around us contains an enormous variety of living organisms, but none tends to fascinate us as much as ourselves and our bodies. The scientific study of living organisms, including humans, is called **biology**. This text describes two important aspects of human biology: body structure, or *anatomy*, and body function, or *physiology*. As you read through this book, you will learn for yourself why the human body has often been called the "incredible machine."

▶ THE SCIENCES OF ANATOMY AND PHYSIOLOGY

The words *anatomy* and *physiology* originated in ancient Greece. **Anatomy** (a-NAT-o-mē), which comes from Greek words that mean "to cut open," is the study of the body's internal and external structures and the physical relationships among body parts. **Physiology** (fiz-ē-OL-o-jē), the study of body function, examines the physical and chemical processes that keep us alive and healthy. As you will see throughout your study of anatomy and physiology, structure and function are closely linked. An understanding of anatomy gives clues to likely functions, and physiology can be explained only in terms of the parts of the body involved.

The link between structure and function is always present but not always understood. The anatomy of the heart, for example, was clearly described in the fifteenth century. Almost 200 years passed, however, before the pumping action of the heart was demonstrated. On the other hand, many important cell functions were known decades before people first used microscopes to study cellular structure.

▶ LEVELS OF ORGANIZATION IN THE BODY

One distinct difference between living and nonliving things is the complexity of their structural organization: living things are much more complex. The human body contains several *levels of organization*. Structures in the simpler levels combine to create structures in the more complex levels. Understanding how the functions of one level affect other levels allows us to predict how the the body will respond to external or internal changes. Look now at Figure 2-1, which shows the various levels of organization in the human body, using the cardiovascular system as an example. The following list describes the structures from simplest to most complex:

- *Molecules*: As you'll discover in the next chapter, *atoms* are the smallest stable units of matter, and atoms combine to form *molecules*. Some molecules have only two atoms, but others consist of many dozens of atoms that form complex shapes. Even at this simplest level, the specialized shape of a molecule often determines its function. This is the *molecular level* of organization.
- *Cells*: *Cells* are the smallest living units in the body. Each cell contains numerous *organelles*, which in turn are composed of many different molecules. Heart muscle cells contain large numbers of special molecules that give these cells the ability to contract, or shorten.
- *Tissues*: A *tissue* is composed of a group of similar cells working together to perform a specific function. The muscle cells of the heart make up one form of *muscle tissue*, whose function is to contract and thereby cause movement. In this case, the movement causes the heart to pump blood.
- *Organs*: An *organ* consists of several different tissues that work together to perform specific functions. For example, the heart is a hollow, three-dimensional organ. Its walls contain layers of muscle and other tissues.
- *Organ System*: Each time the heart contracts, it pushes blood into a network of blood vessels. The heart, blood, and blood vessels form the *cardiovascular system*, an example of an *organ system*. Organ systems are also sometimes called *body systems*.
- *Organism*: All 11 organ systems of the body work together to maintain the highest level of organization, that of the individual *organism*—in this case, a human being.

FIGURE 2-1

Levels of Organization.

Interacting atoms form molecules that combine to form cells, such as heart muscle cells. Groups of cells combine to form tissues with specific functions, such as heart muscle. Two or more tissues combine to form an organ, such as the heart. The heart is one component of the cardiovascular system, which also includes the blood and blood vessels. All the organ systems combine to create an organism, a living human being.

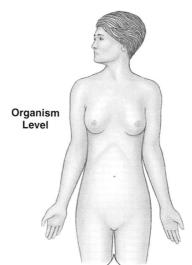

Organism Level

Organ System Level

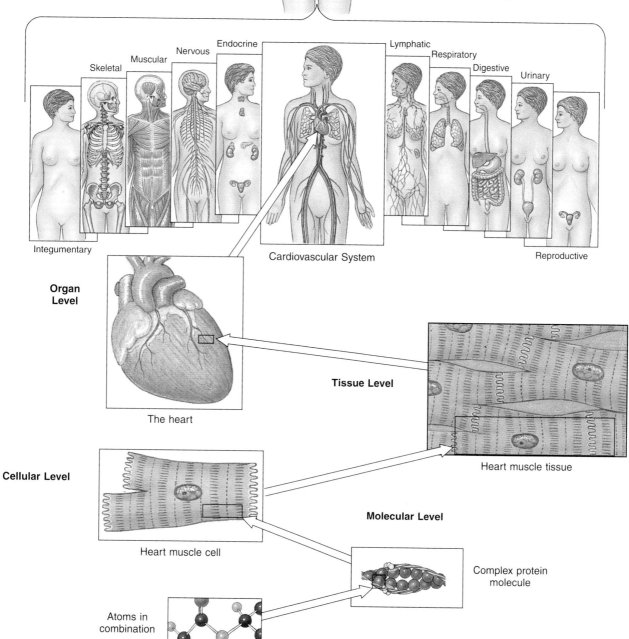

Skeletal Muscular Nervous Endocrine Lymphatic Respiratory Digestive Urinary

Integumentary Cardiovascular System Reproductive

Organ Level

The heart

Tissue Level

Heart muscle tissue

Cellular Level

Heart muscle cell

Molecular Level

Complex protein molecule

Atoms in combination

Each level of structural organization is totally dependent on the others. For example, damage at the cellular, tissue, or organ level may affect an entire organ system. A molecular change in heart muscle cells can cause abnormal contractions or even stop the heartbeat. Physical damage to the heart muscle tissue, as in a chest wound, can make the heart ineffective—even when most of the heart muscle cells are structurally intact. Abnormal structure at the organ level can make the heart an ineffective pump even if the muscle cells and muscle tissue are perfectly normal.

Finally, something that affects an organ system will sooner or later affect all its components. The heart, for example, cannot pump blood effectively if the organism has experienced massive blood loss. If the heart cannot pump and blood cannot flow, the tissues will begin to break down as cells suffocate or starve. These changes will not be restricted to the cardiovascular system. All the cells, tissues, and organs in the body will be damaged.

Concept Questions

✔ What is the smallest living unit in the human body?

✔ What is the difference between an organ and a tissue?

▶ HOMEOSTASIS

Organ systems in the human body are packed together in a relatively small space. The cells, tissues, organs, and organ systems exist together in a shared environment like people in a large city. Just as city dwellers breathe the city air and eat food from local restaurants, cells absorb oxygen and nutrients from their environment. All living cells are in contact with blood or some other body fluid. Within this fluid environment, factors such as temperature, volume, salt levels, or acidity (pH) must remain within a relatively narrow range for the body to function properly. If body fluids become abnormal, cells may become injured or die.

Although very small changes do occur regularly in the fluid environment of the cells, our bodies have many ways of preventing drastic changes. **Homeostasis** (hō-mē-ō-STĀ-sis), derived from the root words *homeo* (unchanging) and *stasis* (standing), refers to the relatively constant internal environment of the body. Our body's systems normally maintain homeostasis regardless of our ongoing activities. But when mechanisms that control homeostasis fail, organ systems begin to malfunction, and the individual then experiences symptoms of illness, or **disease**.

Do you use a thermostat in your house or apartment to control room temperature? If so, you are probably already familiar with the basic principles of homeostatic control, although you may not realize it. A thermostat monitors room temperature, and its function is to keep room temperature within a degree or two of the set point you select. In the summertime, the thermostat does this by controlling an air conditioner. The principle is simple: the thermostat turns on the air conditioner if the room becomes warmer than the set point, and turns it off when the temperature reaches the set point again.

The mechanisms that control homeostasis are activated in response to a *stimulus*. A **stimulus** is anything in the surroundings that produces a *response*—that is, a change in the activities of cells, tissues, organs, or organ systems. In the thermostat analogy, the stimulus is an increase in room temperature. The response produced is the activation of the air conditioner. The air conditioner cools the room and removes the stimulus. This type of homeostatic control is called *negative feedback*.

NEGATIVE FEEDBACK

In **negative feedback**, the response reverses the effect of a stimulus. Most homeostatic control in the body involves negative feedback. One such example is the control of body temperature, a process called *thermoregulation* (ther-mō-reg-ye-LĀ-shun). Thermoregulation balances the amount of heat lost with the amount of heat produced. In the human body, heat is lost mostly through the skin, whereas body heat is produced mainly by the skeletal muscles.

The cells of the the body's "thermostat," the *thermoregulatory center*, are located in the brain (Figure 2-2). The thermoregulatory center has a set point near 37° C (98.6°F). When your body temperature rises above 37.2° C (99° F), the brain cells of the thermoregulatory center send signals that result in the widening, or *dilation* (dī-LĀ-shun), of the blood vessels in the

therme, heat
thermoregulation: the control of body temperature

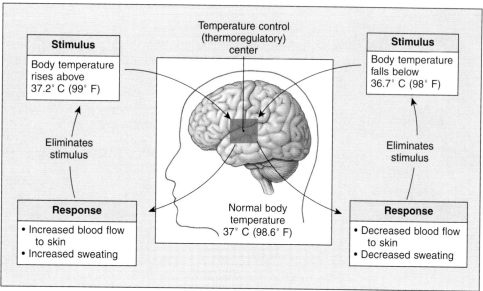

FIGURE 2-2

Negative Feedback.

In negative feedback, a stimulus produces a response that eliminates the original stimulus. Body temperature is regulated by a control center in the brain that functions as a thermostat with a set point of 37ºC. If body temperature climbs above 37.2ºC, heat loss is increased through enhanced blood flow to the skin and increased sweating.

skin, and this increases blood flow to the body surface. Your skin then acts like a radiator, losing heat to the environment. In addition, sweat glands are stimulated, so you begin to perspire. The evaporation of sweat helps carry heat away from the skin surface. When your body temperature returns to normal, the thermoregulatory center reduces blood flow to the skin surface, and sweat gland activity decreases.

POSITIVE FEEDBACK

Not all homeostatic mechanisms work to reverse the effects of a stimulus. In **positive feedback**, the initial stimulus produces a response that *magnifies* the stimulus. For example, suppose that the thermostat in your home was accidentally wired so that when the temperature rose it would turn on the heater, rather than the air conditioner. In that case, the initial stimulus (rising room temperature) would cause a response (heater turning on) that would exaggerate the stimulus, rather than reverse it. The room temperature would continue to rise until some external factor turned off the thermostat or unplugged the heater (or the house burned down).

Remember that negative feedback provides long-term control that results in relatively unchanging internal conditions. Positive feedback, on the other hand, controls less frequent or unusual (but necessary) changes that, once begun, need to be completed quickly. For example, the process of birth can be dangerous to a baby if it continues for too long a time. The primary stimulus that begins labor and delivery is the stretching of the womb, or *uterus*, by the growing fetus. This stimulates a control center in the brain to release a chemical that stimulates muscle contractions in the wall of the uterus. These contractions begin moving the fetus toward the birth canal. This movement causes more uterine stretching and, in turn, additional stimulation of the control center. Each time the control center responds, the uterine muscles produce even more movement and stretching. This kind of cycle, a *positive feedback loop*, can be broken only by some external force or process; in this instance, the delivery of the newborn infant eliminates all stretching of the uterus. Homeostasis is then restored.

Concept Questions

✔ Why is homeostasis important to human beings?

✔ How does negative feedback keep internal body conditions within an acceptable range?

✔ What is the difference between negative feedback and positive feedback?

► LEARNING ANATOMY

Early anatomists faced a serious communication problem when describing various parts of the human body: the ordinary terms used to describe the body were too vague. For example, stating that a bump is "on the back" does not give very exact information about its location. So anatomists began to create maps of the human body, using prominent anatomical structures as landmarks and reporting distances in centimeters or inches. These early anatomists spoke Latin or Greek, and many of the names they gave to anatomical structures are still used today.

ANATOMICAL POSITION AND DIRECTIONAL TERMS

Even precise terminology about the body would be confusing without a standard body position to serve as a reference. (Are your eyes above your nose? What if you're standing on your head?) The standard reference position of the body is known as the **anatomical position**. In this position, the arms are at the sides with the palms facing forward (Figure 2-3a). A person is said to be **supine** (SŪ-pīn) when lying faceup, and **prone** when lying facedown.

Table 2-1 and Figure 2-3 give the most important directional terms and examples of their use. Note that the terms *anterior* and *ventral* both refer to the front of the body. Likewise, *posterior* and *dorsal* are terms that refer to the back of the human body. Remember, "left" and "right" always refer to the left and right sides of the subject, not of the observer.

FIGURE 2-3

Directional References.

Important directional terms used in this text are indicated by arrows; definitions and descriptions are included in Table 2-1.

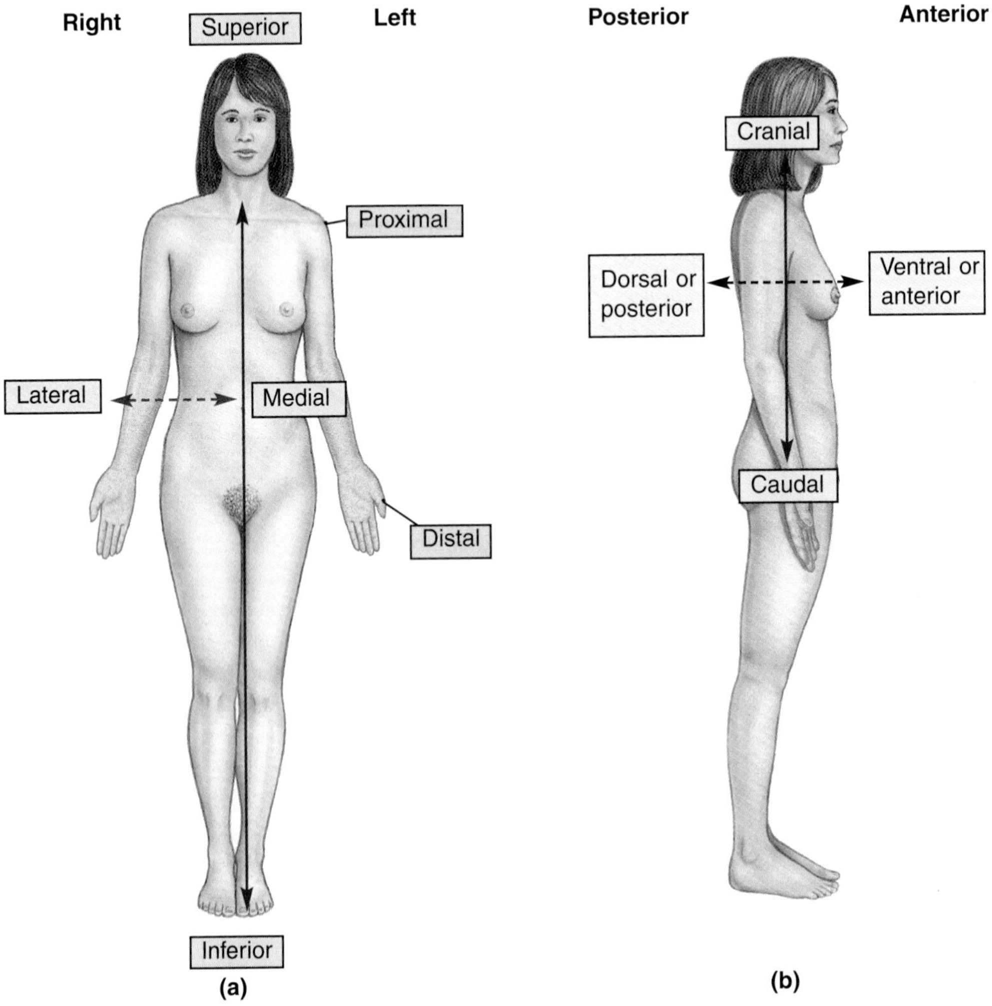

(a)

(b)

Table 2-1	Directional Terms (see Figure 2-3)	
Term	**Region or Reference**	**Example**
Anterior	The front; before	The navel is on the *anterior* (ventral) surface of the trunk
Ventral	The belly side (equivalent to anterior when referring to human body)	
Posterior	The back; behind	The shoulder blade is located *posterior* (dorsal) to the rib cage
Dorsal	The back (equivalent to posterior when referring to human body)	The *dorsal* body cavity encloses the brain and spinal cord
Cranial or cephalic	The head	The *cranial*, or *cephalic*, border of the pelvis is *superior* to the thigh
Superior	Above; at a higher level (in human body, toward the head)	
Caudal	The tail (coccyx in humans)	The hips are *caudal* to the waist
Inferior	Below; at a lower level	The knees are *inferior* to the hips
Medial	Toward the body's longitudinal axis	The *medial* surfaces of the thighs may be in contact; moving medially from the arm across the chest surface brings you to the sternum
Lateral	Away from the body's longitudinal axis	The thigh articulates with the *lateral* surface of the pelvis; moving laterally from the nose brings you to the eyes
Proximal	Toward an attached base	The thigh is *proximal* to the foot; moving proximally from the wrist brings you to the elbow
Distal	Away from an attached base	The fingers are *distal* to the wrist; moving distally from the elbow brings you to the wrist
Superficial	At, near, or relatively close to the body surface	The skin is *superficial* to underlying structures
Deep	Farther from the body surface	The bone of the thigh is *deep* to the surrounding skeletal muscles

REGIONS OF THE HUMAN BODY

To avoid confusion, anatomists and healthcare professionals use very specific names for body structures and for the general area, or region, around each. For example, rather than say "arm," we can say *brachium* to refer specifically to the upper arm, or *brachial* (the adjective form) to refer to something in the region of the upper arm. These regional names are listed in Table 2-2 and, as adjectives, in Figure 2-4. Mastering these terms will be helpful as you learn about the various organs and systems of the body. For example, the term *cranium* refers to the skull, and later chapters will discuss the *cranial nerves*, the *cranial arteries*, and so forth.

Because of the many organs lying within the lower part of the trunk of the body, two types of more detailed surface maps of this area, the *abdominopelvic region*, have been developed. The first approach separates this region into **abdominopelvic quadrants**: four segments divided by imaginary lines that intersect at the *umbilicus* (navel) (Figure 2-5a). This method provides useful references for the description of aches, pains, and injuries. The location of pain can help a healthcare provider determine the possible cause. For example, tenderness in the right lower quadrant (RLQ)

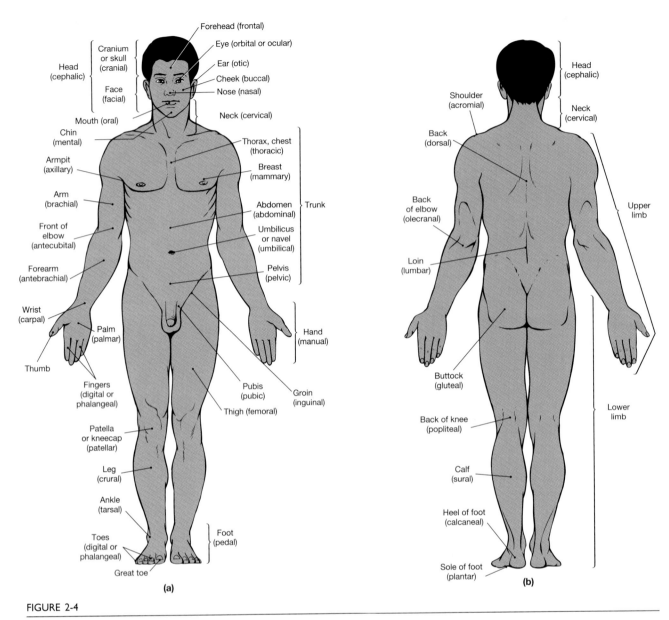

FIGURE 2-4

Anatomical Landmarks.

The common names of anterior and posterior body landmarks are listed first; the anatomical adjectives (in parentheses) follow.

Table 2-2	Regions of the Human Body (see Figure 2-4)		
Structure	**Area**	**Structure**	**Area**
Cephalon (head)	Cephalic region	Axilla (armpit)	Axillary region
Cervicis (neck)	Cervical region	Brachium (arm)	Brachial region
Thoracis (chest)	Thoracic region	Antebrachium (forearm)	Antebrachial region
Abdomen	Abdominal region	Manus (hand)	Manual region
Pelvis	Pelvic region	Thigh	Femoral region
Loin (lower back)	Lumbar region	Leg	Crural region
Buttock	Gluteal region	Calf	Sural region
Pubis (anterior pelvis)	Pubic region	Pes (foot)	Pedal region
Groin	Inguinal region		

FIGURE 2-5

Abdominopelvic Quadrants and Regions.

(a) Abdominopelvic quadrants divide the area into four sections. These terms, or their abbreviations, are most often used in clinical discussions. **(b)** More precise regional descriptions are provided by reference to the appropriate abdominopelvic region. **(c)** Quadrants or regions are useful because there is a known relationship between superficial anatomical landmarks and underlying organs.

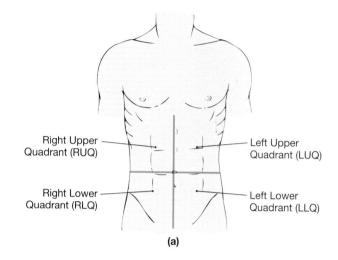

Right Upper Quadrant (RUQ)

Left Upper Quadrant (LUQ)

Right Lower Quadrant (RLQ)

Left Lower Quadrant (LLQ)

(a)

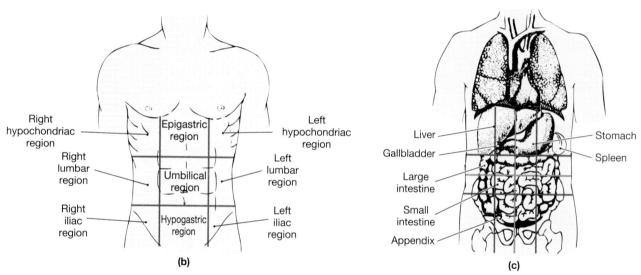

Right hypochondriac region

Epigastric region

Left hypochondriac region

Right lumbar region

Umbilical region

Left lumbar region

Right iliac region

Hypogastric region

Left iliac region

(b)

Liver

Gallbladder

Large intestine

Small intestine

Appendix

Stomach

Spleen

(c)

is a symptom of appendicitis, whereas tenderness in the right upper quadrant (RUQ) may indicate gallbladder or liver problems.

The other approach, which is even more precise, recognizes nine **abdominopelvic regions** (Figure 2-5b). Figure 2-5c shows the relationships among quadrants, regions, and internal organs.

BODY SECTIONS

Many times, the only way to see the inner structure of a body part is to cut a *section* through it. Any slice through a three-dimensional object can be described with reference to three **sectional planes**. These planes, described next, are shown in Figure 2-6 and reviewed in Table 2-3.

1. **Transverse plane.** The **transverse plane** lies at right angles to the long axis (head-to-foot) of the body, dividing it into **superior** and **inferior** sections. A cut in this plane is called a **horizontal section**, a *transverse section*, or a *cross section*.
2. **Frontal plane.** The **frontal plane**, or **coronal plane**, parallels the long axis of the body. The frontal plane extends from side to side, dividing the body into **anterior** and **posterior** sections.
3. **Sagittal plane.** The **sagittal plane** also parallels the long axis of the body, but it divides the body into *left* and *right* sections. A cut that passes along the midline and divides the body into equal left and right halves is a *midsagittal section*. Because they parallel the long axis of the body, frontal and sagittal sections are also often called *longitudinal sections*.

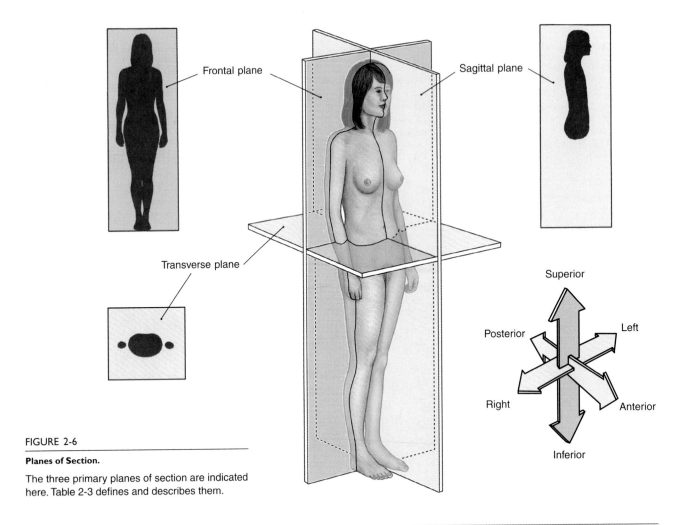

FIGURE 2-6

Planes of Section.

The three primary planes of section are indicated here. Table 2-3 defines and describes them.

Table 2-3	Terms That Indicate Planes of Sections (see Figure 2-6)	
Orientation of Plane	**Adjective**	**Description**
Parallel to long axis	Sagittal Midsagittal	A *sagittal* section separates right and left portions In a *midsagittal* section, the plane passes through the midline, dividing the body in half and separating right and left sides
	Frontal or coronal	A *frontal*, or *coronal*, section separates anterior and posterior portions of the body; *coronal* usually refers to sections passing through the skull
Perpendicular to long axis	Transverse or horizontal	A *transverse*, or *horizontal*, section separates superior and inferior portions of the body

An understanding of sectional views has become increasingly important since the development of electronic imaging techniques that enable us to see inside the living body without resorting to surgery. Figure 2-7 presents examples of CT and MRI scans of a transverse section through the abdomen.

BODY CAVITIES AND BODY LININGS

Many vital organs of the body are suspended within internal chambers called *body cavities*. These cavities have two essential functions: (1) They cushion delicate organs, such as the brain and spinal cord,

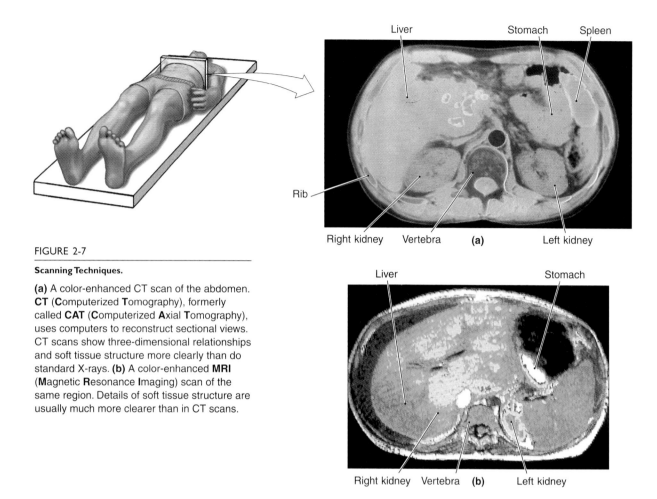

Liver   Stomach   Spleen

Rib

Right kidney   Vertebra   **(a)**   Left kidney

Liver   Stomach

Right kidney   Vertebra   **(b)**   Left kidney

FIGURE 2-7

Scanning Techniques.

(a) A color-enhanced CT scan of the abdomen. **CT** (**C**omputerized **T**omography), formerly called **CAT** (**C**omputerized **A**xial **T**omography), uses computers to reconstruct sectional views. CT scans show three-dimensional relationships and soft tissue structure more clearly than do standard X-rays. **(b)** A color-enhanced **MRI** (**M**agnetic **R**esonance **I**maging) scan of the same region. Details of soft tissue structure are usually much more clearer than in CT scans.

from the thumps and bumps that occur during walking, jumping, and running; and (2) they permit changes in the size and shape of internal organs. Because the lungs, heart, stomach, intestines, urinary bladder, and many other organs are situated within body cavities, they can expand and contract without disrupting the activities of nearby organs.

The two main body cavities are the **dorsal body cavity**, which surrounds the brain and spinal cord, and the much larger **ventral body cavity**, which surrounds the organs of the respiratory, cardiovascular, digestive, urinary, and reproductive systems.

The dorsal body cavity (Figure 2-8a) is a fluid-filled space that contains the brain and spinal cord and is surrounded by the **cranium** (the bones of the skull) and the **vertebrae** (the bones of the spine). The dorsal body cavity is subdivided into the *cranial cavity*, which encloses the brain, and the *spinal cavity*, which surrounds the spinal cord.

The **diaphragm** (DĪ-a-fram), a flat muscular sheet, divides the ventral body cavity into an upper (superior) **thoracic cavity**, enclosed by the chest wall, and a lower (inferior) **abdominopelvic cavity** (Figure 2-8a). The abdominopelvic cavity has two continuous subdivisions: the upper **abdominal cavity** and the lower **pelvic cavity**.

The surfaces of organs and their respective body cavities are covered by shiny, slippery linings called *serous membranes*. The *parietal* portion of a serous membrane forms the outer wall of the body cavity. The *visceral* portion covers the surfaces of internal organs, or **viscera** (VIS-e-ra), where they project into the body cavity. The space between these opposing portions of a serous membrane is very small, but the space contains a thin layer of lubricating fluid. Many visceral organs undergo periodic changes in size and shape. For example, the lungs inflate and deflate with each breath, and the volume of the heart changes during each heartbeat. A covering of serous membrane prevents friction of adjacent organs and between the organs and the body wall.

diaphragma, a partition wall
diaphragm: a muscular sheet that separates the thoracic cavity from the abdominopelvic cavity

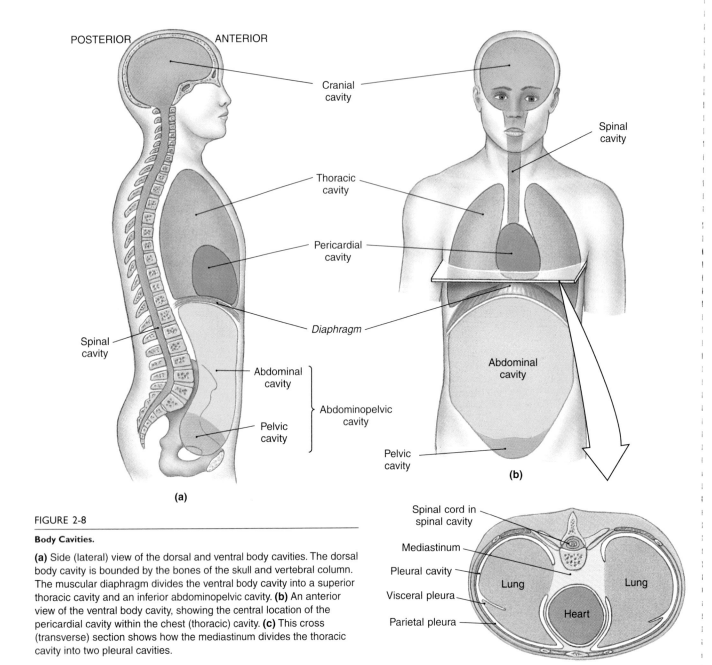

POSTERIOR   ANTERIOR

Cranial cavity

Spinal cavity

Thoracic cavity

Pericardial cavity

Diaphragm

Spinal cavity

Abdominal cavity

Abdominal cavity

Abdominopelvic cavity

Pelvic cavity

Pelvic cavity

(a)   (b)

Spinal cord in spinal cavity

Mediastinum

Pleural cavity

Visceral pleura

Parietal pleura

Lung   Lung

Heart

(c)

FIGURE 2-8

Body Cavities.

(a) Side (lateral) view of the dorsal and ventral body cavities. The dorsal body cavity is bounded by the bones of the skull and vertebral column. The muscular diaphragm divides the ventral body cavity into a superior thoracic cavity and an inferior abdominopelvic cavity. **(b)** An anterior view of the ventral body cavity, showing the central location of the pericardial cavity within the chest (thoracic) cavity. **(c)** This cross (transverse) section shows how the mediastinum divides the thoracic cavity into two pleural cavities.

Concept Questions

✔ Is the elbow proximal or distal to the wrist?

✔ What type of section would divide the body into right and left portions?

✔ If a surgeon makes an incision just inferior to the diaphragm, what body cavity will be opened?

peri, around + *kardia*, heart
pericardial cavity: a cavity that surrounds the heart

The thoracic (chest) cavity contains the heart and lungs. The heart projects into a space known as the **pericardial cavity**. The serous membrane lining this space is called the *pericardium*, a term that means "around the heart." Each lung is surrounded by a **pleural cavity**. The serous membrane lining the pleural cavities is called the *pleura* (PLOO-ra). The region between the two pleural cavities contains a large mass of tissue known as the *mediastinum* (mē-dē-as-TĪ-num or mē-dē-AS-ti-num) (Figure 2-8c). The mediastinum contains the thymus, trachea, esophagus, the large arteries and veins attached to the heart, and the pericardial cavity.

Most of the abdominopelvic cavity and the organs it contains are covered by a serous membrane called the *peritoneum* (pe-ri-tō-NĒ-um). This lined portion of the abdominopelvic cavity is known as the *peritoneal* (per-i-tō-NĒ-al) *cavity*. Organs such as the stomach, small intestine, and portions of the large intestine are suspended within the peritoneal cavity by double sheets of peritoneum, called *mesenteries* (MES-en-ter-ēs).Mesenteries provide support and stability while permitting limited movement.

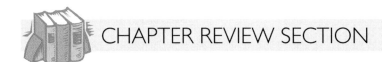

CHAPTER REVIEW SECTION

KEY WORDS

anatomy (a-NAT-o-mē):	The study of the structures of the body.
anatomical position:	The standard reference position of the body; the body viewed from the anterior surface with the palms facing forward.
frontal plane:	A sectional plane that divides the body into anterior and posterior portions.
homeostasis (hō-mē-ō-STĀ-sis):	A relatively stable or constant internal environment.
negative feedback:	Correcting process in which the body's response reverses the effect of a stimulus and restores homeostasis.
organ:	A combination of different tissues that perform complex functions.
physiology (fiz-ē-OL-o-jē):	The study of how the body functions.
positive feedback:	Mechanism that increases a deviation from normal limits following an initial stimulus.
sagittal plane:	Sectional plane that divides the body into left and right portions.
serous membrane:	Slippery, delicate tissue sheet, consisting of *parietal* and *visceral* portions, that lines body cavities and covers internal organs to prevent friction.
tissue:	A collection of specialized cells that perform a specific function.
transverse plane:	Sectional plane that divides the body into superior and inferior portions.
viscera:	Organs in the ventral body cavity.

STUDY OUTLINE

THE SCIENCES OF ANATOMY AND PHYSIOLOGY

1. **Anatomy** is the study of internal and external structure and the physical relationships among body parts. **Physiology** is the study of body function.

LEVELS OF ORGANIZATION IN THE BODY

1. Anatomical structures and physiological mechanisms are arranged in a series of interacting levels of organization. (*Figure 2-1*)

HOMEOSTASIS

1. **Homeostasis** is the maintenance of a relatively stable internal environment.
2. Symptoms of **disease** appear when failure of homeostatic regulation causes organ systems to malfunction.

NEGATIVE FEEDBACK

3. **Negative feedback** is a corrective mechanism involving an action that directly opposes a variation from normal limits. (*Figure 2-2*)

POSITIVE FEEDBACK

4. In **positive feedback**, the initial stimulus produces a response that enhances the stimulus.

LEARNING ANATOMY

ANATOMICAL POSITION AND DIRECTIONAL TERMS

1. Standard anatomical illustrations show the body in the upright **anatomical position**. If the figure is shown lying down, it can be either **supine** (faceup) or **prone** (facedown).

2. The use of special directional terms provides clarity when describing relative locations of anatomical structures. (*Figure 2-3; Table 2-1*)

REGIONS OF THE HUMAN BODY

3. In addition to common names, different regions of the body are also known by specific Latin or Greek names. (*Figure 2-4; Table 2-2*)

4. **Abdominopelvic quadrants** and **abdominopelvic regions** are two different terms used in describing anatomical regions of the body. (*Figure 2-5*)

BODY SECTIONS

5. The three **sectional planes** (**frontal**, or **coronal**, **plane**, **sagittal plane**, and **transverse plane**) describe relationships between the parts of the three-dimensional human body. (*Figures 2-6, 2-7; Table 2-3*)

BODY CAVITIES AND BODY LININGS

6. **Body cavities** protect delicate organs and permit changes in the size and shape of visceral organs. The **dorsal body cavity** contains the *cranial cavity* (enclosing the brain) and *spinal cavity* (surrounding the spinal cord). The **ventral body cavity** surrounds respiratory, cardiovascular, digestive, urinary, and reproductive organs. (*Figure 2-8*)

7. The **diaphragm** divides the ventral body cavity into the superior **thoracic** and inferior **abdominopelvic cavities**. The thoracic cavity contains two *pleural cavities* (each containing a lung) and a *pericardial cavity* (which surrounds the heart). The **abdominopelvic cavity** consists of the **abdominal cavity** and the **pelvic cavity**. (*Figure 2-8*)

8. *Serous membranes* line the surfaces of the thoracic and abdominopelvic cavities and the organs they contain.

REVIEW QUESTIONS

MATCHING

Match each item in Column A with the most closely related item in Column B. Use letters for answers in the spaces provided.

Column A	Column B
J 1. physiology	a. constant internal environment
K 2. homeostasis	b. lying faceup
G 3. supine	c. study of structure
L 4. prone	d. positive feedback
A 5. temperature regulation	e. back of the body
C 6. anatomy	f. tissue
M 7. dorsal body cavity	g. lying facedown
N 8. heart	h. negative feedback
C 9. muscle	i. serous membrane
H 10. birth	j. study of body functions
B 11. ventral body cavity	k. front of the body
H 12. pericardium	l. brain and spinal cord
E 13. anterior	m. thoracic and abdominopelvic
E 14. posterior	n. organ

MULTIPLE CHOICE

15. ____C____ are terms that apply to the front of the body when in the anatomical position.
    (a) anterior, ventral   (b) medial, lateral
    (c) posterior, dorsal   (d) back, front

16. A ____B____ section separates superior and inferior portions of the body.
    (a) sagittal   (b) midsagittal
    (c) frontal   (d) transverse

17. The relative stability of an organism's internal environment is called ____A____
    (a) uniformity   (b) homeostasis
    (c) equilibrium   (d) constancy

18. The umbilicus is ____C____ to the chest.
    (a) anterior   (b) superior
    (c) posterior   (d) inferior

19. The ____D____ region refers to the thigh.
    (a) brachial   (b) femoral
    (c) thoracic   (d) cervical

20. The diaphragm is a flat, muscular sheet that divides the ventral body cavity into a superior ____B____ cavity and an inferior ____B____ cavity.
    (a) pleural, pericardial   (b) abdominal, pelvic
    (c) thoracic, abdominopelvic   (d) cranial, thoracic

21. The mediastinum is the region between the ____A____
    (a) lungs and heart   (b) two pleural cavities
    (c) thorax and abdomen   (d) heart and pericardial cavity

22. The membrane that lines the abdominopelvic cavity is the _C_____.
    (a) mesenteries   (b) pleura
    (c) pericardium   (d) peritoneum

TRUE/FALSE

_____ 23. Organs consist of more than one type of tissue.

_____ 24. The study of anatomy and physiology together is extremely useful in biology because structure and function are closely related.

_____ 25. The simplest living structural and functional units of the human body are tissues.

_____ 26. When the body is in the anatomical position, the palms of the hands touch the lateral surface of the body.

_____ 27. Failure of homeostatic regulation in the body results in disease.

SHORT ESSAY

28. Beginning with the molecular level, list in correct sequence the levels of organization from the simplest level to the most complex level.

29. How does negative feedback differ from positive feedback?

30. Describe the position of the body when it is in the anatomical position.

31. You are awakened in the middle of the night by a mosquito in your otic region. Where is the mosquito?

32. In which body cavity would each of the following organs or systems be found?
    (a) brain and spinal cord   (b) cardiovascular, digestive, and urinary systems
    (c) heart, lungs   (d) stomach, intestines

33. If you begin at the elbow and move proximally 25 cm, medially 20 cm, and inferiorly 30 cm, what surface anatomical landmark will you be near?

✔ ANSWERS TO CONCEPT CHECK QUESTIONS

(p. 36) **1.** A *cell* is the smallest structural and functional unit of life in all living organisms, including humans. **2.** An *organ* is composed of different tissues that work together to perform specific functions; a tissue is composed of a group of similar cells that perform a specific function.

(p. 37) **1.** The cells making up the human body can function normally only under a narrow range of environmental conditions. *Homeostasis* is the process that prevents potentially harmful changes in the body's internal environment. **2.** *Negative feedback* is the major process that maintains homeostasis in the human body. Negative feedback acts by reversing the effect of a stimulus to maintain constant internal conditions in the body. **3.** *Positive feedback* works in a manner opposite to negative feedback. It produces a response that magnifies the initial stimulus.

(p. 44) **1.** The elbow is *proximal* to the wrist. The wrist is *distal* to the elbow. **2.** A sagittal section would divide the body into right and left portions. **3.** The surgeon is making an opening into the *abdominopelvic* (or *peritoneal*) cavity.

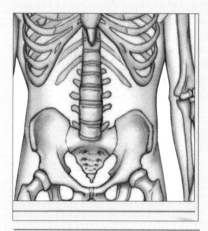

3

MEDICAL TERMINOLOGY OF THE SKELETAL SYSTEM

OBJECTIVES

On completion of this chapter, you should be able to:

- Describe the skeletal system.
- Describe various types of body movement.
- Describe the vertebral column.
- Identify abnormal curvatures of the spine.
- Describe the male and female pelvis.
- Describe various types of fractures.
- Describe skeletal differences of the child and the older adult.
- Analyze, build, spell, and pronounce medical words that relate to surgical procedures and pathology.
- Identify and give the meaning of selected vocabulary words.
- Identify and define selected abbreviations.
- Review Drug Highlights presented in this chapter.
- Provide the description of diagnostic and laboratory tests related to the skeletal system.
- Successfully complete the study and review section.

► ANATOMY AND PHYSIOLOGY OVERVIEW

The skeletal system is composed of 206 *bones* that, together with *cartilage* and *ligaments,* make up the *framework* or skeleton of the body. The skeleton can be divided into two main groups of bones: the *axial skeleton* consisting of 80 bones and the *appendicular skeleton* with the remaining 126 bones (see Fig. 3–1). The principal bones of the axial skeleton are the skull, spine, ribs, and sternum. The shoulder girdle, arms, and hands and the pelvic girdle, legs, and feet are the primary bones of the appendicular skeleton (Fig. 3–2).

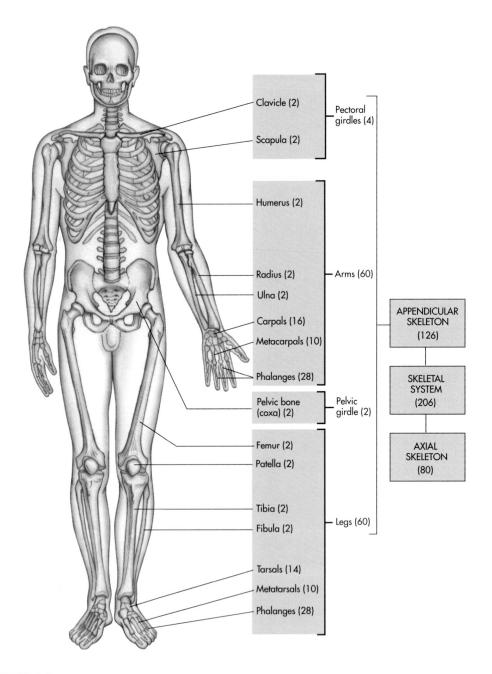

FIGURE 3–1

The principal bones of the appendicular skeleton.

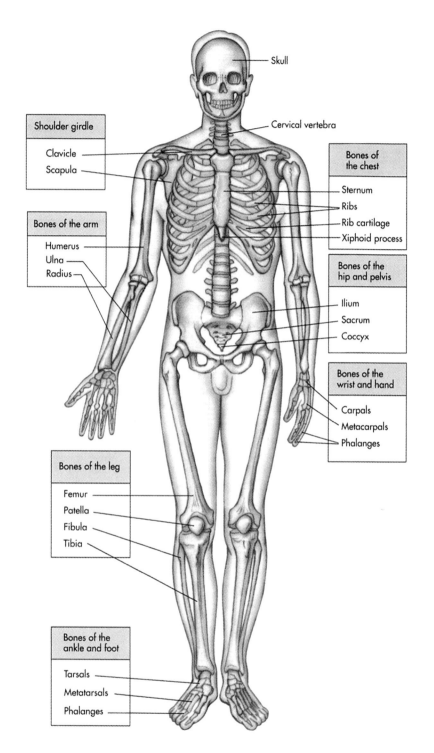

FIGURE 3–2

The skull, cervical vertebra, and principal bones of the axial and appendicular skeleton.

THE SKELETAL SYSTEM

ORGAN/STRUCTURE	PRIMARY FUNCTIONS
Bones	Provide shape, support, protection, and the framework of the body
	Serve as a storage place for mineral salts, calcium, and phosphorus
	Play an important role in the formation of blood cells
	Provide areas for the attachment of skeletal muscles
	Help make movement possible
Cartilages	Form the major portion of the embryonic skeleton and part of the skeleton in adults
Ligaments	Connect the articular ends of bones, binding them together and facilitating or limiting motion
	Connect cartilage and other structures
	Serve to support or attach fascia or muscles

▶ BONES

The *bones* are the primary organs of the skeletal system and are composed of about 50% water and 50% solid matter. The solid matter in bone is a calcified, rigid substance known as *osseous tissue.*

CLASSIFICATION OF BONES

Bones are classified according to their shapes. The following table classifies the bones and gives an example of each type:

SHAPE	EXAMPLE OF THIS CLASSIFICATION
Flat	Ribs, scapula, parts of the pelvic girdle, bones of the skull
Long	Tibia, femur, humerus, radius
Short	Carpal, tarsal
Irregular	Vertebrae, ossicles of the ear
Sesamoid	Patella

FUNCTIONS OF BONES

The following are the main functions of bones:

1. Provide shape and support and form the framework of the body
2. Provide protection for internal organs
3. Serve as a storage place for mineral salts, calcium, and phosphorus
4. Play an important role in the formation of blood cells as *hemopoiesis* takes place in the bone marrow
5. Provide areas for the attachment of skeletal muscles
6. Help to make movement possible through *articulation*

THE STRUCTURE OF A LONG BONE

Long bones, such as the tibia, femur, humerus, or radius, have most of the features found in all bones. These features are shown in Figure 3–3.

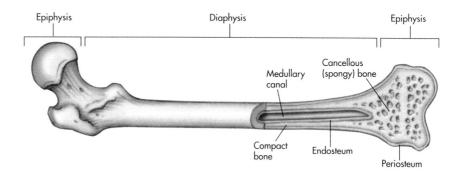

FIGURE 3–3

The features found in a long bone.

Epiphysis. The ends of a developing bone

Diaphysis. The shaft of a long bone

Periosteum. The membrane that forms the covering of bones except at their articular surfaces

Compact bone. The dense, hard layer of bone tissue

Medullary canal. A narrow space or cavity throughout the length of the diaphysis

Endosteum. A tough, connective tissue membrane lining the medullary canal and containing the bone marrow

Cancellous or spongy bone. The reticular tissue that makes up most of the volume of bone

BONE MARKINGS

There are certain commonly used terms that describe the *markings of bones*. These markings are listed for your better understanding of their role in joining bones together, providing areas for muscle attachments, and serving as a passageway for blood vessels, ligaments, and nerves.

MARKING	DESCRIPTION OF THE BONE STRUCTURE
Condyle	A rounded process that enters into the formation of a joint, articulation
Crest	A ridge on a bone
Fissure	A slit-like opening between two bones
Foramen	An opening in the bone for blood vessels, ligaments, and nerves
Fossa	A shallow depression in or on a bone
Head	The rounded end of a bone
Meatus	A tube-like passage or canal
Process	An enlargement or protrusion of a bone
Sinus	An air cavity within certain bones
Spine	A pointed, sharp, slender process
Sulcus	A groove, furrow, depression, or fissure
Trochanter	A very large process of the femur
Tubercle	A small, rounded process
Tuberosity	A large, rounded process

► JOINTS AND MOVEMENT

A *joint* is an articulation, a place where two or more bones connect. The manner in which bones connect determines the type of movement allowed at the joint. Joints are classified as:

Synarthrosis. Does not permit movement. The bones are in close contact with each other and there is no joint cavity. An example is the *cranial sutures.*

Amphiarthrosis. Permits very slight movement. An example of this type of joint is the *vertebrae.*

Diarthrosis. Allows free movement in a variety of directions. Examples of this type of joint are the *knee, hip, elbow, wrist,* and *foot.*

The following terms describe types of body movement that occur at the *diarthrotic joints* (Fig. 3–4):

Abduction. The process of moving a body part away from the middle

Adduction. The process of moving a body part toward the middle

Circumduction. The process of moving a body part in a circular motion

Dorsiflexion. The process of bending a body part backward

Eversion. The process of turning outward

Extension. The process of straightening a flexed limb

Flexion. The process of bending a limb

Inversion. The process of turning inward

Pronation. The process of lying prone or face downward; also the process of turning the hand so the palm faces downward

Protraction. The process of moving a body part forward

Retraction. The process of moving a body part backward

Rotation. The process of moving a body part around a central axis

Supination. The process of lying supine or face upward; also the process of turning the palm or foot upward

► THE VERTEBRAL COLUMN

The *vertebral column* is composed of a series of separate bones *(vertebrae)* connected in such a way as to form four spinal curves. These curves have been identified as the cervical, thoracic, lumbar, and sacral. The *cervical curve* consists of the first 7 vertebrae, the *thoracic curve* consists of the next 12 vertebrae, the *lumbar curve* consists of the next 5 vertebrae, and the *sacral curve* consists of the sacrum and coccyx (tailbone) (Fig. 3–5).

It is known that a curved structure has more strength than a straight structure. The spinal curves of the human body are most important, as they help support the weight of the body and provide the balance that is necessary to walk on two feet.

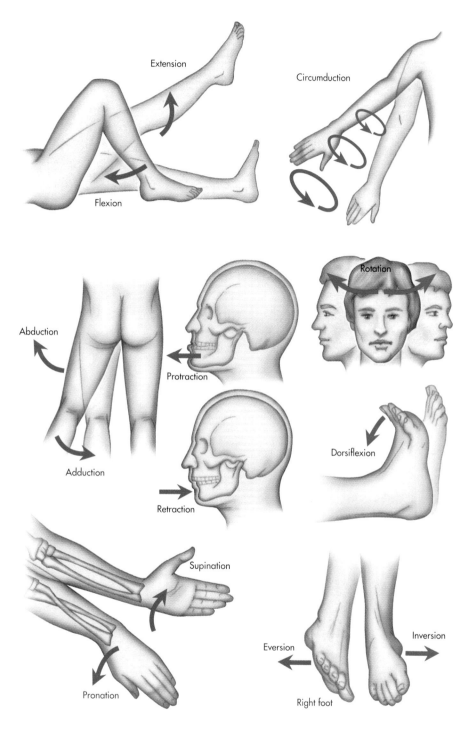

FIGURE 3–4

Types of body movements.

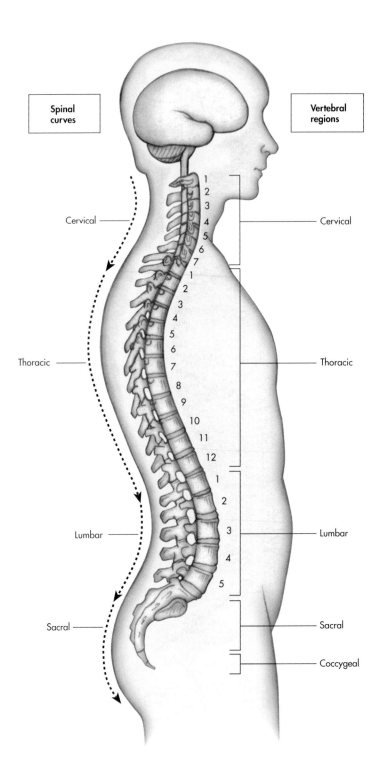

FIGURE 3–5

Vertebral regions, showing the four spinal curves.

▶ ABNORMAL CURVATURES OF THE SPINE

SCOLIOSIS, LORDOSIS, AND KYPHOSIS

In *scoliosis,* there is an abnormal lateral curvature of the spine. This condition usually appears in adolescence, during periods of rapid growth. Treatment modalities may include the application of a cast, brace, traction, electrical stimulation, and/or surgery. See Figure 3–6A.

In *lordosis,* there is an abnormal anterior curvature of the spine. This condition may be referred to as *"swayback"* as the abdomen and buttocks protrude due to an exaggerated lumbar curvature. See Figure 3–6B.

In *kyphosis,* the normal thoracic curvature becomes exaggerated, producing a *"humpback"* appearance. This condition may be caused by a congenital defect, a disease process such as tuberculosis and/or syphilis, a malignancy, compression fracture, faulty posture, osteoarthritis, rheumatoid arthritis, rickets, osteoporosis, or other conditions. See Figure 3–6C.

▶ THE MALE AND FEMALE PELVIS

The *pelvis* is the lower portion of the trunk of the body. It forms a basin bound anteriorly and laterally by the hip bones and posteriorly by the sacrum and coccyx.

The bony pelvis is formed by the sacrum, the coccyx, and the bones that form the hip and pubic arch, the ilium, pubis, and ischium. These bones are separate in the child, but become fused in adulthood.

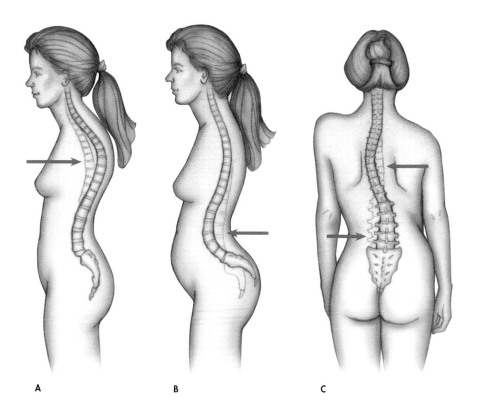

A   B   C

FIGURE 3–6

Abnormal curvatures of the spine: **(A)** kyphosis, **(B)** lordosis, **(C)** scoliosis.

THE MALE PELVIS

The *male pelvis* is shaped like a *funnel,* forming a narrower outlet than the female. It is heavier and stronger than the female pelvis; therefore, it is more suited for lifting and running. See Figure 3–7A.

THE FEMALE PELVIS

The *female pelvis* is shaped like a *basin.* It may be oval to round, and it is wider than the male pelvis. The female pelvis is constructed to accommodate the fetus during pregnancy and to facilitate its downward passage through the pelvic cavity in childbirth. In general the female pelvis is broader and lighter than the male pelvis. See Figure 3–7B.

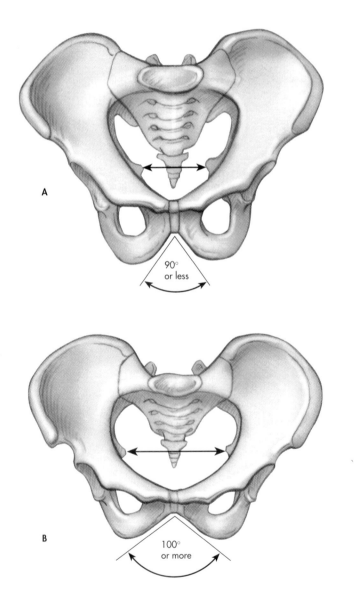

FIGURE 3–7

(A) The male pelvis is shaped like a funnel, forming a narrower outlet than the female. **(B)** The female pelvis is shaped like a basin.

► FRACTURES

Fractures are classified according to their external appearance, the site of the fracture, and the nature of the crack or break in the bone. Important fracture types are indicated in Figure 3–8 and several have been paired with representative x-rays. Many fractures fall in more than one category. For example, Colles' fracture is a transverse fracture, but depending on the injury it may also be a comminuted fracture that can be either open or closed.

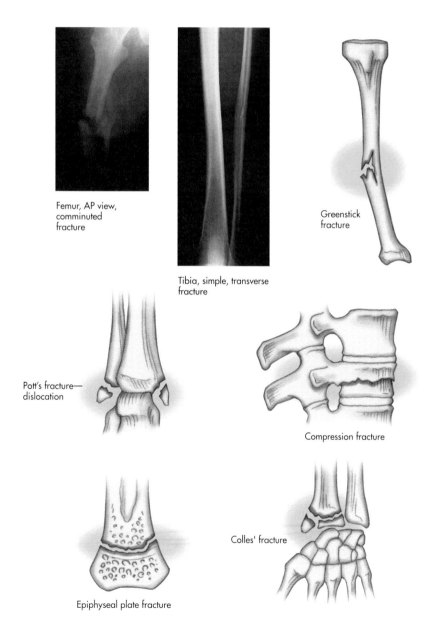

Femur, AP view, comminuted fracture

Tibia, simple, transverse fracture

Greenstick fracture

Pott's fracture—dislocation

Compression fracture

Epiphyseal plate fracture

Colles' fracture

FIGURE 3–8

Various types of fractures.

TYPES OF FRACTURES (SEE FIGURE 3–8)

- **Closed,** or **simple,** fractures do not involve a break in the skin; they are completely internal.

- **Open,** or **compound,** fractures are more dangerous because the fracture projects through the skin and there is a possibility of infection or hemorrhage.

- **Comminuted** fractures shatter the affected part into a multitude of bony fragments.

- **Transverse** fractures break the shaft of a bone across its longitudinal axis.

- **Greenstick** fractures usually occur in children whose long bones have not fully ossified; only one side of the shaft is broken, and the other is bent (like a green stick).

- **Spiral** fractures are spread along the length of a bone and are produced by twisting stresses.

- **Colles'** fracture is often the result of reaching out to cushion a fall; there is a break in the distal portion of the radius.

- **Pott's** fracture occurs at the ankle and affects both bones of the lower leg (fibula and tibia).

- **Compression** fractures occur in vertebrae subjected to extreme stresses, as when one falls and lands on his/her bottom.

- **Epiphyseal** fractures usually occur where the matrix is undergoing calcification and chondrocytes (cartilage cells) are dying; this type of fracture is seen in children.

Life Span Considerations

▶ THE CHILD

Bone begins to develop during the second month of fetal life as cartilage cells enlarge, break down, disappear, and are replaced by bone-forming cells called **osteoblasts.** Most bones of the body are formed by this process, known as **endochondral ossification.** In this process, the bone cells deposit organic substances in the spaces vacated by cartilage to form bone matrix. As this process proceeds, blood vessels form within the bone and deposit salts such as calcium and phosphorus that serve to harden the developing bone.

The **epiphyseal plate** is the center for longitudinal bone growth in children. See Figure 3–9. It is possible to determine the biological age of a child from the development of epiphyseal ossification centers as shown radiographically.

About 3 years from the onset of puberty the ends of the long bones **(epiphyses)** knit securely to their shafts **(diaphysis),** and further growth can no longer take place.

The bones of children are more resilient, tend to bend, and before breaking may become deformed. Fracture healing occurs more quickly in children because there is a rich blood supply to bones and their periosteum is thick and osteogenic activity is high.

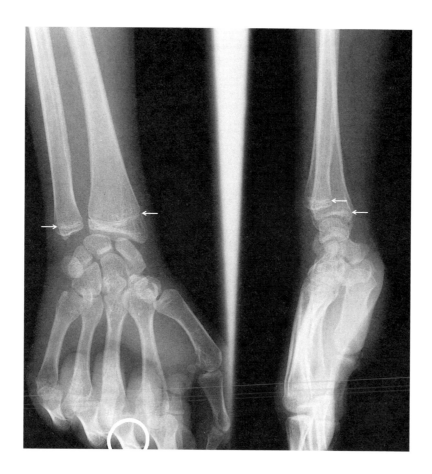

FIGURE 3–9

Epiphyseal plate (arrows). *(Courtesy of Teresa Resch.)*

Calcium is critical to the strength of bones. The daily recommendations of calcium by age group are:

- 1 to 3 years   500 mg
- 4 to 8 years   800 mg
- 9 to 13 years   1300 mg
- 14 to 18 years   1300 mg

▶ THE OLDER ADULT

Women build bone until about age 35, then begin to lose about 1% of bone mass annually. Men usually start losing bone mass 10 to 20 years later. Most of the skeletal system changes that take place during the aging process involve changes in connective tissue. There is a loss of bone mass and bone strength due to the loss of bone mineral content during later life. Calcium salts may be deposited in the matrix and cartilage becomes hard and brittle.

Age-related **osteoporosis,** loss of bone mass, is often seen in older women and men. Other changes that may occur involve the joints as there is diminished viscosity of the synovial fluid, degeneration of collagen and elastin cells, outgrowth of cartilaginous clusters in response to continuous wear and tear, and formation of scar tissues and calcification in the joint capsules.

Low levels of calcium can make people more susceptible to osteoporosis and stress fractures, especially those that are commonly seen in the older adult. Bone healing in the older adult is slower and impaired due to osteoblasts being less able to use calcium to restructure bone tissue. The National Academy of Sciences suggests that people 51 and older consume 1200 mg of calcium per day to help strengthen their bones. See Table 3–1 for good sources of calcium.

TABLE 3–1   Good Sources of Calcium

1 cup skim milk	300 mg
1 cup yogurt	450 mg
1 cup calcium-fortified orange juice	300 mg
1 ounce cheddar cheese	205 mg
1 ounce Swiss cheese	270 mg
1 cup tofu (processed with calcium sulfate)	520 mg
1 cup turnip greens, cooked	200 mg
3 ounces canned salmon (with bones)	205 mg
7-inch homemade waffle	179 mg
1 cup broccoli, cooked	90 mg

Dairy foods supply 75% of all the calcium in the U.S. food supply. People who get 2 to 3 servings of dairy products a day are most likely meeting the recommended requirements. For those who do not like milk or dairy products, there are other ways of getting enough calcium per day.

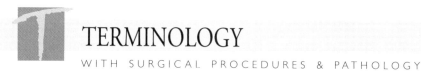

TERMINOLOGY

WITH SURGICAL PROCEDURES & PATHOLOGY

TERM	WORD PARTS			DEFINITION
acetabular (ăs″ ĕ-tăb′ ū-lăr)	acetabul ar	R S	vinegar cup pertaining to	The cup-shaped socket of the hipbone into which the thighbone fits
achillobursitis (ă-kil″ ō-bŭr-sī′ tĭs)	achillo burs itis	CF R S	achilles, heel a pouch inflammation	Inflammation of the bursa lying over the Achilles' tendon
achondroplasia (ă-kŏn″ drō-plā′ sĭ-ă)	a chondro plasia	P CF S	without cartilage formation	A defect in the formation of cartilage at the epiphyses of long bones
acroarthritis (ăk″ rō-ăr-thrī′ tĭs)	acro arthr itis	CF R S	extremity joint inflammation	Inflammation of the joints of the hands or feet
acromion (ă-krō′ mĭ-ŏn)	acr omion	R S	extremity, point shoulder	The projection of the spine of the scapula that forms the point of the shoulder and articulates with the clavicle
ankylosis (ăng″ kĭ-lō′ sĭs)	ankyl osis	R S	stiffening, crooked condition of	A condition of stiffening of a joint
arthralgia (ăr-thrăl′ jĭ-ă)	arthr algia	R S	joint pain	Pain in a joint
arthrectomy (ăr-thrĕk′ tō-mē)	arthr ectomy	R S	joint excision	Surgical excision of a joint
arthredema (ăr″ thrĕ-dē′ mă)	arthr edema	R S	joint swelling	Swelling of a joint
arthritis (ăr-thrī′ tĭs)	arthr itis	R S	joint inflammation	Inflammation of a joint
arthrocentesis (ăr″ thrō-sĕn-tē′ sĭs)	arthro centesis	CF S	joint surgical puncture	Surgical puncture of a joint for removal of fluid
arthrodesis (ăr″ thrō-dē′ sĭs)	arthro desis	CF S	joint binding	The surgical binding of a joint for immobilization
arthropathy (ăr-thrŏp′ ă-thē)	arthro pathy	CF S	joint disease	Any joint disease

continued

Terminology - continued

TERM	WORD PARTS			DEFINITION
arthroplasty (ăr″ thrō-plăs′ tē)	arthro plasty	CF S	joint surgical repair	Surgical repair of a joint
arthropyosis (ăr″ thrō-pī-ō′ sĭs)	arthro py osis	CF R S	joint pus condition of	A condition of pus at a joint
bursectomy (bŭr-sĕk′ tō-mē)	burs ectomy	R S	a pouch excision	Surgical excision of a bursa
bursitis (bŭr-sī′ tĭs)	burs itis	R S	a pouch inflammation	Inflammation of a bursa
calcaneal (kăl-kā′ nē-ăl)	calcane al	R S	heel bone pertaining to	Pertaining to the heel bone
calcaneodynia (kăl-kā″ nē-ō-dĭn′ ĭ-ă)	calcaneo dynia	CF S	heel bone pain	Pain in the heel bone
carpal (kär′ pəl)	carp al	R S	wrist pertaining to	Pertaining to the wristbone
carpopedal (kär″ pō-pēd′ ăl)	carpo ped al	CF R S	wrist foot pertaining to	Pertaining to the wrist and the foot
carpoptosis (kär″ pŏp-tō′ sĭs)	carpo ptosis	CF S	wrist drooping	Wrist drop
chondral (kŏn′ drăl)	chondr al	R S	cartilage pertaining to	Pertaining to cartilage
chondralgia (kŏn-drăl′ jĭ-ă)	chondr algia	R S	cartilage pain	Pain in or around cartilage
chondrectomy (kŏn-drĕk′ tō-mē)	chondr ectomy	R S	cartilage excision	Surgical excision of a cartilage
chondroblast (kŏn′ drō-blăst)	chondro blast	CF S	cartilage immature cell, germ cell	A cell that forms cartilage
chondrocostal (kŏn″ drō-kŏs′ tăl)	chondro cost al	CF R S	cartilage rib pertaining to	Pertaining to the rib cartilage
chondropathology (kŏn″ drō-pă-thŏl′ ō-jē)	chondro patho logy	CF CF S	cartilage disease study of	The study of the diseases of cartilage

Terminology - continued

TERM	WORD PARTS			DEFINITION
clavicular (klă-vĭk′ ū-lăr)	clavicul ar	R S	little key pertaining to	Pertaining to the clavicle
cleidorrhexis (klī″ dō-rĕks′ sĭs)	cleido rrhexis	CF S	clavicle rupture	Rupture of the clavicle of the fetus to facilitate delivery
coccygeal (kŏk-sĭj′ ĭ-ăl)	coccyge al	CF S	tailbone pertaining to	Pertaining to the coccyx
coccygodynia (kŏk-sĭ-gō-dĭn′ ĭ-ă)	coccygo dynia	CF S	tailbone pain	Pain in the coccyx
collagen (kŏl′ ă-jĕn)	colla gen	CF S	glue formation, produce	A fibrous insoluble protein found in the connective tissue, skin, ligaments, and cartilage
connective (kə′ nĕk′ tĭv)	connect ive	R S	to bind together nature of	That which connects or binds together
costal (käst′ əl)	cost al	R S	rib pertaining to	Pertaining to the rib
costosternal (kŏs″ tō-stĕr′ năl)	costo stern al	CF R S	rib sternum pertaining to	Pertaining to a rib and the sternum
coxalgia (kŏk-săl′ jĭ-ă)	cox algia	R S	hip pain	Pain in the hip
coxofemoral (kŏk″ sō-fĕm′ ŏ-răl)	coxo femor al	CF R S	hip femur pertaining to	Pertaining to the hip and femur
craniectomy (krā″ nĭ-ĕk′ tŏ-mē)	crani ectomy	R S	skull excision	Surgical excision of a portion of the skull
cranioplasty (krā′ nĭ-ō-plăs″ tē)	cranio plasty	CF S	skull surgical repair	Surgical repair of the skull
craniotomy (krā″ nĭ-ŏt′ ō-mē)	cranio tomy	CF S	skull incision	Incision into the skull
dactylic (dăk′ tĭl′ ĭk)	dactyl ic	R S	finger or toe pertaining to	Pertaining to the finger or toe
dactylogram (dăk-til′ə grăm)	dactylo gram	CF S	finger or toe mark, record	A fingerprint

continued

Terminology - continued

TERM	WORD PARTS			DEFINITION
dactylogryposis (dăk″ tĭ-lō-grĭ-pō′ sĭs)	dactylo gryp osis	CF R S	finger or toe curve condition of	Permanent contraction of the fingers
dactylomegaly (dăk″ tĭ-lō-mĕg′ ă-lē)	dactylo megaly	CF S	finger or toe enlargement, large	Enlargement of the fingers and toes
epicondyle (ĕp-ĭ-kŏn′ dīl)	epi condyle	P R	upon, above knuckle	A projection from a long bone near the articular extremity above or upon the condyle
femoral (fĕm′ ŏr-ăl)	femor al	R S	femur pertaining to	Pertaining to the femur; the thighbone
fibular (fĭb′ ū-lăr)	fibul ar	R S	fibula pertaining to	Pertaining to the fibula
humeral (hū′ mĕr-ăl)	humer al	R S	humerus pertaining to	Pertaining to the humerus
hydrarthrosis (hi″ drăr-thrō′ sĭs)	hydr arthr osis	P R S	water joint condition of	Condition of fluid in a joint
iliac (ĭl′ ē-ăk)	ili ac	R S	ilium pertaining to	Pertaining to the ilium
iliosacral (ĭl″ ĭ-ō-sā′ krăl)	ilio sacr al	CF R S	ilium sacrum pertaining to	Pertaining to the ilium and the sacrum
iliotibial (ĭl″ ĭ-ō-tĭb′ ĭ-ăl)	ilio tibi al	CF R S	ilium tibia pertaining to	Pertaining to the ilium and tibia
intercostal (ĭn″ tēr-kŏs′ tăl)	inter cost al	R R S	between rib pertaining to	Pertaining to between the ribs
ischial (ĭs′ kĭ-al)	ischi al	R S	ischium, hip pertaining to	Pertaining to the ischium, hip
ischialgia (ĭs″ kĭ-ăl′ jĭ-ă)	ischi algia	R S	ischium, hip pain	Pain in the ischium, hip
kyphosis (kī-fō′ sĭs)	kyph osis	R S	a hump condition of	Humpback
laminectomy (lăm″ ĭ-nĕk′ tō-mē)	lamin ectomy	R S	lamina (thin plate) excision	Surgical excision of a vertebral posterior arch

Terminology - continued

TERM	WORD PARTS			DEFINITION
lordosis (lŏr-dō′ sĭs)	lord osis	R S	bending condition of	Abnormal anterior curvature of the spine
lumbar (lŭm′ băr)	lumb ar	R S	loin pertaining to	Pertaining to the loins
lumbodynia (lŭm″ bō-dĭn′ ĭ-ă)	lumbo dynia	CF S	loin pain	Pain in the loins
mandibular (măn-dĭb′ ū-lăr)	mandibul ar	R S	lower jawbone pertaining to	Pertaining to the lower jawbone
maxillary (măk′ sĭ-lĕr″ ē)	maxill ary	R S	jawbone pertaining to	Pertaining to the upper jawbone
metacarpal (mĕt″ ă-kär′ pəl)	meta carp al	P R S	beyond wrist pertaining to	Pertaining to the bones of the hand
metacarpectomy (mĕt″ ă-kăr-pĕk′ tō-mē)	meta carp ectomy	P R S	beyond wrist excision	Surgical excision of one or more bones of the hand
myelitis (mī-ĕ-li′ tĭs)	myel itis	R S	marrow inflammation	Inflammation of the bone marrow
myeloma (mī-ē-lō′ mă)	myel oma	R S	marrow tumor	A tumor of the bone marrow
myelopoiesis (mī′ ĕl-ō-poy-ē′ sĭs)	myelo poiesis	CF S	marrow formation	The formation of bone marrow
olecranal (ō-lĕk′ răn-ăl)	olecran al	R S	elbow pertaining to	Pertaining to the elbow
osteoarthritis (ŏs″ tē-ō-ăr-thrī′ tĭs)	osteo arthr itis	CF R S	bone joint inflammation	Inflammation of the bone and joint
osteoarthropathy (ŏs″ tē-ō-ăr-thrŏp′ ă-thē)	osteo arthro pathy	CF CF S	bone joint disease	Any disease of the bones and joints
osteoblast (ŏs′ tē-ō-blăst″)	osteo blast	CF S	bone immature cell, germ cell	A bone-forming cell
osteocarcinoma (ŏs″ tē-ō-kăr″ sĭn-ō mă)	osteo carcin oma	CF R S	bone cancer tumor	A cancerous tumor of a bone; new growth of epithelial tissue

continued

Terminology - continued

TERM	WORD PARTS			DEFINITION
osteochondritis (ŏs″ tē-ō-kŏn-drī′ tĭs)	osteo chondr itis	CF R S	bone cartilage inflammation	Inflammation of the bone and cartilage
osteoclasia (ŏs″ tē-ō-klā′ zĭ-ă)	osteo clasia	CF S	bone a breaking	Surgical fracture of a bone to correct a deformity
osteodynia (ŏs″ tē-ō-dĭn′ ĭ-ă)	osteo dynia	CF S	bone pain	Pain in a bone
osteofibroma (ŏs″ tē-ō-fĭ-brō′ mă)	osteo fibr oma	CF R S	bone fibrous tumor	A tumor of bone and fibrous tissues
osteogenesis (ŏs″ tē-ō-jĕn′ ĕ-sĭs)	osteo genesis	CF S	bone formation, produce	The formation of bone
osteomalacia (ŏs″ tē- ō-măl-ā′ shĭ-ă)	osteo malacia	CF S	bone softening	Softening of the bones
osteomyelitis (ŏs″ tē-ō-mī″ ĕl-ī′ tĭs)	osteo myel itis	CF R S	bone marrow inflammation	Inflammation of the bone marrow
osteonecrosis (ŏs″ tē-ō-nē-krō′ sĭs)	osteo necr osis	CF R S	bone death condition of	A condition in which there is death of bone tissue
osteopenia (ŏs″ tē-ō-pē′ nĭ-ă)	osteo penia	CF S	bone lack of	A lack of bone tissue
osteoporosis (ŏs″ tē-ō-por-ō′ sĭs)	osteo por osis	CF R S	bone a passage condition of	A condition that results in reduction of bone mass

 TERMINOLOGY SPOTLIGHT

Osteoporosis affects more than 25 million Americans, most of them women 50 to 70 years of age. Each year, the disease leads to 1.4 million bone fractures, including more than 500,000 vertebral fractures, 300,000 hip fractures, and 200,000 wrist fractures. Osteoporosis frequently occurs when there is not enough calcium in the diet. The body then uses calcium stored in bones, weakening them and making them vulnerable to breaking. See Table 3–1 for good sources of calcium.

There are some risk factors involved in developing osteoporosis and these are:

- Family history of osteoporosis
- Lack of exercise
- Thin, petite build
- Never been pregnant
- Early menopause (before 45 years)
- Prone to fractures, and loss of height in the past few years
- Avoided dairy products as a child
- Smoking, drinking alcoholic beverages
- Diet high in salt, caffeine, or fat

Terminology - continued

TERM	WORD PARTS			DEFINITION
osteorrhagia (ŏs″ tē-ō-ră′ jĭ-ă)	osteo rrhagia	CF S	bone to burst forth	Hemorrhage from a bone
osteorrhaphy (ŏs-tē-or′ ă-fē)	osteo rrhaphy	CF S	bone suture	Suture of a bone
osteosarcoma (ŏs″ tē-ō-săr-kō′ mă)	osteo sarc oma	CF R S	bone flesh tumor	A malignant tumor of the bone; cancer arising from connective tissue
osteosclerosis (ŏs″ tē-ō-sklĕ-rō′ sĭs)	osteo scler osis	CF R S	bone hardening condition of	A condition of hardening of the bone
osteotome (ŏs′ tē-ō-tōm″)	osteo tome	CF S	bone instrument to cut	An instrument used for cutting bone
patellapexy (pă-těl′ ă-pěk″ sē)	patella pexy	R S	kneecap fixation	Surgical fixation of the patella
patellar (pă-těl′ ăr)	patell ar	R S	kneecap pertaining to	Pertaining to the patella
pedal (pěd ′l)	ped al	R S	foot pertaining to	Pertaining to the foot
perichondral (pěr″ i-kŏn′ drăl)	peri chondr al	P R S	around cartilage pertaining to	Pertaining to the membrane that covers cartilage
periosteoedema (pěr″ ĭ-ŏs″ tē-ō- ĕ-dē′ mă)	peri osteo edema	P CF S	around bone swelling	Swelling around a bone
phalangeal (fā-lăn′ jē-ăl)	phalange al	CF S	closely knit row pertaining to	Pertaining to the bones of the fingers and the toes
polyarthritis (pŏl″ ē-ăr-thrī′ tĭs)	poly arthr itis	P R S	many, much joint inflammation	Inflammation of more than one joint
rachialgia (rā″ kĭ-ăl′ jĭ-ă)	rachi algia	CF S	spine pain	Pain in the spine
rachigraph (rā′ kĭ-grăf)	rachi graph	CF S	spine to write	An instrument used to measure the curvature of the spine
rachiotomy (rā″ kĭ-ŏt′ ō-mē)	rachio tomy	CF S	spine incision	Surgical incision of the spine

continued

Terminology - continued

TERM	WORD PARTS			DEFINITION
radial (rā′ dĭ-ăl)	radi al	CF S	radius pertaining to	Pertaining to the radius
scapular (skăp′ ū-lăr)	scapul ar	R S	shoulder blade pertaining to	Pertaining to the shoulder blade
scoliosis (skō″ lĭ-ō′ sĭs)	scoli osis	R S	curvature condition of	A condition of lateral curvature of the spine
scoliotone (skō′ lĭ-ō-tōn)	scolio tone	CF S	curvature tension	A device for correcting the curve in scoliosis by stretching the spine
spinal (spī′ năl)	spin al	R S	spine pertaining to	Pertaining to the spine
spondylitis (spŏn-dĭl-ī′ tĭs)	spondyl itis	R S	vertebra inflammation	Inflammation of one or more vertebrae
sternal (stēr′ năl)	stern al	R S	sternum pertaining to	Pertaining to the sternum
sternalgia (stĕr-năl′ jĭ-ă)	stern algia	R S	sternum pain	Pain in the sternum
sternotomy (stĕr-nŏt′ ō-mē)	sterno tomy	CF S	sternum incision	Surgical incision of the sternum
subclavicular (sŭb″ klă-vĭk′ ū-lăr)	sub clavicul ar	P R S	under, beneath a little key pertaining to	Pertaining to beneath the clavicle
subcostal (sŭb-kŏs′ tăl)	sub cost al	P R S	under, beneath rib pertaining to	Pertaining to beneath the ribs
submaxilla (sŭb″ măk-sĭl′ ă)	sub maxilla	P R	under, beneath jaw	The lower jaw or mandible
symphysis (sĭm′ fĭ-sĭs)	sym physis	P S	together growth	A growing together
syndesis (sĭn′ dē-sĭs)	syn desis	P S	together binding	Binding together; surgical fixation or ankylosis of a joint
tendoplasty (tĕn′ dō-plăs″ tē)	tendo plasty	CF S	tendon surgical repair	Surgical repair of a tendon
tenonitis (tĕn″ ō-nī′ tĭs)	tenon itis	R S	tendon inflammation	Inflammation of a tendon

Terminology - continued

TERM	WORD PARTS			DEFINITION
tibial (tĭb′ ĭ-ăl)	tibi al	R S	tibia pertaining to	Pertaining to the tibia
ulnar (ŭl′ năr)	uln ar	R S	elbow pertaining to	Pertaining to the elbow
ulnocarpal (ŭl″ nō-kăr′ păl)	ulno carp al	CF R S	elbow wrist pertaining to	Pertaining to the ulna side of the wrist
ulnoradial (ŭl″ nō-rā′ dĭ-ăl)	ulno radi al	CF CF S	elbow radius pertaining to	Pertaining to the ulna and radius
vertebral (vĕr′ tĕ-brăl)	vertebr al	R S	vertebra pertaining to	Pertaining to a vertebra
vertebrectomy (vĕr″ tĕ-brĕk′ tō-mē)	vertebr ectomy	R S	vertebra excision	Surgical excision of a vertebra
vertebrosternal (vĕr″ tĕ-brō-ster′ năl)	vertebro stern al	CF R S	vertebra sternum pertaining to	Pertaining to a vertebra and the sternum
xiphoid (zĭf′ oyd)	xiph oid	R S	sword resemble	Resembling a sword

VOCABULARY WORDS

Vocabulary words are terms that have not been divided into component parts. They are common words or specialized terms associated with the subject of this chapter. These words are provided to enhance your medical vocabulary.

WORD	DEFINITION
arthroscope (ăr-thrŏs′ kōp)	An instrument used to examine the interior of a joint
bone marrow transplant (bōn măr′ ō trăns′ plånt)	The surgical process of transferring bone marrow from a donor to a patient

continued

Vocabulary - continued

WORD	DEFINITION
breakbone fever (brāk′ bōn fē′ vėr)	An acute febrile disease characterized by intense, arthritis-like pain; also known as *dengue fever*
bursa (bŭr′ sah)	A small space between muscles, tendons, and bones that is lined with synovial membrane and contains a fluid, *synovia*
calcium (kăl′ sĭ-ŭm)	A mineral that is essential for bone growth, teeth development, blood coagulation, and many other functions
carpal tunnel syndrome (kär′ pĕl tŭn′ ĕl sĭn′ drōm)	A condition caused by compression of the median nerve by the carpal ligament; symptoms: soreness, tenderness, weakness, pain, tingling, and numbness at the wrist
cartilage (kär′ tĭ-lĭj)	A specialized type of fibrous connective tissue present in adults, which forms the major portion of the embryonic skeleton
cast (kȧst)	A type of material, made of plaster of paris, sodium silicate, starch, or dextrin used to immobilize a fractured bone, a dislocation, or a sprain
clawfoot (klō fȯt)	A deformity of the foot characterized by an abnormally high arch; *also known as pes cavus*
dislocation (dĭs″ lō-kā′ shŭn)	The displacement of a bone from a joint
fixation (fĭks-ā′ shŭn)	The process of holding or fastening in a fixed position; making rigid, immobilizing
flatfoot (flăt fȯt)	An abnormal flatness of the sole and arch of the foot; *also known as pes planus*
genu valgum (jē′ nū văl′ gŭm)	Knock-knee
genu varum (jē′ nū vā′ rŭm)	Bowleg
gout (gowt)	A hereditary metabolic disease that is a form of acute arthritis; usually begins in the knee or foot but can affect any joint
hallux (hăl″ ŭks)	The big or great toe
hammertoe (hăm′ er-tō)	An acquired flexion deformity of the interphalangeal joint

Vocabulary - continued

WORD	DEFINITION
ligament (lĭg' ă-mĕnt)	A band of fibrous connective tissue that connects bones, cartilages, and other structures; also serves as a place for the attachment of fascia or muscle
meniscus (mĕn-ĭs'kŭs)	Crescent-shaped interarticular fibrocartilage found in certain joints, especially the lateral and medial *menisci* (semilunar cartilages) of the knee joint
phosphorus (fŏs' fō-rŭs)	A mineral that is essential in bone formation, muscle contraction, and many other functions
radiograph (rā' dĭ-ō-grăf)	An x-ray photograph of a body part
reduction (rē-dŭk' shŭn)	The manipulative or surgical procedure used to correct a fracture or hernia
rheumatoid arthritis (roo' mă-toyd ăr-thrī' tĭs)	A chronic systemic disease characterized by inflammation of the joints, stiffness, pain, and swelling that results in crippling deformities. See Figure 3–10.
rickets (rĭk' ĕts)	A deficiency condition in children primarily caused by a lack of vitamin D; may also result from inadequate intake or excessive loss of calcium
sequestrum (sē-kwĕs' trŭm)	A fragment of a dead bone that has become separated from its parent bone
splint (splĭnt)	An appliance used for fixation, support, and rest of an injured body part
sprain (sprān)	Twisting of a joint that causes pain and disability
spur (spər)	A sharp or pointed projection, as on a bone
tennis elbow (tĕn' ĭs ĕl' bō)	A chronic condition characterized by pain caused by excessive pronation and supination activities of the forearm; usually caused by strain, as in playing tennis
traction (trăk' shŭn)	The process of drawing or pulling on bones or muscles to relieve displacement and facilitate healing

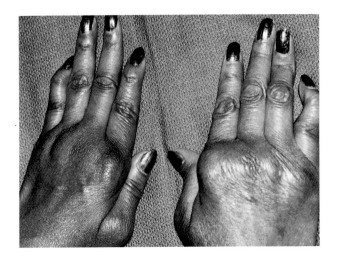

FIGURE 3–10

Rheumatoid arthritis. *(Courtesy of Jason L. Smith, MD.)*

 ABBREVIATIONS

AP	anteroposterior	**C-1**	cervical vertebra, first
CDH	congenital dislocation of hip	**C-2**	cervical vertebra, second
C-3	cervical vertebra, third	**ortho**	orthopedics, orthopaedics
Ca	calcium	**OA**	osteoarthritis
DJD	degenerative joint disease	**PEMFs**	pulsing electromagnetic fields
Fx	fracture	**PWB**	partial weight bearing
JRA	juvenile rheumatoid arthritis	**RA**	rheumatoid arthritis
jt	joint	**SAC**	short arm cast
KJ	knee jerk	**SLC**	short leg cast
L-1	lumbar vertebra, first	**SPECT**	single-photon emission
L-2	lumbar vertebra, second		computed tomography
L-3	lumbar vertebra, third	**T-1**	thoracic vertebra, first
LAC	long arm cast	**T-2**	thoracic vertebra, second
lig	ligament	**T-3**	thoracic vertebra, third
LLC	long leg cast	**TMJ**	temporomandibular joint
LLCC	long leg cylinder cast	**Tx**	traction

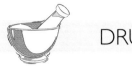

DRUG HIGHLIGHTS

Drugs that are generally used for skeletal system diseases and disorders include anti-inflammatory drugs, antirheumatic drugs, and analgesics. Fractures, arthritis, rheumatoid arthritis, bursitis, carpal tunnel syndrome, dislocation, and pain are some of the conditions involving the skeletal system and the need for pharmacologic therapy.

Anti-inflammatory Agents

Relieve the swelling, tenderness, redness, and pain of inflammation. These agents may be classified as steroidal (corticosteroids) and nonsteroidal.

Corticosteroids

Steroid substance with potent anti-inflammatory effects.
Examples: Depo-Medrol (methylprednisolone acetate), Aristocort (triamcinolone), Celestone (betamethasone), and Decadron (dexamethasone).

Nonsteroidal (NSAIDs)

Agents that are used in the treatment of arthritis and related disorders.
Examples: Bayer Aspirin (acetylsalicylic acid), Motrin (ibuprofen), Feldene (piroxicam), and Orudis (ketoprofen).

Antirheumatic Drugs

Prevent or relieve rheumatism. Rheumatism is defined as an acute or chronic condition characterized by inflammation, soreness and stiffness of muscles, and pain in joints and associated structures. *Gold therapy* and *Rheumatrex (methotrexate)* are used in the treatment of rheumatoid arthritis.

Gold therapy (chrysotherapy)

Used in the long-term treatment of rheumatoid arthritis. Gold preparations have been shown to be effective in reducing the progression of the disease, as well as relieving inflammation, but its use is limited by the toxicity of the gold compound.
Examples: Ridaura (auranofin), Myochrysine (gold sodium thiomalate), and Solganal (aurothioglucose).

Rheumatrex

A low-dose form of *methotrexate* approved for adult rheumatoid arthritis. It is recommended for selected adults with severe, active, classical, or definite rheumatoid arthritis who have had insufficient response to other forms of treatment. The patient may see improvement within 3 to 6 weeks.

Analgesics

Agents that relieve pain without causing loss of consciousness. They are classified as narcotic or non-narcotic.

Narcotic
Non-narcotic

Examples: Demerol (meperidine HCl) and morphine sulfate.
Examples: Tylenol (acetaminophen), aspirin, ibuprofen (Advil, Motrin, Nuprin), and Naprosyn (naproxen).

DIAGNOSTIC AND LABORATORY TESTS

Test	Description
arthrography (ăr-thrŏg′ ră-fē)	A diagnostic examination of a joint (usually the knee) in which air and, then, a radiopaque contrast medium are injected into the joint space, x-rays are taken, and internal injuries of the meniscus, cartilage, and ligaments may be seen, if present.
arthroscopy (ăr-thrŏs′ kō-pē)	The process of examining internal structures of a joint via an arthroscope; usually done after an arthrography and before joint surgery.
goniometry (gō″ nē-ŏm′ ĕt-rē)	The measurement of joint movements and angles via a goniometer.
photon absorptiometry (fō′ tŏn ăb-sorp′ shē-ŏm′ ĕt-rē)	A bone scan that uses a low beam of radiation to measure bone-mineral density and bone loss in the lumbar vertebrae; useful in monitoring osteoporosis.
thermography (thĕr-mŏg′ ră-fē)	The process of recording heat patterns of the body's surface; can be used to investigate the pathophysiology of rheumatoid arthritis.
x-ray (ĕks′ rā)	The examination of bones by use of an electromagnetic wave of high energy produced by the collision of a beam of electrons with a target in a vacuum tube; used to identify fractures and pathologic conditions of the bones and joints such as rheumatoid arthritis, spondylitis, and tumors.
alkaline phosphatase blood test (ăl′ kă-līn fŏs′ fă-tās)	A blood test to determine the level of alkaline phosphatase; increased in osteoblastic bone tumors, rickets, osteomalacia, and during fracture healing.
antinuclear antibodies (ANA) (ăn″ tĭ-nū′ klē-ăr ăn′ tĭ-bŏd″ ēs)	Present in a variety of immunologic diseases; positive result may indicate rheumatoid arthritis.
calcium (Ca) blood test (kăl′ sē- ŭm)	The calcium level of the blood may be increased in metastatic bone cancer, acute osteoporosis, prolonged immobilization, and during fracture healing; may be decreased in osteomalacia and rickets.
C-Reactive protein blood test (sē-rē-ăk″ tĭv prō′ tē-in)	Positive result may indicate rheumatoid arthritis, acute inflammatory change, and widespread metastasis.
phosphorus (P) blood test (fŏs′ fō-rŭs)	Phosphorus level of the blood may be increased in osteoporosis and fracture healing.

Test	Description
serum rheumatoid factor (RF) (sĕ′ rŭm roo′ mă-toyd făk′ tōr)	An immunoglobulin present in the serum of 50 to 95% of adults with rheumatoid arthritis.
uric acid blood test (ū′ rĭk ăs′ ĭd)	Uric acid is increased in gout, arthritis, multiple myeloma, and rheumatism.

COMMUNICATION ENRICHMENT

This segment is provided for those who wish to enhance their ability to communicate in either English or Spanish.

► **Related Terms**

English	Spanish	English	Spanish
fracture	fractura (frăc-*tŭ*-ră)	plaster	yeso (*jĕ*-sō)
sprain	torcer (*tōr*-sĕ r)	ray	rayo (*ră*-jō)
bones	huesos (*wĕ*-sŏs)	crutches	muletas (mŭ-*lĕ*-tăs)
shoulder	hombros (*ōm*-brōs)	foot	pie (*pĭ*-ĕ)
elbow	codo (*kō*-dō)	hands	manos (*mă*-nōs)
wrist	muñeca (mŭ-*ñĕ*-kă)	joint	cojuntura (kō-jŭn-*tŭ*-ră)
fingers, toes	dedos (*dĕ*-dōs)	leg	pierna (pĭ-*ĕr*-nă)
hip	cadera (kă-*dĕ*-ră)	neck	cuello (*kū*-ĕ-jŏ)
knee	rodilla (rō-*dĭ*-jă)	chest x-ray	radiografia del tórax (*nă*-dĭ-ō-gră-fĭ-ă dĕl *tō*-răx)
ankle	tobillo (tō-*bĭ*-jō)	rib	costilla (kōs-*tĭ*-jă)

English	Spanish	English	Spanish
cartilage	cartilago (*kăr*-tĭ-lă-gō)	water	agua (*ă*-gŭ-ă)
ligament	ligamento (*lĭ*-gă-mĭẽn-tō)	thigh	muslo (*mŭs*-lō)
skeleton	esqueleto (*ĕs*-kĕ-lĕ-tō)	pelvis	pelvis (*pĕl*-vĭs)
skull	craneo (*kră*-nĕ-ō)	shape	forma (*fŏr*-mă)
spine	espinazo (ĕs-pĭ-*nă*-zō)	support	sustento (*sŭs*-tĕn-tō)
calcium	calcio (*kăl*-sĭ-ō)	protection	protección (*prō*-tĕk-sĭ-ōn)
phosphorus	fósforo (*fŏs*-fō-rō)	reduction	reducción (*rĕ*-dŭk-sĭ-ōn)

CHAPTER REVIEW SECTION

LEARNING EXERCISES

▶ **Anatomy and Physiology**

Write your answers to the following questions. Do not refer back to the text.

1. The skeletal system is composed of _____ bones.

2. Name the two main divisions of the skeletal system.

    a. _____   b. _____

3. Name the five classifications of bone and give an example of each.

    a. _____   Example _____

    b. _____   Example _____

    c. _____   Example _____

    d. _____   Example _____

    e. _____   Example _____

4. State the six main functions of the skeletal system.

    a. _____   b. _____

    c. _____   d. _____

    e. _____   f. _____

5. Define the following features of a long bone:

    a. Epiphysis _____

    b. Diaphysis _____

    c. Periosteum _____

    d. Compact bone _____

    e. Medullary canal _____

    f. Endosteum _____

    g. Cancellous or spongy bone _____

6. Match the term in column one with its definition from column two. Place the correct number from column two in the space provided in column one.

    _____ a. Meatus   1. An air cavity within certain bones
                                  2. A shallow depression in or on a bone
    _____ b. Head   3. A pointed, sharp, slender process
                                  4. A large, rounded process
    _____ c. Tuberosity   5. A groove, furrow, depression, or fissure
                                  6. A tube-like passage or canal
    _____ d. Process   7. An opening in the bone for blood vessels,
                                      ligaments, and nerves
    _____ e. Condyle   8. A rounded process that enters into the formation of a
                                      joint, articulation
    _____ f. Tubercle   9. A ridge on a bone
                                  10. A small, rounded process
    _____ g. Crest   11. The rounded end of a bone
                                  12. A slit-like opening between two bones
    _____ h. Trochanter   13. An enlargement or protrusion of a bone
                                  14. A very large process of the femur
    _____ i. Sinus

    _____ j. Fissure

    _____ k. Fossa

    _____ l. Spine

    _____ m. Foramen

    _____ n. Sulcus

7. Name the three classifications of joints.

    a. _____   b. _____

    c. _____

8. _____ is the process of moving a body part away from the middle.

9. Adduction is _____.

10. _____ is the process of moving a body part in a circular motion.

11. Dorsiflexion is _____.

12. _____ is the process of turning outward.

13. Extension is _____.

14. _____ is the process of bending a limb.

15. Inversion is _____.

16. _____ is the process of lying face downward.

17. Protraction is _____.

18. _____ is the process of moving a body part backward.

19. Rotation is _____.

20. _____ is the process of lying face upward.

▶   Word Parts

1. In the spaces provided, write the definition of these prefixes, roots, combining forms, and suffixes. Do not refer to the listings of terminology words. Leave blank those terms you cannot define.

2. After completing as many as you can, refer back to the terminology word listings to check your work. For each word missed or left blank, write the term and its definition several times on the margins of these pages or on a separate sheet of paper.

3. To maximize the learning process, it is to your advantage to do the following exercises as directed. To refer to the terminology listings before completing these exercises invalidates the learning process.

Prefixes

Give the definitions of the following prefixes:

1. a- _____   2. epi- _____

3. hydr- _____   4. inter- _____

5. meta- _____   6. peri- _____

7. poly- _____   8. sub- _____

9. sym- _____   10. syn- _____

Roots and Combining Forms

Give the definitions of the following roots and combining forms:

1. acetabul _____
2. achillo _____
3. acr _____
4. acro _____
5. ankyl _____
6. arthr _____
7. arthro _____
8. burs _____
9. calcane _____
10. calcaneo _____
11. carcin _____
12. carp _____
13. carpo _____
14. chondr _____
15. chondro _____
16. clavicul _____
17. cleido _____
18. coccyge _____
19. coccygo _____
20. colla _____
21. condyle _____
22. connect _____
23. cost _____
24. costo _____
25. cox _____
26. coxo _____
27. crani _____
28. cranio _____
29. dactyl _____
30. dactylo _____
31. femor _____
32. fibr _____
33. fibul _____
34. gryp _____
35. humer _____
36. ili _____
37. ilio _____
38. ischi _____
39. kyph _____
40. lamin _____
41. lord _____
42. lumb _____
43. lumbo _____
44. mandibul _____
45. maxill _____
46. maxilla _____
47. myel _____
48. myelo _____
49. necr _____
50. olecran _____
51. osteo _____
52. patell _____
53. patella _____
54. patho _____
55. ped _____
56. phalange _____

57. por _____   58. py _____

59. rachi _____   60. rachio _____

61. radi _____   62. sacr _____

63. sarc _____   64. scapul _____

65. scler _____   66. scoli _____

67. scolio _____   68. spin _____

69. spondyl _____   70. stern _____

71. sterno _____   72. tendo _____

73. tenon _____   74. tibi _____

75. uln _____   76. ulno _____

77. vertebr _____   78. vertebro _____

79. xiph _____

Suffixes

Give the definitions of the following suffixes:

1. -ac _____   2. -al _____

3. -algia _____   4. -ar _____

5. -ary _____   6. -blast _____

7. -centesis _____   8. -clasia _____

9. -desis _____   10. -dynia _____

11. -ectomy _____   12. -edema _____

13. -gen _____   14. -genesis _____

15. -gram _____   16. -graph _____

17. -ic _____   18. -itis _____

19. -ive _____   20. -logy _____

21. -malacia _____   22. -megaly _____

23. -oid _____   24. -oma _____

25. -omion _____   26. -osis _____

27. -pathy _____   28. -penia _____

29. -pexy _____   30. -physis _____

31. -plasia _____   32. -plasty _____

33. -poiesis _____   34. -ptosis _____

35. -rrhagia _____   36. -rrhaphy _____

37. -rrhexis _____   38. -tome _____

39. -tomy _____   40. -tone _____

▶ **Identifying Medical Terms**

In the spaces provided, write the medical term for the following meanings:

1. _____   Inflammation of the joints of the hands or feet

2. _____   The condition of stiffening of a joint

3. _____   Surgical excision of a joint

4. _____   Inflammation of a joint

5. _____   Any joint disease

6. _____   Pertaining to the heel bone

7. _____   Wrist drop

8. _____   Pertaining to cartilage

9. _____   Study of the diseases of cartilage

10. _____   Pain in the coccyx

11. _____   Pertaining to the rib

12. _____   Surgical excision of a portion of the skull

13. _____   Pertaining to the finger or toe

14. _____   Condition of fluid in a joint

15. _____   Pertaining to between the ribs

16. _____   Pain in the hip

17. _____   Pertaining to the loins

18. _____   A tumor of the bone marrow

19. _____   Inflammation of the joint and bone

20. _____   Pain in a bone

21. _____   Inflammation of the bone marrow

22. _____   A lack of bone tissue

23. _____   Pertaining to the foot

24. _____   Pain in the sternum

25. _____   Resembling a sword

▶ Spelling

In the spaces provided, write the correct spelling of these misspelled terms:

1. acrmoin _____
2. arthedema _____
3. buritis _____
4. chondblast _____
5. conective _____
6. cranplasty _____
7. dactlomegaly _____
8. ischal _____
9. melyitis _____
10. ostchonditis _____
11. ostnecrosis _____
12. patelar _____
13. phalangal _____
14. rachgraph _____
15. scolosis _____
16. spondlitis _____
17. symphsis _____
18. tennitis _____
19. ulncarpal _____
20. vertbral _____

WORD PARTS STUDY SHEET

Word Parts	Give the Meaning
epi-	_____
hydr-	_____
inter-	_____
meta-	_____
peri-	_____
poly-	_____
sym-, syn-	_____
acr-, acro-	_____
arthr-, arthro-	_____

burs- _____

chondr-, chondro- _____

dactyl-, dactylo- _____

fibr- _____

ischi- _____

kyph- _____

lord- _____

myel-, myelo- _____

osteo- _____

ped- _____

por- _____

scoli- _____

-algia _____

-al, -ic _____

-blast _____

-centesis _____

-clasia _____

-desis _____

-dynia _____

-ectomy _____

-itis _____

-ive _____

-logy _____

-malacia _____

-omnion _____

-osis _____

-pathy _____

-plasty _____

-tomy _____

REVIEW QUESTIONS

▶ **Matching**

Select the appropriate lettered meaning for each numbered line.

_____ 1. arthroscope

_____ 2. carpal tunnel syndrome

_____ 3. clawfoot

_____ 4. gout

_____ 5. hammertoe

_____ 6. kyphosis

_____ 7. metacarpal

_____ 8. rickets

_____ 9. tennis elbow

_____ 10. ulnar

a. A deficiency condition in children primarily caused by a lack of vitamin D
b. An acquired flexion deformity of the interphalangeal joint
c. A hereditary metabolic disease that is a form of acute arthritis
d. A chronic condition characterized by pain that is caused by excessive pronation and supination activities of the forearm
e. A deformity of the foot characterized by an abnormally high arch
f. Pertaining to the elbow
g. Pertaining to the bones of the hand
h. Humpback
i. An instrument used to examine the interior of a joint
j. A condition caused by compression of the median nerve by the carpal ligament
k. Pertaining to the knee

▶ **Abbreviations**

Place the correct word, phrase, or abbreviation in the space provided.

1. congenital dislocation of hip _____

2. degenerative joint disease _____

3. LLC _____

4. OA _____

5. pulsing electromagnetic fields _____

6. RA _____

7. single-photon emission computed tomography _____

8. T-1 _____

9. TMJ _____

10. traction _____

► **Diagnostic and Laboratory Test**

Select the best answer to each multiple choice question. Circle the letter of your choice.

1. _____ is a diagnostic examination of a joint in which air and, then, a radiopaque contrast medium are injected into the joint space, x-rays are taken, and internal injuries of the meniscus, cartilage, and ligaments may be seen, if present.
   a. Arthroscopy
   b. Goniometry
   c. Arthrography
   d. Thermography

2. The process of recording heat patterns of the body's surface is:
   a. arthrography
   b. arthroscopy
   c. goniometry
   d. thermography

3. _____ is increased in gout, arthritis, multiple myeloma, and rheumatism.
   a. Calcium
   b. Phosphorus
   c. Uric acid
   d. Alkaline phosphatase

4. _____ level of the blood may be increased in osteoporosis and fracture healing.
   a. Antinuclear antibodies
   b. Phosphorus
   c. Uric acid
   d. Alkaline phosphatase

5. _____ is/are present in a variety of immunologic diseases.
   a. Alkaline phosphatase
   b. Antinuclear antibodies
   c. C-Reactive protein
   d. Uric acid

CRITICAL THINKING ACTIVITY

▶ **Case Study**

Osteoporosis

Please read the following case study and then answer the questions that follow.

A 62-year-old female was seen by a physician, and the following is a synopsis of her visit.

Present History: The patient states that she seems to be shorter, her back "hurts" all the time, and she has developed a humpback.

Signs and Symptoms: Loss of height, kyphosis, and pain in the back.

Diagnosis: Osteoporosis (postmenopausal)

Treatment: Estrogen replacement therapy (ESTRADERM—Estradiol Transdermal System), begin a regular exercise program, a diet rich in calcium, phosphorus, magnesium, and vitamins A, C, D, the B-complex vitamins, and analgesics for pain.

Prevention: Know the risk factors involved in developing osteoporosis, follow a regular exercise program, and include a diet rich in calcium, phosphorus, magnesium, and vitamins A, C, D, and the B-complex vitamins. For more information on osteoporosis you can call the National Osteoporosis Foundation at 1–800–464–6700.

Good sources of **vitamin A** are dairy products, fish, liver oils, animal liver, green and yellow vegetables. Good sources of **vitamin D** are ultraviolet rays, dairy products, and commercial foods that contain supplemental vitamin D (milk and cereals). Good sources of **vitamin C** are citrus fruits, tomatoes, melons, fresh berries, raw vegetables, and sweet potatoes. Good sources of the **B-complex vitamins** are organ meats, dried beans, poultry, eggs, yeast, fish, whole grains, and dark-green vegetables. Good sources of **calcium** are dairy products, beans, cauliflower, egg yolk, molasses, leafy green vegetables, tofu, sardines, clams, and oysters. Good sources of **phosphorus** are dairy products, eggs, fish, poultry, meats, dried peas and beans, whole grain cereals, and nuts. Good sources of **magnesium** are whole grain cereals, fruits, milk, nuts, vegetables, seafood, and meats.

Critical Thinking Questions

1. Signs and symptoms of osteoporosis include loss of height, _____, and pain in the back.

2. _____ is an Estradiol Transdermal System.

3. Good sources of vitamin A are dairy products, fish, liver oils, _____ _____, green and yellow vegetables.

4. Good sources of magnesium are whole grain cereals, fruits, milk, _____, vegetables, seafood, and meats.

4

ANATOMY AND PHYSIOLOGY OF THE SKELETAL SYSTEM

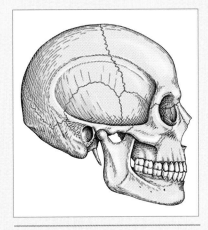

OBJECTIVES

- Describe the functions of bones and the skeletal system.

- Compare the structure and function of compact and spongy bones.

- Discuss the processes by which bones develop and grow.

- Describe how the activities of the bone cells constantly remodel bones.

- Discuss the effects of aging on the bones of the skeletal system.

- Contrast the structure and function of the axial and appendicular skeletons.

- Identify the bones of the skull.

- Discuss the differences in structure and function of the various vertebrae.

- Identify the bones of the limbs.

- Describe the three basic types of joints.

- Relate body movements to the action of specific joints.

The skeletal system includes the bones of the skeleton and the specialized tissues that interconnect them. Besides supporting the weight of the body and protecting delicate internal organs, bones work together with muscles to produce the movements that let you walk, run, or turn the pages of this book.

This chapter examines the skeletal system from the cellular structure of bone and cartilage to the individual bones themselves. Finally, we show how two or more bones interact at joints, or *articulations*, to permit normal movements.

► SYSTEM BRIEF

The skeletal system performs the following functions:

1. **Support**: Bones and cartilages provide structural support for the entire body.
2. **Protection**: Delicate tissues and organs are often surrounded by bones. The ribs protect the heart and lungs; the skull encloses the brain; the vertebrae shield the spinal cord; and the pelvis cradles delicate digestive and reproductive organs.
3. **Leverage**: When a skeletal muscle contracts, it pulls on a bone and produces movement at a specific joint. The location of the muscle attachment site relative to the joint determines the speed and power of the resulting movement.
4. **Storage**: Bones store valuable minerals such as calcium and phosphate. In addition, fat cells within the internal cavities of many bones store lipids as an energy reserve.
5. **Blood cell production**: Red blood cells and other blood elements are produced within the internal cavities of many bones.

► BONE STRUCTURE

Bone, or **osseous tissue**, is one of the two supporting connective tissues. (Can you name the other supporting connective tissue?) Like other connective tissues, osseous tissue contains specialized cells in a *matrix* containing extracellular fibers and a ground substance. Remember, it is the matrix that determines the consistency of a connective tissue, and the matrix of bone is dominated by calcium deposits. These compounds account for almost two thirds of a bone's mass and give the tissue its characteristic solid, stony feel. The remaining bone mass is mainly collagen fibers, with living cells providing only around 2 percent of the mass of a bone.

GENERAL FEATURES OF BONE

Human bones have four general shapes: *long, short, flat,* and *irregular.* **Long bones** are longer than they are wide, whereas short bones are of roughly equal dimensions. Examples of long bones include bones of the limbs such as the arm (*humerus*) and thigh (*femur*). **Short bones** include the bones of the wrist (*carpals*) and ankle (*tarsals*). **Flat bones** are thin and relatively broad, such as the *parietal bones* of the skull, the ribs, and the shoulder blades (*scapulae*). **Irregular bones** have shapes that do not fit easily into any other category. An example would be one of the *vertebrae*, the bones of the spinal column.

dia, through + physis, growth
diaphysis, growing between; the shaft that separates the two epiphyses of a long bone

The typical features of a long bone are shown in Figure 4-1. A long bone has a central shaft, or **diaphysis** (dī-AF-i-sis), and expanded ends, or **epiphyses** (ē-PIF-i-sēs; singular; *epiphysis*). The diaphysis surrounds a central *marrow cavity*. **Marrow** is the name given to the loose connective tissue that fills such cavities. *Red marrow* is blood-forming tissue, and *yellow marrow* is adipose tissue. The epiphyses of adjacent bones interact at a joint. Within many joints the opposing bony surfaces are covered by smooth and slippery *articular cartilages.*

epi, upon + *physis*, growth
epiphysis: one expanded end of a long bone

Figure 4-1 also shows the two types of bone tissue: *compact bone* and *spongy bone.* **Compact bone** is relatively solid, whereas **spongy bone** is porous and less dense. Both types are present in long bones. Compact bone forms the diaphysis and covers the surfaces of the epiphyses. Each epiphysis contains a core of spongy bone.

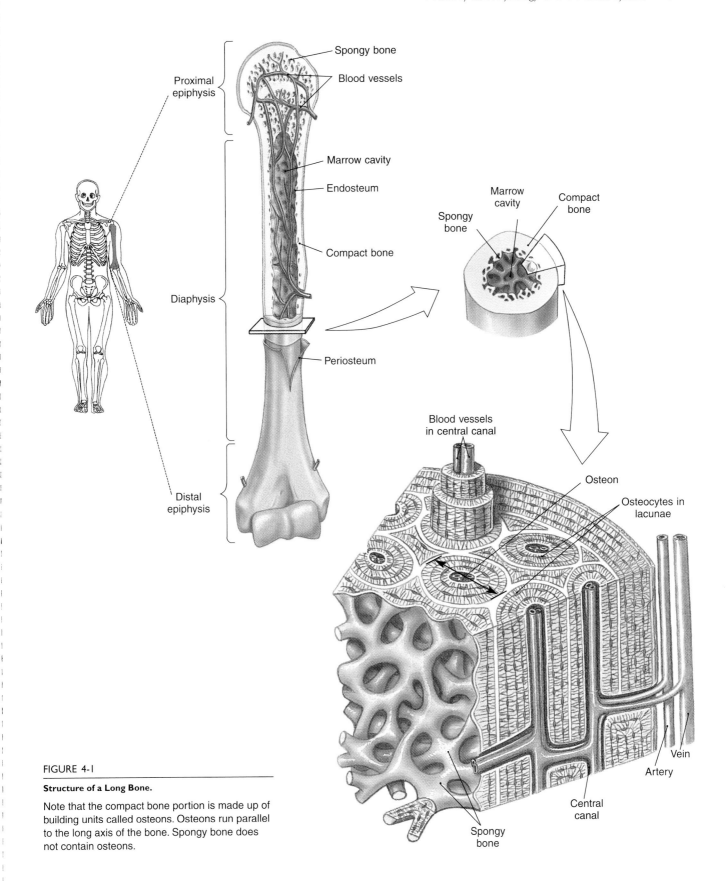

FIGURE 4-1

Structure of a Long Bone.

Note that the compact bone portion is made up of building units called osteons. Osteons run parallel to the long axis of the bone. Spongy bone does not contain osteons.

peri, around + *osteon*, bone
periosteum: the connective tissue sheath around a bone

endo, inside + *osteon*, bone
endosteum: a layer of cells that lines the internal surfaces of bones

The outer surface of a bone is covered by a **periosteum** (per-ē-OS-tē-um), a term that means "around the bone" (Figure 4-1). The periosteum consists of a fibrous outer layer and an inner cellular layer. A cellular **endosteum** (en-DOS-te-um) (*endo-* means "inside") lines the marrow cavity inside the bone. Blood vessels and nerves penetrate the periosteum to supply the bone and tissues of the bone marrow, and both the periosteum and endosteum are important for bone growth and repair.

MICROSCOPIC FEATURES OF BONE

Bone Cells

There are three different types of bone cells, each with its own function in the growth or maintenance of bone:

osteon, bone + *cyte*, cell
osteocyte: a mature bone cell

1. **Osteocytes** (OS-tē-ō-sīts) are mature bone cells that are embedded in the matrix. As you will recall, the solid matrix in bone tissue provides strength and rigidity. Osteocytes maintain the density and composition of the bone matrix by removing and replacing the calcium compounds in the surrounding matrix. They also help repair damaged bone. In a mature adult, whose bones are no longer growing, osteocytes are the most numerous bone cells.

osteon, bone + *blastos*, a germ (like a seed)
osteoblast: immature bone cells responsible for bone growth

2. **Osteoblasts** (OS-tē-ō-blasts) are immature bone cells that can develop into osteocytes (the term *blast* means "precursor"). Osteoblasts are bone builders that are responsible for the production of new bone. This process is called *osteogenesis* (os-tē-ō-JEN-e-sis). Osteoblasts produce the matrix of bone. When they become surrounded by this matrix, they become osteocytes.

osteon, bone + *klastos*, broken
osteoclast: a cell that dissolves bone matrix and releases the stored minerals

3. **Osteoclasts** (OS-tē-ō-klasts) are the demolition team of bone tissue. The term *clast* means "to break," an appropriate name for their function. Osteoclasts within the endosteum and periosteum break down and remove bony matrix. This process is essential for bone remodeling and growth. Osteoclast activity also releases the minerals stored in bone. This process adds calcium and phosphate ions to body fluids. The release of stored minerals from bone is called *resorption*.

Bone is a very dynamic tissue, and at any given moment osteoclasts are removing matrix while osteoblasts are adding to it. If osteoblasts add matrix faster than osteoclasts remove it, the bones grow thicker and stronger. If osteoclasts remove matrix faster than osteoblasts deposit it, the bones grow thinner and weaker.

Concept Questions

✔ A sample of bone shows concentric layers surrounding a central canal. Is it from the shaft (diaphysis) or the end (epiphysis) of a long bone?

✔ If the activity of osteoclasts exceeds the activity of osteoblasts in a bone, how will the mass of the bone be affected?

Bone Tissue

Within both compact and spongy bone, osteocytes exist within microscopic pockets called **lacunae** (la-KOO-nē), which means "little lakes." The lacunae are found between thin sheets of calcified matrix. Adjacent lacunae are interconnected by small channels that also link them to nearby blood vessels. Nutrients from the blood and waste products from the osteocytes diffuse through the fluid within these channels, which also contain slender extensions of the osteocytes.

Within compact bone, the basic functional unit is the **osteon** (OS-tē-on), or *Haversian system* (Figure 4-1). In each osteon, the calcified matrix is arranged in concentric layers around a **central canal** (also known as a *Haversian canal*). The central canal always contains one or more blood vessels, and it may also contain nerves that supply the bone. The central canals are usually oriented along the long axis of the bone. Smaller, transverse canals link the blood vessels of the central canals with those of the periosteum or the marrow cavity.

Unlike compact bone, spongy bone has no osteons. It consists of an open network of interconnecting calcified rods or plates. These open areas of spongy bone provide space for red marrow or yellow marrow.

► BONE DEVELOPMENT AND MAINTENANCE

A person's height and general body proportions are determined by his or her skeleton. Bone formation is called **ossification**. Ossification begins about 6 weeks after fertilization, when the embryo is approximately 12 mm (1/2 in.) long. Bone formation and growth continue through adolescence, and parts of the skeleton usually do not stop growing until ages 18 to 25.

BONE GROWTH

endo, inside + *chondros*, cartilage
endochondral ossification: bone formation within an existing cartilage

Before bone formation begins, an embryo has a cartilaginous skeleton. As development proceeds, many of these cartilages are replaced by bones. This process is called **endochondral ossification** (en-dō-KON-dral). Endochondral ossification begins as cartilage cells within a cartilaginous model break down and are then replaced by osteoblasts that begin producing bone matrix. As more cartilage breaks down, the number of osteoblasts increases, and more and more of the cartilage is replaced by bone. Steps in the growth and ossification of a limb bone are diagrammed in Figure 4-2. Bone formation starts at the shaft surface and then begins within the shaft before it occurs in the ends of the bone.

This process continues until the cartilaginous model has been almost completely replaced. However, until growth is completed, zones of cartilage remain between the bone of the shaft and the bone of each epiphysis. These cartilaginous connections are known as the **epiphyseal plates** (see Figure 4-2). The cartilage at an epiphyseal plate is continually being remodeled. On the shaft side of the epiphyseal plate, osteoblasts are invading the cartilage and converting it to bone. But on the epiphyseal side of the plate, new cartilage is being produced at the same rate. As a result, the epiphyseal plate persists, but the shaft grows longer. This process can be compared to a jogger chasing

FIGURE 4-2

Endochondral Ossification.

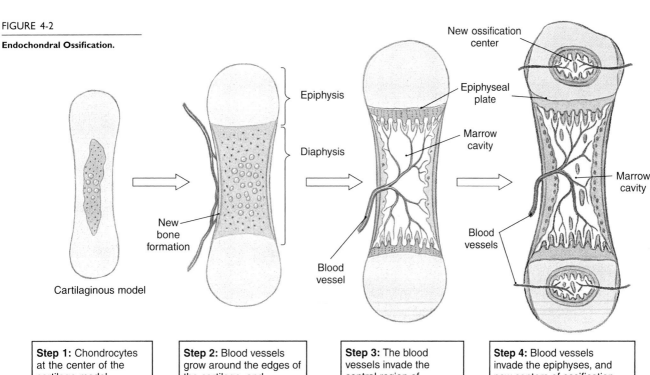

Step 1: Chondrocytes at the center of the cartilage model begin to disintegrate.

Step 2: Blood vessels grow around the edges of the cartilage, and osteoblasts form within and around the diaphysis (shaft). The shaft then becomes covered in a layer of bone.

Step 3: The blood vessels invade the central region of cartilage, growing toward the epiphysis at either end. The bone of the shaft becomes thicker, and the cartilage near each epiphysis is replaced by bone.

Step 4: Blood vessels invade the epiphyses, and new centers of ossification form. The surfaces at the ends of the bone will remain cartilaginous, and the thin epiphyseal plate will separate the spongy bone of the epiphysis from the marrow cavity of the shaft.

someone on a bicycle. As long as the jogger and the bicycle are moving at the same speed, the jogger will keep advancing but never catch the cyclist.

When sex hormone production increases at puberty, bone growth accelerates, and the rate of bone production by osteoblasts exceeds the rate of new epiphyseal cartilage formation. In effect, the jogger speeds up and begins to overtake the bicycle. Soon the osteoblasts have completely replaced the cartilage of the epiphyseal plate. This marks the end of the period of sudden growth that accompanies adolescence, and the person becomes physically as well as sexually mature. The location of what was once an epiphyseal plate can still be detected in an X-ray of an adult bone as a distinct *epiphyseal line* that remains after it has stopped growing.

While the bone lengthens, it also grows larger in diameter. The increase in width occurs as osteoblasts form in the cellular layer of the periosteum. These cells begin producing additional bone, and as they become surrounded with calcified matrix, the osteoblasts become osteocytes. As new bone is deposited on the outer surface of the shaft, the inner surface is eroded by osteoclasts in the endosteum. This combination of bone formation on the outside and resorption in the inside increases the diameter of the bone and enlarges the marrow cavity.

BONE MAINTENANCE

The support and storage functions of the skeleton depend on the dynamic nature of bone tissue. Even after the epiphyseal plates have closed, each bone is constantly being modified by the activities of its various cells. Osteocytes, for example, maintain the bony matrix by continually removing and replacing calcium. Osteoclasts and osteoblasts also remain active, continually forming and destroying bony tissue. Normally these activities are balanced, and in adults, about one-fifth of the protein and mineral components of the skeleton are removed and then replaced each year.

Constant mineral turnover gives each bone the ability to adapt to new stresses. When stresses are applied, osteoblasts are stimulated. As a result, heavily stressed bones become thicker, stronger, and develop more pronounced surface ridges. When bones are not stressed, they get thin and brittle because osteoblast activity decreases. One of the benefits of regular exercise is that it stresses the skeleton and helps keep bones strong.

Despite its mineral strength, bone can crack or even break if subjected to extreme loads, sudden impacts, or stresses from unusual directions. Any crack or break in a bone is called a **fracture**.

Fractures are classified according to their external appearance, the site of the fracture, and the type of crack or break in the bone. In a *closed fracture*, or *simple fracture*, the broken bones do not penetrate the skin. In an *open fracture*, or *compound fracture*, the skin is broken. Open fractures are more dangerous than closed fractures because the opening in the skin increases the chances for severe bleeding and bacterial infection.

Fractured bones will usually heal as long as the circulatory supply remains and the cells of the endosteum and periosteum survive the injury. The repair process may take from 4 months to well over a year. In some cases, the repair may be "good as new," with no sign that a fracture ever occurred. Often, however, the bone will be slightly thicker than normal at the fracture site.

Concept Questions

✔ How could X-rays of the femur be used to determine whether a person had reached full height?

✔ In the Middle Ages, choirboys were sometimes castrated (had their testes removed) before puberty, to prevent their voices from changing. How would this have affected their height?

✔ Why would you expect the arm bones of a weight lifter to be thicker and heavier than those of a jogger?

✚ Clinical Note

What Is Osteoporosis?

Osteoporosis (os-tē-ō-por-Ō-sis) is a disease condition caused by an abnormal loss of bone mass that results in extremely fragile bones. Because bones are more fragile, they break easily and do not repair well. For example, a hip fracture may occur when an individual simply stands up, or vertebrae may collapse, distorting the joints between them and putting pressure on spinal nerves.

Sex hormones are important in maintaining normal rates of bone deposition. A significant percentage of women over age 45 suffer from osteoporosis. The condition becomes more common after menopause due to a decline in the levels of estrogen. Because men continue to produce sex hormones until relatively late in life, severe osteoporosis is less common in males below age 60.

Therapies that boost estrogen levels, dietary changes that elevate calcium levels in the blood, and exercise that stresses bones and stimulates osteoblast activity appear to slow, but not completely prevent, the development of osteoporosis.

AGING AND THE SKELETAL SYSTEM

The bones of the skeleton become thinner and relatively weaker as a normal part of the aging process. A reduction in bone mass begins to occur between the ages of 30 and 40. It begins when the rate of bone formation by osteoblasts begins to fall below the rate of bone breakdown by osteoclasts. Once the reduction in bone mass begins, a woman loses roughly 8 percent of her skeletal mass every decade. The rate of bone loss in men is somewhat lower, averaging around 3 percent per decade. Not all parts of the skeleton are equally affected. Epiphyses, vertebrae, and the jaws lose more than their fair share, resulting in fragile limbs, a reduction in height, and the loss of teeth. If the bones become so thin that they can no longer withstand normal stresses, the condition of *osteoporosis* exists.

▶ THE SKELETON

The skeletal system consists of 206 separate bones and a number of associated cartilages. There are two skeletal divisions: the **axial skeleton**, whose 80 bones form the vertical axis of the body, and the **appendicular skeleton**, which includes the bones of the limbs as well as those bones that attach the limbs to the trunk (Figure 4-3). All together, there are 126 appendicular bones: 32 are associated with each upper limb, and 31 with each lower limb.

SKELETAL TERMS

In addition to its shape, each bone in the skeleton has a variety of other identifying external features. These features, called *bone markings*, are the attachments of tendons and ligaments, or passageways for nerves and blood vessels. A group of specialized terms are commonly used in describing bone markings. For example, a *process* is a general term for a projection or bump on a bone. Table 4-1 contains a short list of these terms, and many specific examples will be seen in the bone illustrations that follow.

Table 4-1	External Features of Bones	
Description	**Term**	**Definition**
Processes formed where tendons or ligaments attach	Trochanter	A large, rough projection
	Tuberosity	A smaller, rough projection
	Tubercle	A small, rounded projection
	Crest	A prominent ridge
	Spine	A pointed process
Processes formed at articulations	Head	Distinct epiphysis, separated from the shaft of a long bone by a narrow neck
	Condyle	A smooth, rounded bump
	Facet	A small, flat surface
Depressions and openings	Fossa	A shallow depression
	Sulcus	A narrow groove
	Foramen	A rounded passageway for blood vessels and/or nerves
	Sinus	A chamber within a bone, normally filled with air

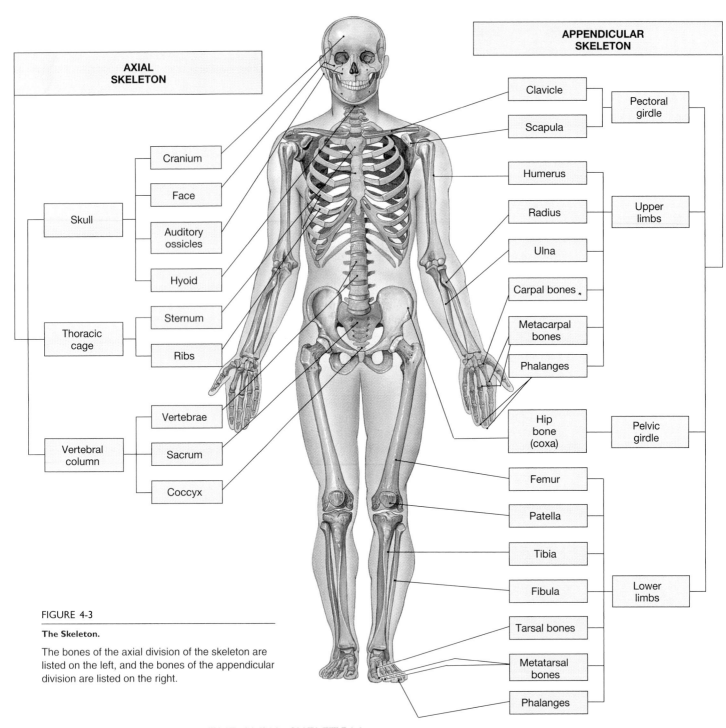

AXIAL
SKELETON

Cranium

Face

Skull

Auditory
ossicles

Hyoid

Sternum

Thoracic
cage

Ribs

Vertebrae

Vertebral
column

Sacrum

Coccyx

APPENDICULAR
SKELETON

Clavicle

Scapula

Pectoral
girdle

Humerus

Radius

Upper
limbs

Ulna

Carpal bones

Metacarpal
bones

Phalanges

Hip
bone
(coxa)

Pelvic
girdle

Femur

Patella

Tibia

Fibula

Lower
limbs

Tarsal bones

Metatarsal
bones

Phalanges

FIGURE 4-3

The Skeleton.

The bones of the axial division of the skeleton are listed on the left, and the bones of the appendicular division are listed on the right.

THE AXIAL SKELETON

The axial skeleton creates a framework that supports and protects organ systems in the dorsal and ventral body cavities. In addition, it provides an extensive surface area for the attachment of muscles that adjust the positions of the head, neck, and trunk. Its 80 bones include the **skull** and other bones associated with the skull, the **vertebral column**, and the **thoracic** (*rib*) **cage**.

The Skull

The bones of the skull protect the brain and support delicate sense organs involved with vision, hearing, balance, smell, and taste. The skull is made up of 22 bones: 8 form the **cranium** (which encloses the brain), and 14 are associated with the *face*. Seven additional bones are associated with the skull: 6 *auditory ossicles*, tiny bones involved in sound detection, and the *hyoid bone*, which is connected by ligaments to the inferior surface of the skull.

Figure 4-4 presents the cranial and facial portions of the skull. External views of the skull are shown in Figure 4-5. Figure 4-6 reveals internal features through horizontal (transverse) and sagittal sections. Table 4-2 provides a summary of the names and descriptions of the bones of the skull.

The bones of the cranium include the **frontal**, **parietal** (pa-RĪ-e-tal), **occipital**, **temporal**, **sphenoid** (SFĒ-noid), and **ethmoid bones** (see Table 4-2). These bones form the **cranial cavity** that encloses and protects the brain. The outer surface of the cranium provides attachment points for muscles that move the eyes, jaws, and head.

The 14 facial bones protect and support the entrances to the digestive and respiratory tracts. The superficial facial bones (the **lacrimal** (LAK-ri-mal), **nasal**, **maxillary**, and **zygomatic bones**, and the **mandible**) also provide areas for the attachment of muscles that control facial expressions and manipulate food. Of all the facial bones, only the mandible, or lower jaw, is movable. The deeper bones of the face include the **palatines bones**, the **vomer**, and the **inferior nasal conchae** (see Table 4-2).

Sutures are immovable joints between bones. Except for the mandible and its joint with the cranium, all the joints between the skull bones of adults are sutures. At a suture the bones are joined together by dense fibrous connective tissue. The illustrations of the different views of the skull show its four major cranial sutures; the **lambdoidal** (lam-DOYD-al), **coronal**, **sagittal**, and **squamosal sutures**.

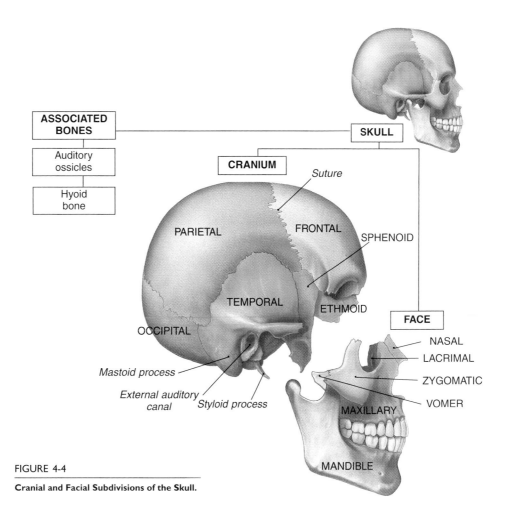

FIGURE 4-4

Cranial and Facial Subdivisions of the Skull.

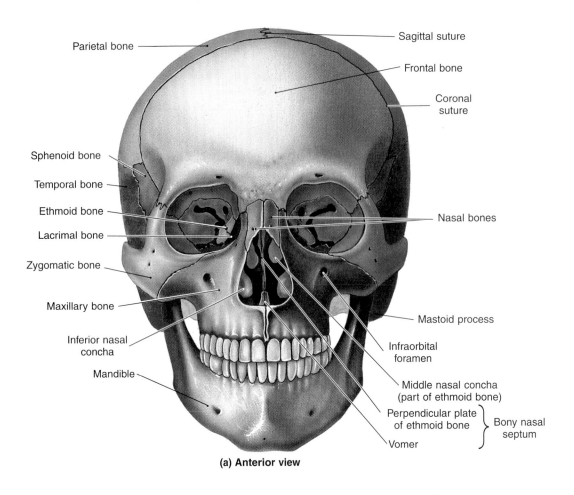

Parietal bone

Sagittal suture

Frontal bone

Coronal suture

Sphenoid bone

Temporal bone

Ethmoid bone

Lacrimal bone

Zygomatic bone

Maxillary bone

Inferior nasal concha

Mandible

Nasal bones

Mastoid process

Infraorbital foramen

Middle nasal concha (part of ethmoid bone)

Perpendicular plate of ethmoid bone

Vomer

Bony nasal septum

(a) Anterior view

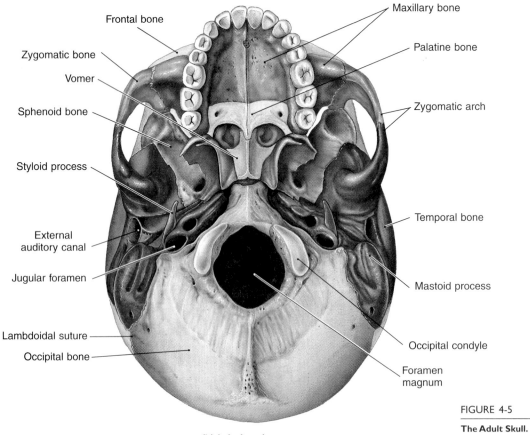

Frontal bone

Zygomatic bone

Vomer

Sphenoid bone

Styloid process

External auditory canal

Jugular foramen

Lambdoidal suture

Occipital bone

Maxillary bone

Palatine bone

Zygomatic arch

Temporal bone

Mastoid process

Occipital condyle

Foramen magnum

(b) Inferior view

FIGURE 4-5

The Adult Skull.

(a) Anterior view and **(b)** inferior view.

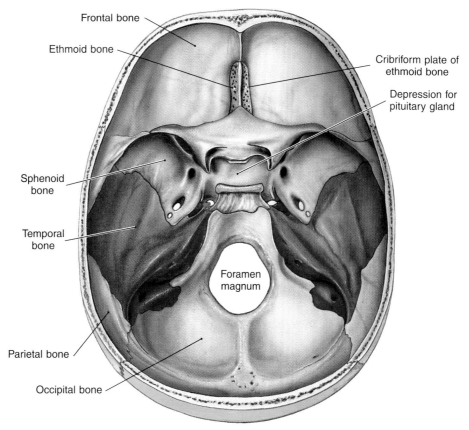

Frontal bone

Ethmoid bone

Cribriform plate of
ethmoid bone

Depression for
pituitary gland

Sphenoid
bone

Temporal
bone

Foramen
magnum

Parietal bone

Occipital bone

(a) Horizontal section

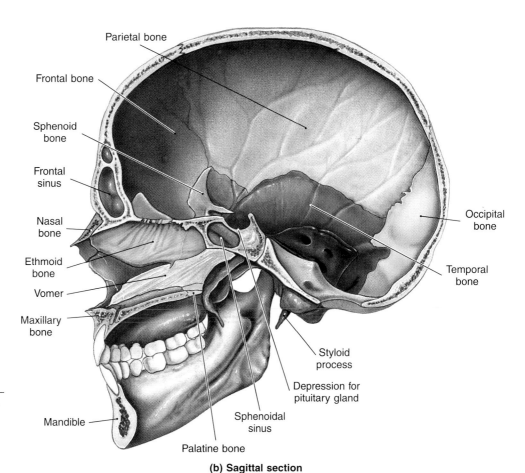

Parietal bone

Frontal bone

Sphenoid
bone

Frontal
sinus

Nasal
bone

Ethmoid
bone

Vomer

Maxillary
bone

Mandible

Occipital
bone

Temporal
bone

Styloid
process

Depression for
pituitary gland

Sphenoidal
sinus

Palatine bone

(b) Sagittal section

FIGURE 4-6

Internal Structure of the Skull.

(a) Horizontal section
through the skull, looking
down on the floor of the
cranial cavity. **(b)** Sagittal
section through the skull.

Table 4-2	Bones of the Skull	
Bone	**Number**	**Comments**
Cranium		
Frontal bone	1	Forms the forehead and the upper surface of each eye socket; contains *frontal sinuses*
Parietal bones	2	Form the roof and the upper walls of the cranium
Occipital bone	1	Forms the posterior and inferior portions of the cranium; contains the *foramen magnum*, the opening through which the spinal cord connects to the brain
Temporal bones	2	Make up the sides and base of the cranium; each contains an *external auditory canal* that leads to the eardrum; contains the auditory ossicles, or ear bones
Sphenoid bone	1	Forms part of the cranial floor and also acts as a bridge uniting the cranial and facial bones; contains a pair of *sphenoidal sinuses*
Ethmoid bone	1	Forms narrow part of the anterior floor of the cranium and part of nasal cavity roof; projections called the *superior* and *middle conchae* extend into the nasal cavity; forms upper portion of the nasal septum; contains the *ethmoidal sinuses*
Face		
Maxillary bones	2	Form (1) the floor and medial portion of the rim of the orbit, (2) the walls of the nasal cavity, and (3) the anterior roof of the mouth, or *hard palate*; contain large *maxillary sinuses*
Palatine bones	2	Form the posterior surface of the *hard palate*, or roof of the mouth
Vomer	1	Forms the inferior portion of the nasal septum
Zygomatic bones	2	Slender bony extension curves laterally and posteriorly to meet a process from the temporal bone to form the *zygomatic arch*, or cheekbone
Nasal bones	2	Form the bridge of the nose
Lacrimal bones	2	Contain the opening for the passageway of the tear duct to the nasal cavity
Inferior nasal conchae	2	Project from the lateral walls of the nasal cavity; with superior and middle conchae of the ethmoid slows and deflects arriving air toward the olfactory (smell) receptors located near the upper portions of the nasal cavity
Mandible	1	Bone of the lower jaw; articulates with the temporal bones
Associated Bones		
Auditory ossicles	6	Three tiny bones enclosed within each temporal bone; transfer sound vibrations from eardrum to hearing receptors in the inner ear
Hyoid bone	1	Suspended under skull by ligaments from the styloid processes of the temporal bones; base for muscles associated with the tongue and *larynx* (voicebox); supports the larynx

Concept Questions

✔ What is the name of the cranial bone of the forehead?

✔ The occipital bone contains a large opening. What is the name of this cranial feature, and what is its function?

✔ What are the functions of the paranasal sinuses?

The sutures so characteristic of the adult skull were not always immovable. At birth, infant skulls lack sutures. Instead, their cranial bones are connected by areas of fibrous connective tissue known as **fontanels** (fon-tah-NELS) (Figure 4-7). These fontanels, or "soft spots," are quite flexible and permit distortion of the skull without damage. Such distortion normally occurs during delivery and eases the passage of the infant along the birth canal. The fontanels disappear as the cranial bones fuse and interlock during the first 4 years of life.

The frontal, temporal, sphenoid, ethmoid, and maxillary bones contain air-filled internal chambers called **sinuses** (Figure 4-6b). The *paranasal sinuses*—all the sinuses except for those in the temporal bone—empty into the nasal cavity.

Sinuses make the bones of the face lighter. In addition, the paranasal sinuses are lined by an extensive area of mucous epithelium. Here, mucous secretions are released into the nasal cavities, and the ciliated epithelium passes the mucus back toward the throat, where it is eventually swallowed. Incoming air is moisturized and warmed as it flows across this carpet of mucus, and foreign particles, such as dust or bacteria, become trapped in the sticky mucus and swallowed. This mechanism helps protect more delicate portions of the respiratory tract.

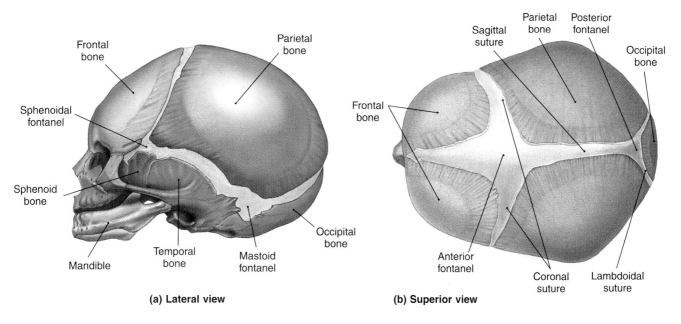

FIGURE 4-7

The Skull of an Infant.

(a) Lateral view. The bones of the infant skull are separated by areas of fibrous connective tissue called fontanels. **(b)** Superior view. The large anterior fontanel closes when a child is about 18 months old.

The Vertebral (Spinal) Column

The axial skeleton consists of the vertebral (spinal) column and the thoracic (rib) cage. The spinal column protects the spinal cord and provides attachment sites for the ribs as well as the muscles that move the *trunk* (the part of the body to which the limbs are attached) and maintain body posture. The vertebral column is divided into regions based on the structure of the vertebrae, as indicated in Figure 4-8. Just below the skull are the 7 **cervical vertebrae** of the neck (abbreviated C_1 to C_7). Next, are the 12 **thoracic vertebrae** (T_1 to T_{12}), each of which articulates with one or more pairs of **ribs**. The 5 **lumbar vertebrae** (L_1 to L_5) continue toward the base of the spine, the fifth lumbar vertebra articulating with the **sacrum**, a single bone formed by the fusion of 5 vertebrae. The small **coccyx** (KOK-siks) also consists of fused vertebrae.

Although it may seem like a straight and rigid structure, the spinal column is surprisingly flexible. A side view of the adult spinal column reveals that the vertebrae align to form four **spinal curves** (see Figure 4-8). These curves add strength to the spine, increasing the skeleton's balance and ability to hold the body upright. The *thoracic* and *sacral curves*, known as the **primary curves**, are present at birth. The *cervical* and *lumbar curves* are known as **secondary curves** because they do not appear until months later. The cervical curve develops as an infant learns to balance its head upright, and the lumbar curve develops with the ability to stand. All four spinal curves are fully developed by the time a child is 10 years old.

All vertebrae share some common features: a relatively massive, weight-bearing **body**; **transverse processes** that project laterally and serve as sites for muscle attachment; and a **spinous** (or *spinal*) **process**. Each vertebra also has an opening called the **vertebral foramen**, through which the spinal cord passes. Viewed collectively, the vertebral foramina of adjacent vertebrae form the *vertebral canal* that encloses the spinal cord. Despite basic structural similarities throughout the vertebrae of the spine, some regional differences reflect important differences in function. Figure 4-9 shows typical vertebrae from each region.

Vertebrae form joints with each other at specialized flattened areas called *facets* and at their vertebral bodies. The vertebral bodies, however, usually do not contact one another directly because an **intervertebral disc** of cartilage lies between them. An intervertebral disc consists of a thick outer

Spinal curves

Vertebral regions

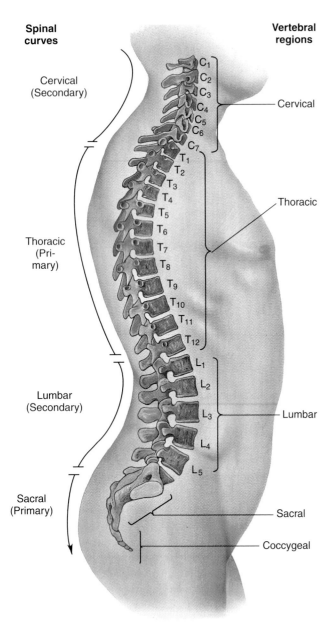

Cervical (Secondary)

Thoracic (Primary)

Lumbar (Secondary)

Sacral (Primary)

Cervical

Thoracic

Lumbar

Sacral

Coccygeal

FIGURE 4-8

The Vertebral Column.

The major divisions of the vertebral column, showing the four spinal curves.

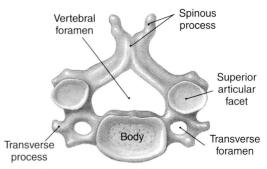

(a) Typical cervical vertebra, superior view

All cervical vertebrae contain transverse foramina that protect important blood vessels supplying the brain.

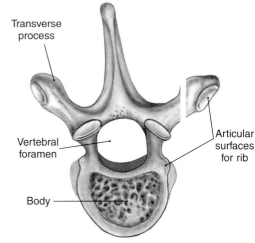

(b) Thoracic

A distinctive feature of thoracic vertebrae are articular surfaces on the body and on most of the transverse processes for articulation with one or more pairs of ribs.

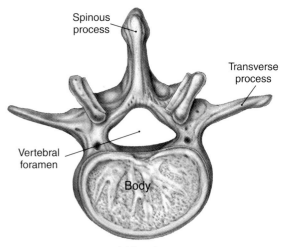

(c) Lumbar

The lumbar vertebrae are the most massive and least mobile, for they support most of the body weight. All have a wide and thick vertebral body.

FIGURE 4-9

Typical Cervical, Thoracic, and Lumbar Vertebrae.

All vertebrae are shown in superior view.

layer of fibrous cartilage surrounding a soft, gelatinous core. The intervertebral discs act as shock absorbers, compressing and distorting when stressed. Part of the loss of height that comes with aging results from the decreasing size and resiliency of the intervertebral discs.

The Thoracic Cage

The skeleton of the chest, or *thorax*, consists of the thoracic vertebrae, the ribs, and the sternum. The ribs and the sternum form the **thoracic cage**, or *rib cage*, and establish the shape of the thoracic cavity. The thoracic cage protects the heart, lungs, and other internal organs and serves as an attachment base for muscles involved with breathing (Figure 4-10).

The adult sternum has three parts: the broad, triangular **manubrium** (ma-NOO-brē-um); an elongate **body**; and the slender, inferior tip of the body, called the **xiphoid** (ZĪ-foid) **process**. Impact or strong pressure can drive the xiphoid process into the liver, causing severe damage. That is why proper hand position is so important when someone is performing cardiopulmonary resuscitation (CPR).

There are 12 pairs of ribs, or *costal bones*. Each pair of ribs is connected posteriorly to one of the 12 thoracic vertebrae. The first seven pairs, called **true ribs**, extend around the entire thoracic cavity and are connected to the sternum by cartilaginous extensions, the **costal cartilages**. Ribs 8 to 12 are called the **false ribs** because rather than attaching directly to the sternum, they attach to the costal cartilage of the seventh rib. The last two pairs of ribs are called **floating ribs** because they have no connection with the sternum at all.

Table 4-3 lists and describes the bones making up the vertebral column and thoracic cage.

Concept Questions

✔ Intervertebral discs are not found between the first and second cervical vertebrae. How does this fact relate to the function of these vertebrae?

✔ In adults, five large vertebrae fuse to form what single structure?

✔ What bones make up the thoracic cage?

FIGURE 4-10

The Thoracic Cage.

Anterior view of the rib cage and sternum.

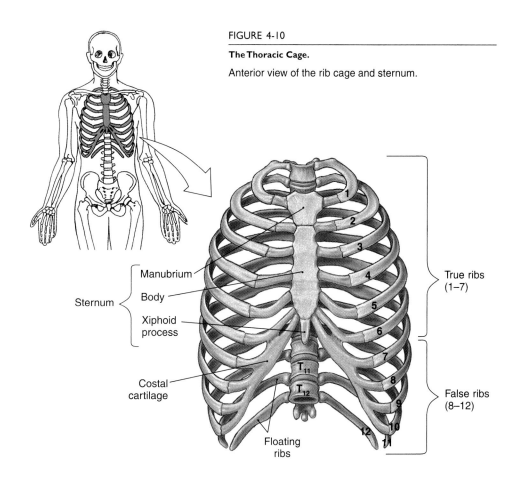

Manubrium

Body

Sternum

Xiphoid process

Costal cartilage

Floating ribs

True ribs (1–7)

False ribs (8–12)

Table 4-3		Bones of the Vertebral Column and Thoracic Cage
Bone (Region)	**Number**	**Comments**
Vertebral Column		
Cervical vertebrae	7	The bones of the neck; contain *transverse foramina* for protection of blood vessels that supply the brain
Thoracic vertebrae	12	Characteristics include large, slender spinous process that points inferiorly; articular surfaces on the vertebral body and, in most cases, on transverse processes for forming joints with one or more pairs of ribs
Lumbar vertebrae	5	Thicker and more oval vertebral body than thoracic vertebrae; stumpy spinous process points posteriorly
Sacrum	1	Made up of five fused vertebrae; protects internal organs; articulates with appendicular skeleton; site of muscle attachment for movement of lower limbs
Coccyx	1	Made up of three to five fused vertebrae; fusion not complete until adulthood
Thoracic Cage		
Sternum	1	Made up of three fused bones: the manubrium, body, and xiphoid process; xiphoid process is usually the last to ossify and fuse
Ribs	24	Same number in each sex
True ribs	14	Each forms portion of anterior body wall and connects to sternum by separate *costal cartilages*
False ribs	6	Do not attach directly to sternum; costal cartilages fuse together and then merge with that of rib 7
Floating ribs	4	Do not attach directly to sternum; no costal cartilages

THE APPENDICULAR SKELETON

The appendicular skeleton includes the bones of the upper and lower limbs as well as the pectoral and pelvic girdles that connect the limbs to the trunk. These bones are all listed and described in Table 4-4.

The Pectoral Girdle

Each upper limb articulates with the trunk at the *shoulder girdle*, or **pectoral girdle**. The pectoral girdle consists of a broad, flat **scapula** (*shoulder blade*) and the short **clavicle** (*collarbone*). The bones of the pectoral girdle are illustrated in Figure 4-11.

The S-shaped clavicle bone is small, light, and relatively fragile. Furthermore, the joint between the clavicle and sternum forms the *only* direct connection between the axial skeleton and the shoulder girdle. Pressure stress from a simple fall on the hand of an outstretched arm or a sudden jolt to the shoulder is often focused on the clavicle. As a result, broken or fractured clavicles are very common injuries.

The anterior face of the scapula forms a broad triangle. Muscles attach along the edges. Its posterior surface is divided by a long, and easily felt, spine. The shallow, cup-shaped *glenoid cavity* of the scapula articulates with the proximal end of the humerus to form the *shoulder joint*. Two processes of the scapula extend over the glenoid cavity. The **acromion** (a-KRŌ-mē-on) **process** forms the tip of the shoulder and a point of attachment for ligaments that interconnect the scapula and the clavicle. The underlying **coracoid process** provides another attachment site for muscles and ligaments.

The Upper Limb

The upper limb consists of the arm, forearm, wrist, and hand. You will notice that the anatomical term *arm* refers only to the proximal segment, rather than to the entire upper limb. The arm contains a single bone, the **humerus**, which extends from the shoulder joint to the elbow joint. At the elbow

FIGURE 4-11

The Pectoral Girdle.

The clavicle and scapula are the bones of the pectoral girdle.

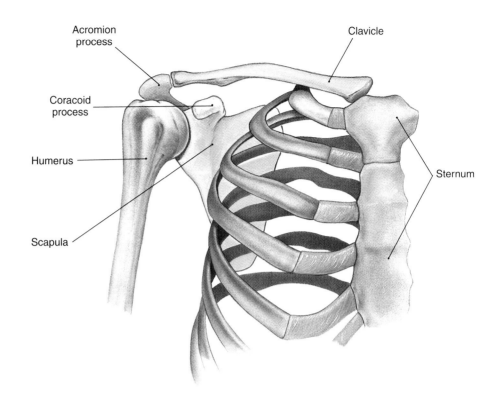

Table 4-4	Bones of the Pectoral Girdle and Upper Limb		
Bone (Region)	**Number**	**Comments**	
Pectoral Girdle			
Clavicle	2	Articulates with the sternum and the *acromion process* of the scapula; forms the only connection between the pectoral girdle and the axial skeleton	
Scapula	2	Provides attachment sites for muscles of the shoulder and arm; the humerus articulates with the scapula at its glenoid cavity, forming the shoulder joint	
Upper Limb			
Humerus	2	Various projections mark the attachments of different muscles; depressions at its distal end accept processes of the ulna as the elbow reaches its limits of motion	
Radius	2	The lateral bone of the forearm; the proximal joint with the ulna allows the distal radius to roll across the ulna and rotate the hand.	
Ulna	2	The medial bone of the forearm; the olecranon process forms the elbow	
Wrist and Hand Carpal bones	16	The 8 carpal bones of each wrist form two rows. The proximal row contains (1) *scaphoid*, (2) *lunate*, (3) *triangular* (or *triquetral*), and (4) *pisiform* (PI-si-form). There are also four distal carpal bones: (1) *trapezium*, (2) *trapezoid*, (3) *capitate*, and (4) *hamate*	
Metacarpal bones	10	Five metacarpal bones form the palm of each hand	
Phalanges Carpal Bones	28	Each finger contains three phalanges, and the thumb (*pollex*) contains two	

joint, the humerus articulates with the two bones of the forearm, the **radius** (lateral) and **ulna** (medial). These bones are shown in Figure 4-12.

In the anatomical position, with the palm facing forward, the radius lies along the lateral (thumb) side of the forearm. When turning the forearm so that the palm faces backward, the distal portion of the radius rolls across the ulna (see Figure 4-12). In life, a fibrous membrane connects the lateral margin of the ulna to the radius along its entire length. This thin sheet provides added stability to the forearm as this movement occurs. It also provides a large surface area for the attachment of muscles that control movements of the wrist and hand.

The point of the elbow is formed by a superior projection of the ulna, the **olecranon** (ō-LEK-ra-non) **process**. The distal end of the ulna is separated from the wrist joint by a pad of cartilage,

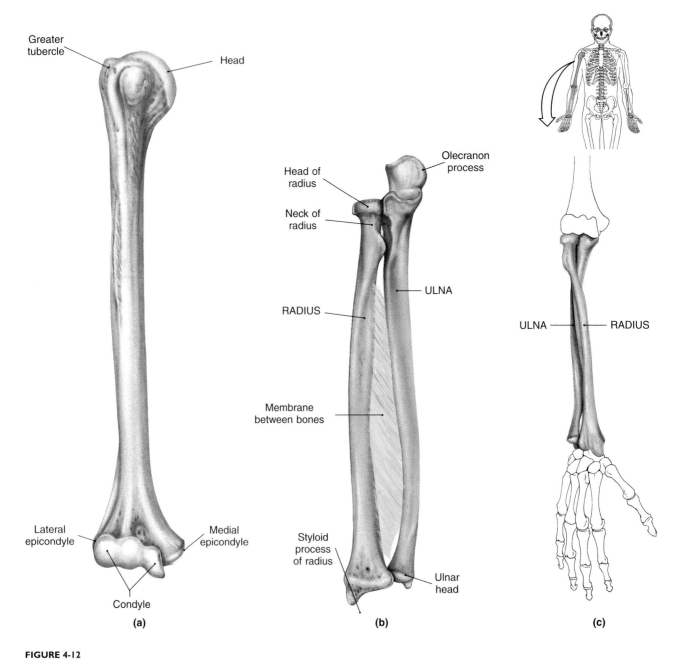

FIGURE 4-12

Bones of the Upper Limb.

Landmarks of the anterior surfaces of the **(a)** right humerus, and **(b)** right radius and ulna. **(c)** Note how the radius crosses over the ulna in a movement called *pronation*.

and only the wide distal portion of the radius articulates with the bones of the wrist. The *styloid process* of the radius helps in stabilizing the wrist joint by keeping the small wrist bones from sliding laterally.

Concept Questions

✔ Where does the only direct connection occur between the pectoral girdle and the axial skeleton?

✔ Which forearm bone is directly involved in the wrist joint?

There are 27 bones in the wrist and hand (Figure 4-13). The 8 bones known as **carpal bones** form the wrist. A fibrous capsule, reinforced by broad ligaments, surrounds the wrist and stabilizes the positions of the individual carpals. Five **metacarpal bones** (met-a-KAR-pals) articulate with the distal carpals and form the palm of the hand. The metacarpals in turn articulate with the finger bones, or **phalanges** (fa-LAN-jēs).There are 14 phalangeal bones in each hand. The thumb has only two phalanges (proximal and distal), whereas the other fingers contain three each (proximal, middle, and distal).

The Pelvic Girdle

The **pelvic girdle** articulates with the thigh bones of the lower limbs. Because of the stresses involved in weight bearing and locomotion, the bones of the pelvic girdle and lower limbs are more massive than those of the pectoral girdle and upper limbs. The pelvic girdle is also much more firmly attached to the axial skeleton. Dorsally, the two halves of the pelvic girdle attach to the sacrum. Ventrally, the pelvic bones are interconnected by a fibrocartilage pad.

The pelvic girdle consists of two large hip bones, or **coxae** (see Figures 4-3, 4-14a). Each coxa forms through the fusion of three bones: an **ilium** (IL-ē-um), an **ischium** (IS-kē-um), and a **pubis** (PŪ-bis). At the hip joint on either side, the head of the femur (thighbone) articulates with the curved surface of the **acetabulum** (as-e-TAB-ū-lum).

The **pelvis** consists of the two coxae, the sacrum, and the coccyx (see Figure 4-14). The pelvis is a composite structure that includes portions of both the appendicular and axial skeletons. An extensive network of ligaments interconnects these structures and increases the strength of the pelvis.

FIGURE 4-13

Bones of the Wrist and Hand.

Anterior view of the right wrist and hand.

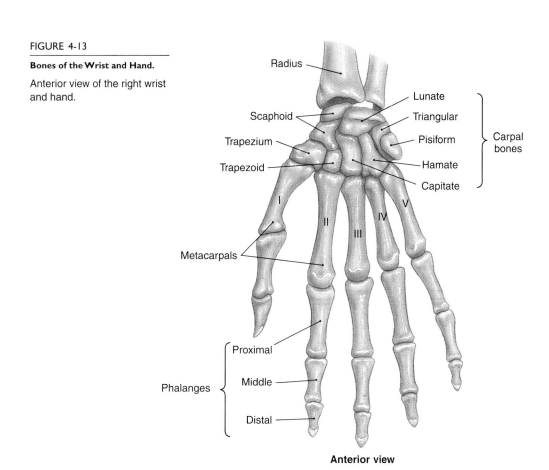

Anterior view

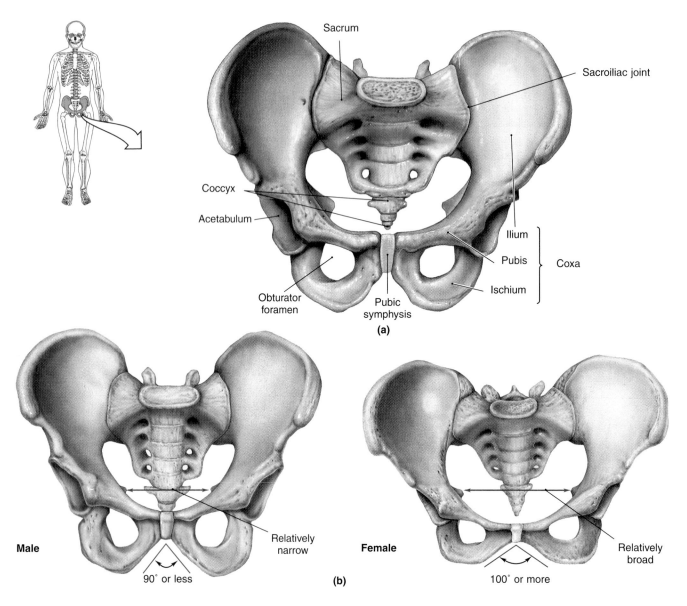

FIGURE 4-14

The Pelvis.

(a) Anterior view of the pelvis. **(b)** Anatomical differences in the pelvis of a male and female.

The shapes of the male pelvis and female pelvis are somewhat different (Figure 4-14b). Although some of the differences can be explained by variations between men and women in terms of body size and muscle mass, some features of the female pelvis are necessary adaptations for childbearing. A broader, flatter pelvis helps support the weight of the developing fetus, and a wider pelvic inlet helps ease passage of the newborn through the pelvis during delivery.

The Lower Limb

The lower limb consists of the thigh, the leg, the ankle, and the foot. Notice that the arrangement of bones in the lower limb is similar to that in the upper limb: one bone attaches to the girdle, two bones form the more distal portion, and a number of small bones combine to form the ankle and foot. Also note that the term *leg* refers only to the distal portion of the lower limb, rather than to the limb as a whole.

The **femur**, or *thighbone*, is the longest, heaviest, and strongest bone in the body (Figure 4-15a). Distally, the femur articulates with the *tibia*, the larger bone of the leg, at the knee joint. The rounded head of the femur joins the pelvis at the acetabulum.

Figure 4-15b shows the structure of the *tibia* and *fibula*. The **tibia** is the large medial bone of the leg. It is also known as the shinbone. The slender **fibula** parallels the lateral border of the tibia. The fibula does not participate in the knee joint, and it does not distribute weight to the ankle and foot. However, it is an important surface for muscle attachment, and it helps keep the ankle bones from sliding laterally. A fibrous membrane between the tibia and fibula helps lock the fibula in position and provides additional area for the attachment of muscles that move the ankle and foot.

The ankle includes seven separate **tarsal bones** (Figure 4-15c). Only the proximal tarsal bone, the **talus**, articulates with the tibia and fibula. The talus then passes the weight to the other tarsals, and ultimately to the ground. When standing normally, most of your weight is supported by the large **calcaneus** (kal-KĀ-nē-us), or *heel bone*. The rest of the body weight is passed through other tarsal bones to the **metatarsal bones** that support the sole of the foot. Powerful muscles on the back of the leg are attached to the posterior portion of the calcaneus by the *Achilles tendon*. Contraction of these calf muscles raises the heel and depresses the sole of the foot, as when you stand on tiptoes.

Concept Questions

✔ What three bones make up the coxa?

✔ The fibula does not participate in the knee joint nor does it bear weight, but when the fibula is fractured, it is difficult to walk. Why?

✔ While jumping off the back steps at his house, 10-year-old Joey lands on his right heel and breaks his foot. What foot bone is most likely broken?

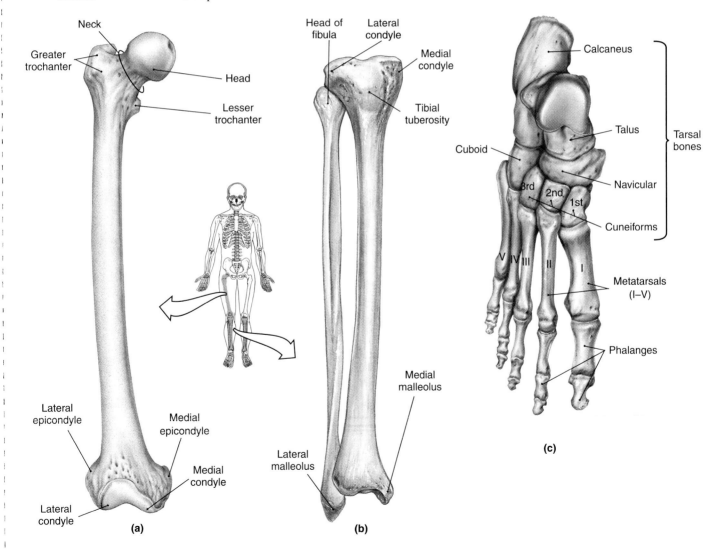

FIGURE 4-15

Bones of the Lower Limb.

Some features of the anterior surfaces of the right (a) femur and (b) tibia and fibula. (c) Bones of the right foot as viewed from above.

The basic organization of the metatarsal bones and phalanges of the foot resembles that of the metacarpals and phalanges of the hand. The metatarsal bones are numbered 1 to 5 (from medial to lateral). The big toe contains two phalanges, whereas each of the other toes contains three phalanges. Table 4-5 provides a summary of the bones of the pelvic girdle and lower limb.

▶ JOINTS

Joints, or **articulations**, exist wherever two bones meet. The function of each joint is closely related to its structure. Each joint reflects a workable compromise between the need for strength and the need for mobility. When movement is not required, joints can be very strong. For example, joints such as the sutures of the skull lock its separate elements together as if they were a single bone. At other joints, movement is more important than strength. At highly mobile joints, the interconnections between bones are looser and the joints weaker. For example, the shoulder joint permits a great variety of arm movements. The range of motion is limited more by the surrounding muscles than by joint structure. The joint itself is relatively weak, however, and shoulder injuries are rather common.

TYPES OF JOINTS

Three types of joints are recognized, based on the range of motion they permit: (1) An immovable joint is a **synarthrosis** (sin-ar-THRŌ-sis; *syn*, together + *arthros*, joint); (2) a slightly movable joint is an **amphiarthrosis** (am-fē-ar-THRŌ-sis; *amphi*, on both sides); and (3) a freely movable joint is a

Table 4-5	Bones of the Pelvic Girdle and Lower Limb.		
Bone (Region)	**Number**	**Comments**	
Pelvic Girdle			
Coxa (hip bone)	2	Each coxa forms through the fusion of three bones; the ilium, ischium, and pubis	
Ilium	2	The most superior and largest coxal bone; provides an extensive area for the attachment of muscles, tendons, and ligaments	
Ischium	2	The *ilium* fuses with the *ischium* near the superior and posterior margin of the acetabulum; the inferior surface of the ischium supports the body's weight when sitting	
Pubis	2	An opening formed by the pubis and ischium, the *obturator foramen*, is covered by connective tissue fibers to which muscles and internal organs attach; the *pubic symphysis* marks the articulation with the pubis of the opposite side; it limits movement between the two pubic bones	
Lower Limb			
Femur	2	The longest, heaviest, and strongest bone in the body; the *greater trochanter* and *lesser trochanter* provide attachment sites for large tendons; the distal shaft ends in two large *articular condyles* (*lateral* and *medial*)	
Patella	2	The patella, or kneecap, glides over the anterior surface of the articular condyles of the femur	
Tibia	2	The large medial bone of the leg; the inferior surface forms a joint with the proximal bone of the ankle; a large process, the *medial malleolus* (ma-LĒ-o-lus; malleolus, "hammer"), provides medial support for the ankle	
Fibula	2	Lies lateral to the tibia; the distal *lateral malleolus* provides lateral stability to the ankle	
Ankle and Foot			
Tarsal bones	14	Each ankle is made up of seven tarsal bones: the (1) *talus*, (2) *calcaneus*, (3) *navicular*, (4) *cuboid*, (5) *medial cuneiform*, (6) *intermediate cuneiform*, and (7) *lateral cuneiform*	
Metatarsal bones	10	Form the sole and ball of the foot	
Phalanges		Each toe contains three phalanges, and the great toe contains two	

diarthrosis (dī-ar-THRŌ-sis; *dia*, through). Freely movable joints are capable of a wide range of movements. As a result, freely movable joints are further subdivided according to the more specific types of movement they permit.

Immovable Joints (Synarthroses)

At a synarthrosis the bony edges of the articulating bones are quite close together, and they are bound to each other by dense fibrous connective tissue. An example is a suture, an immovable joint between the bones of the skull. Another example of a synarthrosis is the joint between a tooth and its bony socket.

Slightly Movable Joints (Amphiarthroses)

An amphiarthrosis permits very limited movement. The bones at such joints are usually farther apart than they are at a synarthrosis, and they are separated by a cartilage. Examples include (1) the articulations between the bodies of adjacent spinal vertebrae, which are separated by intervertebral discs, and (2) the *pubic symphysis*, where a fibrocartilage pad forms the articulation between the right and left pelvic bones (coxae).

Freely Movable Joints (Diarthroses)

Diarthroses permit a wide range of motion. Diarthroses, or **synovial joints**, take advantage of the great friction-reducing properties of synovial fluid. Figure 4-16a shows the general structure of a synovial joint.

Synovial joints are typically found at the ends of long bones, such as those of the limbs. Under normal conditions the bony surfaces do not contact one another, for they are covered with special **articular cartilages**. The joint is surrounded by a fibrous **joint capsule**, and the inner surfaces of the joint cavity are lined with a synovial membrane. **Synovial fluid** diffuses across the synovial membrane and provides additional lubrication.

FIGURE 4-16

The Structure of a Synovial Joint.

(a) Diagrammatic view of a simple articulation. **(b)** A simplified sectional view of the knee joint.

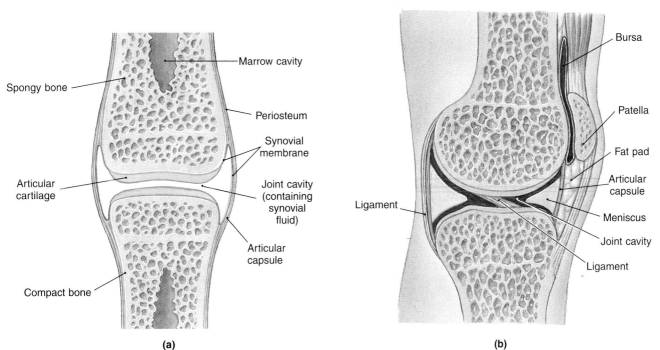

(a)

(b)

In complex joints such as the knee, additional padding in the form of cartilage lies between the opposing articular surfaces. Such shock-absorbing cartilage pads are called **menisci** (men-IS-kē), shown in Figure 4-16b. (*Meniscus* means "crescent," and refers to the shape of these pads.) Also present in such joints are **fat pads** which protect the articular cartilages and act as packing material. When the bones move, the fat pads fill in the spaces created as the joint cavity changes shape.

The joint capsule that surrounds the entire joint is continuous with the per-iosteum of each articulating bone. Ligaments that join one bone to another may be found on the outside or inside of the joint capsule. Where a tendon or ligament rubs against other tissues, small pockets of synovial fluid called **bursae** form to reduce friction and act as shock absorbers. Bursae are characteristic of many synovial joints and may also appear around tendons, beneath the skin covering a bone, or within other connective tissues exposed to friction or pressure.

ACTIONS OF MOVABLE JOINTS

Synovial joints are involved in all our day-to-day body movements. Although we commonly describe our movements with general phrases such as "bend the leg" or "raise the arm," it is sometimes helpful to use more specific descriptive terms.

Types of Movement.

In **gliding**, two opposing surfaces slide past each other. Gliding occurs between the surfaces of articulating carpal bones (and tarsal bones), and between each clavicle and the sternum. Gliding can involve movement in almost any direction, but the amount of movement is slight.

Most **angular movements** are best remembered in opposing pairs: for example, *flexion* and *extension*, or *adduction* and *abduction*. The descriptions of each movement assume that the individual begins in the anatomical position.

Flexion (FLEK-shun) is a movement that *reduces* the angle between the articulating bones. **Extension** *increases* the angle between the articulating bones (Figure 4-17a). When you bring your head toward your chest, you flex the neck. When you bend down to touch your toes, you flex the spine. Extension reverses these movements. Flexion at the shoulder or hip moves a limb forward (anteriorly), whereas extension moves it backward (posteriorly). Flexion of the wrist moves the palm forward, and extension moves it back. In each of these examples, extension can be continued past the anatomical position, in which case **hyperextension** occurs. You can also hyperextend the head, a movement that allows you to gaze at the ceiling. Hyperextension of other joints is usually prevented or severely limited by ligaments, bony processes, or soft tissues.

Abduction (*ab*, from) is movement *away* from the longitudinal axis of the body. For example, swinging the upper limb away from the trunk is abduction of the limb (Figure 4-17b); moving it toward the trunk is **adduction** (*ad*, to). Adduction of the wrist moves the heel of the hand toward the body, whereas abduction moves it farther away. Spreading the fingers or toes apart abducts them, because they move *away* from a central digit (finger or toe), as in Figure 4-17c. Adduction brings the digits together. Abduction and adduction always refer to movements of the appendicular skeleton.

In **circumduction**, the distal portion of a limb moves in a circle while the proximal portion is fixed, as when one is drawing a large circle on a chalkboard (Figure 4-17d). The fingers may circumduct as well, as when you trace a small circle with the tip of your index finger.

Rotational movements are also described with reference to a figure in the anatomical position. Rotation involves turning around the longitudinal axis of the body or limb, as when you rotate your head to look to one side or rotate your arm and forearm to screw in a lightbulb (Figure 4-18a). Moving the wrist and hand from palm-facing-front to palm-facing-back is called **pronation** (prō-NĀ-shun) (Figure 4-18b). The opposing movement, in which the palm is turned forward, is **supination** (sū-pi-NĀ-shun).

There are a number of special terms that apply to specific articulations or unusual types of movement (Figure 4-19).

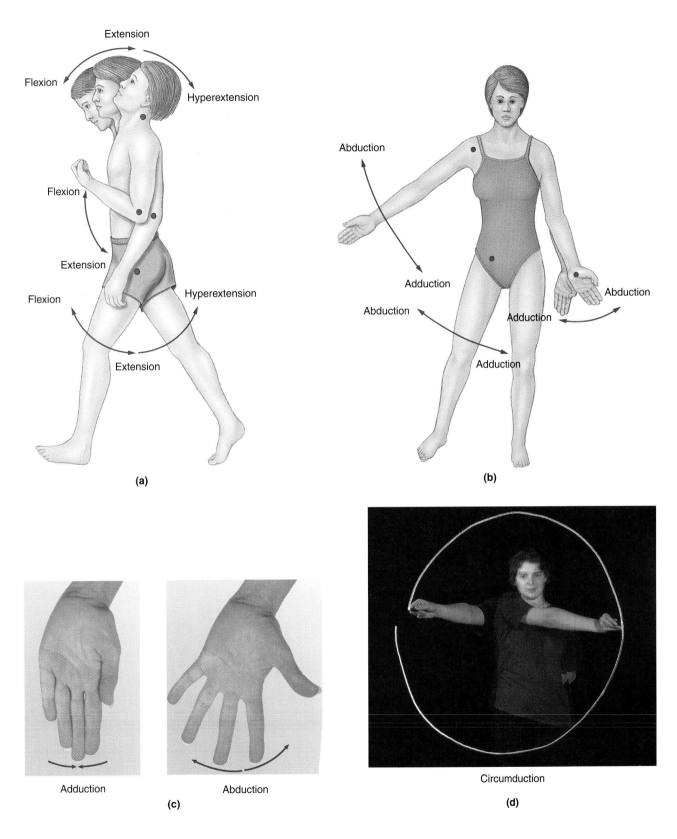

FIGURE 4-17

Angular Movements.

The red dots mark the locations of joints involved in the movements.

FIGURE 4-18

Rotational Movements.

Head rotation

Limb
rotation

(a)

Supination

Pronation

(b)

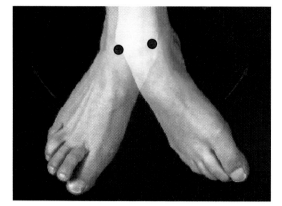

Eversion   Inversion

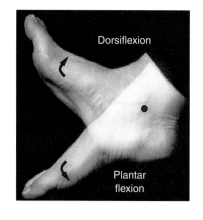

Dorsiflexion

Plantar
flexion

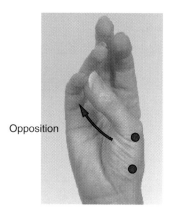

Opposition

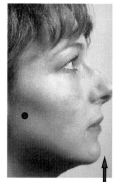

Retraction   Protraction

Elevation

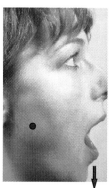

Depression

FIGURE 4-19

Special Movements.

- **Inversion** (*in*, into + *vertere*, to turn), is a twisting motion of the foot that turns the sole inward. The opposite movement is called **eversion** (ē-VER-shun; *e*, out).
- **Dorsiflexion** is flexion of the ankle and elevation of the sole, as when "digging in the heels." The opposite movement, **plantar flexion** (from *planta*, the sole), extends the ankle and elevates the heel, as when standing on tiptoes.
- **Elevation** and **depression** occur when a structure moves in a superior or inferior direction. You depress your mandible when you open your mouth, and elevate it as you close it. Another familiar elevation occurs when you shrug your shoulders.
- **Protraction** involves moving a part of the body anteriorly in the horizontal plane. **Retraction** is the reverse movement. You protract your jaw when you grasp your upper lip with your lower teeth, and you protract your clavicles when you reach for something in front of you.

The Shapes of Movable Joints

Synovial joints can be described as *gliding, hinge, pivot, ellipsoidal, saddle,* or *ball-and-socket* joints based on the shapes of the articulating surfaces. Each type of joint permits a different type and range of motion.

- **Gliding joints** (Figure 4-20a) have flattened or slightly curved faces. The relatively flat articular surfaces slide across one another, but the amount of movement is very slight. Although rotation is theoretically possible at such a joint, ligaments usually prevent or restrict such movement. Gliding joints are found at the ends of the clavicles, between the carpal bones, between the tarsal bones, and between the articular facets of adjacent spinal vertebrae.
- **Hinge joints** (Figure 4-20b) permit angular movement in a single plane, like the opening and closing of a door. Examples include the elbow, knee, ankle, and interphalangeal joints.
- **Pivot joints** (Figure 4-20c) permit rotation only. A pivot joint between the atlas (C_1) and axis (C_2) vertebrae allows you to rotate your head to either side, and another between the radius and the proximal shaft of the ulna permits turning of the hand (pronation and supination).
- In an **ellipsoidal joint** (Figure 4-20d), an oval articular face nestles within a depression on the opposing surface. With such an arrangement, angular motion occurs in two planes, along or across the length of the oval. Ellipsoidal joints connect the fingers and toes with the metacarpal and metatarsal bones, respectively.
- **Saddle joints** (Figure 4-20e) have articular faces that resemble saddles. Each face is concave on one axis and convex on the other, and the opposing faces nest together. This arrangement permits angular motion, including circumduction, but prevents rotation. The carpometacarpal joint at the base of the thumb is the best example of a saddle joint, and "twiddling your thumbs" demonstrates the possible movements.
- In a **ball-and-socket joint** (Figure 4-20f), the round head of one bone rests within a cup-shaped depression in another. All combinations of movements, including circumduction and rotation, can be performed at ball-and-socket joints. Examples include the shoulder and hip joints.

Concept Questions

✔ In a newborn infant the large bones of the skull are joined by fibrous connective tissue. What type of joint is this? These bones later grow, interlock, and form immovable joints. What type of joints are these?

✔ Give the proper term for each of the following types of motion: (a) moving your arm away from the midline of the body, (b) turning your palms so that they face forward, (c) bending your elbow.

FIGURE 4-20

Types of Movable Joints.

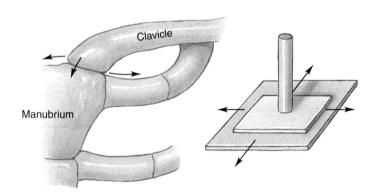

(a) Gliding joint

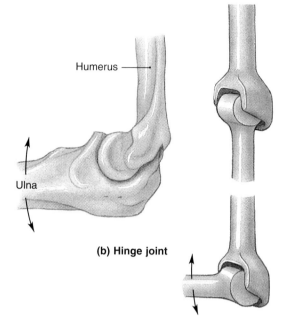

(b) Hinge joint

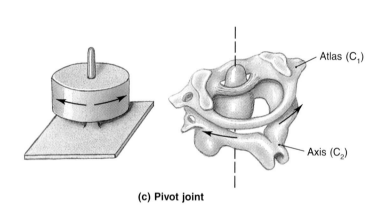

Atlas (C₁)

Axis (C₂)

(c) Pivot joint

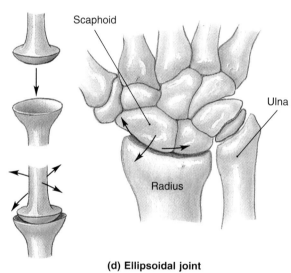

Scaphoid

Ulna

Radius

(d) Ellipsoidal joint

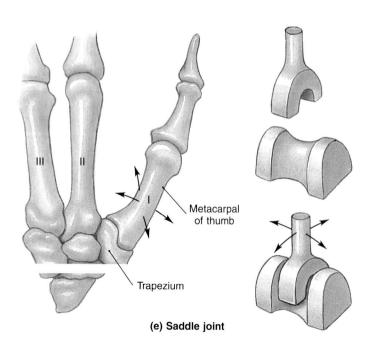

III   II   I

Metacarpal
of thumb

Trapezium

(e) Saddle joint

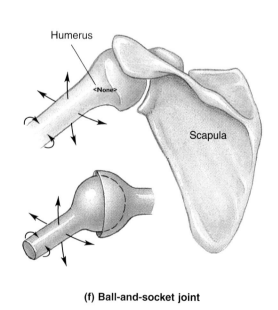

Humerus

<None>

Scapula

(f) Ball-and-socket joint

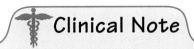

Clinical Note

What Are Rheumatism and Arthritis?

Rheumatism (ROO-ma-tizm) is a general term that indicates pain and stiffness affecting the skeletal and/or muscular systems. There are several major forms of rheumatism. One of them, arthritis (ar-THRĪ-tis), includes all the rheumatic diseases that affect synovial joints.

Proper working of synovial joints depends on healthy articular cartilages. When an articular cartilage has been damaged, the matrix breaks down and the exposed cartilage surface changes from slick and slippery to rough and frayed. The change in surface texture increases the amount of contact and friction between adjacent bones, and eventually the central area of cartilage may be completely worn away.

Arthritis always involves damage to the articular cartilage on the ends of bones, but the specific causes may vary. For example, arthritis can result from bacterial or viral infection, injury to the joint, metabolic problems, or severe physical stresses.

Regular exercise, physical therapy, and drugs that reduce inflammation, such as aspirin, can slow the progress of some forms of arthritis. In others, surgery to realign the joint may be required, or in extreme cases involving the hip, knee, elbow or shoulder, the problem joint may be replaced with an artificial one.

CHAPTER REVIEW SECTION

KEY WORDS

amphiarthrosis:	An articulation that permits a small degree of movement.
appendicular skeleton:	Pertaining to the bones of the upper or lower limbs.
articulation (ar-tik-ū-LĀ-shun):	A joint between bones.
axial skeleton:	Pertaining to the bones of the skull, vertebral column, and rib cage.
diarthrosis:	freely movable joint; a synovial joint.
ligament (LI-ga-ment):	Dense band of connective tissue fibers that attach one bone to another.
marrow:	A tissue that fills the internal cavities in a bone; may be dominated by blood element–forming cells (red marrow) or adipose tissue (yellow marrow).
ossification:	The replacement of other tissue with bone.
osteoblast:	A cell that produces the fibers and matrix of bone.
osteoclast:	A cell that dissolves the fibers and matrix of bone.
osteocyte (OS-tē-ō-sīt):	A bone cell responsible for the maintenance and turnover of the mineral content of the surrounding bone.
osteon (OS-tē-on):	The basic structural unit of compact bone, consisting of osteocytes organized around a central canal and separated by rings of calcified matrix.
periosteum (pe-rē-OS-tē-um):	Layer of fibers and cells that surrounds a bone.
synarthrosis:	A joint that does not permit movement.
synovial (sī-NŌV-ē-ul) **fluid:**	Substance secreted by synovial membranes that lubricates most freely movable joints.

STUDY OUTLINE

SYSTEM BRIEF

1. The skeletal system includes the bones of the skeleton and the cartilages, ligaments, and other connective tissues that stabilize or interconnect bones. Its functions include structural support, protection, leverage, storage, and blood cell production.

BONE STRUCTURE

1. **Osseous tissue** is a supporting connective tissue with a solid **matrix**.

GENERAL FEATURES OF BONE

2. General shapes of bones include long bones, short bones, flat bones, and irregular bones.
3. The features of a long bone include a **diaphysis**, **epiphyses**, and a central marrow cavity. (*Figure 4-1*)
4. There are two types of bone: **compact bone** and **spongy bone**.
5. A bone is covered by a **periosteum** and lined with an **endosteum**.

MICROSCOPIC FEATURES OF BONE

6. There are three types of bone cells. **Osteocytes** maintain the structure of existing bones. **Osteoblasts** produce the matrix of new bone through the process of *osteogenesis*. **Osteoclasts** dissolve the bony matrix and release the stored minerals.
7. Osteocytes occupy **lacunae**, spaces in bone. The lacunae are surrounded by layers of calcified matrix.
8. The basic functional unit of compact bone is the **osteon**, containing osteocytes arranged around a **central canal**. (*Figure 4-1*)

BONE DEVELOPMENT AND MAINTENANCE

1. **Ossification** is the process of converting other tissues to bone.

BONE GROWTH

2. In the process of **endochondral ossification**, a cartilaginous model is gradually replaced by bone. (*Figure 4-2*)
3. There are differences among bones and among individuals regarding the timing of epiphyseal closure.
4. Normal osteogenesis requires a reliable source of minerals, vitamins, and hormones.

BONE MAINTENANCE

5. The organic and mineral components of bone are continually recycled and renewed through the process of remodeling.
6. The shapes and thicknesses of bones reflect the stresses applied to them. Mineral turnover allows bone to adapt to new stresses.
7. Calcium is the most common mineral in the human body, with roughly 99 percent of it located in the skeleton.
8. A **fracture** is a crack or break in a bone.

AGING AND THE SKELETAL SYSTEM

9. The bones of the skeleton become thinner and relatively weaker as aging occurs.

THE SKELETON

1. The skeletal system consists of the axial skeleton and the appendicular skeleton. The **axial skeleton** can be subdivided into the **skull**, the **thoracic** (rib) **cage**, and the **vertebral column**.

2. The **appendicular skeleton** includes the limbs and the pectoral and pelvic girdles that attach the limbs to the trunk. (*Figure 4-3*)

SKELETAL TERMS

3. Bone markings are used to describe and identify specific bones. (*Table 4-1*)

THE AXIAL SKELETON

4. The skull can be divided into *cranial* and *facial* subdivisions. The **cranium** encloses the **cranial cavity**, a division of the dorsal body cavity that encloses the brain. (*Figure 4-4*)

5. The cranial bones include the **frontal bone, parietal bones, occipital bone, temporal bones, sphenoid bone**, and **ethmoid bone**. (*Figures 4-4, 4-5, 4-6; Table 4-2*)

6. The facial bones include the left and right **maxillary bones** (*maxillae*), **palatine bones, vomer, zygomatic bones, nasal bones, lacrimal bones, inferior nasal conchae**, and the **mandible**. (*Figures 4-4, 4-5, 4-6; Table 4-2*)

7. The **auditory ossicles** lie within the temporal bone. The **hyoid bone** is suspended below the skull by ligaments from the styloid processes of the temporal bones. (*Figure 4-4; Table 4-2*)

8. The nasal septum divides the nasal cavities. Together the **frontal**, **sphenoid**, **ethmoid**, and **maxillary sinuses** make up the *paranasal sinuses*, which drain into the nasal cavities. (*Figures 4-5, 4-6*)

9. Fibrous connections at **fontanels** permit the skulls of infants and children to continue growing. (*Figure 4-7*)

10. There are 7 **cervical vertebrae**, 12 **thoracic vertebrae** (which articulate with ribs), and 5 **lumbar vertebrae** (which articulate with the sacrum). The **sacrum** and **coccyx** consist of fused vertebrae. (*Figure 4-8; Table 4-3*)

11. The spinal column has four **spinal curves** that accommodate the unequal distribution of body weight and keep it in line with the body axis. (*Figure 4-8*)

12. A typical vertebra has a **body** and a **vertebral foramen**. Adjacent vertebral bodies are separated by an **intervertebral disc**.

13. Cervical vertebrae are distinguished by the *transverse foramina* on either side. Thoracic vertebrae articulate with the ribs. The lumbar vertebrae are the most massive and least mobile, and they are subjected to the greatest strains. (*Figure 4-9*)

14. The **sacrum** protects reproductive, digestive, and excretory organs. It articulates with the **coccyx**. (*Figures 4-3, 4-8; Table 4-3*)

15. The skeleton of the thorax consists of the thoracic vertebrae, the ribs, and the sternum. The ribs and sternum form the **rib cage**. (*Figure 4-10; Table 4-3*)

16. Ribs 1 to 7 are **true ribs**. Ribs 8 to 12 lack direct connections to the sternum and are called **false ribs**; they include two pairs of **floating ribs**. (*Figure 4-10; Table 4-3*)

17. The sternum consists of a **manubrium**, a **body**, and a **xiphoid process**. (*Figure 4-10; Table 4-3*)

THE APPENDICULAR SKELETON

18. Each upper limb articulates with the trunk at the *shoulder*, or **pectoral**, *girdle*, which consists of the **scapula** and **clavicle**. (*Figures 4-3, 4-11; Table 4-4*)

19. The clavicle and scapula position the shoulder joint, help move the arm, and provide a base for arm movement and muscle attachment.

20. The scapula articulates with the **humerus** at the shoulder joint. (*Figure 4-12a; Table 4-4*)

21. Distally the humerus articulates with the radius and ulna at the elbow joint.

22. The radius and ulna are the bones of the forearm. The **olecranon** process forms the point of the elbow. (*Figure 4-12b,c; Table 4-4*)
23. The bones of the wrist form two rows of **carpal bones**. The distal carpal bones articulate with the **metacarpal bones** of the hand. Four of the fingers contain three **phalanges**; the thumb has only two. (*Figure 4-13; Table 4-4*)
24. The **pelvic girdle** consists of two **coxae**; each coxa forms through the fusion of an **ilium**, an **ischium**, and a **pubis**. (*Figure 4-14; Table 4-5*)
25. The **pelvis** consists of the coxae, the sacrum, and the coccyx.
26. The **femur**, or *thighbone*, is the longest bone in the body. It articulates with the **tibia** at the knee joint. (*Figure 4-15a,b*)
27. The *medial malleolus* of the tibia and the *lateral malleolus* of the fibula articulate with the *talus* at the ankle joint. (*Figure 4-15b*)
28. The ankle includes seven **tarsal bones**; only the **talus** articulates with the tibia and fibula. When we are standing normally, most of our weight is transferred to the ground through the **calcaneus**; the rest is passed through the **metatarsal bones**. (*Figure 4-15c*)

JOINTS

1. **Articulations** (joints) exist wherever two bones interact.

TYPES OF JOINTS

2. Immovable joints are **synarthroses**, slightly movable joints are **amphiarthroses**, and those that are freely movable are called **diarthroses**.
3. An example of a synarthrosis is a *suture*.
4. An example of an amphiarthrosis is the *pubic symphysis*. (*Figure 4-14*)
5. The bony surfaces at diarthroses, or **synovial joints**, are covered by **articular cartilages**, lubricated by **synovial fluid**, and enclosed within a **joint capsule**. Other synovial structures can include **menisci**, **fat pads**, and various ligaments. (*Figure 4-16*)

ACTIONS OF MOVABLE JOINTS

6. Important terms that describe dynamic motion are **flexion**, **extension**, **hyperextension**, **rotation**, **circumduction**, **abduction**, and **adduction**. (*Figure 4-17*)
7. The bones in the forearm permit **pronation** and **supination**. (*Figures 4-12c, 4-18*)
8. The ankle undergoes **dorsiflexion** and **plantar flexion**. Movements of the foot include **inversion** and **eversion**. **Opposition** is the thumb movement that enables us to grasp objects. (*Figure 4-19*)
9. **Protraction** involves moving something forward; **retraction** involves moving it back. **Depression** and **elevation** occur when we move a structure down and up. (*Figure 4-19*)
10. Synovial joints include **gliding joints**, **hinge joints**, **pivot joints**, **ellipsoidal joints**, **saddle joints**, and **ball-and-socket joints**. (*Figure 4-20*)

REVIEW QUESTIONS

MATCHING

Match each item in Column A with the most closely related item in Column B. Use letters for answers in the spaces provided.

	Column A		**Column B**
K	1. elbow and knee	a.	abduction
S	2. diaphysis	b.	heel bone
M	3. auditory ossicles	c.	ball-and-socket joints
L	4. moving the hand into a palm-back position	d.	bone-dissolving cells
A	5. osteoblasts	e.	hinge joints
B	6. C_1	f.	bone covering that increases the thickness of bone
O	7. periosteum	g.	immovable joints
N	8. hip and shoulder	h.	bone shaft
T	9. patella	i.	functional unit of compact bone
B	10. calcaneus	j.	bone-producing cells
E	11. sutures	k.	a cervical vertebra
C	12. moving the hand	l.	pronation into a palm-front position
K	13. osteoclasts	m.	ear bones
M	14. raising the arm laterally	n.	supination
I	15. osteon	o.	kneecap

MULTIPLE CHOICE

16. The bones of the skeleton store energy reserves as lipids in areas of ____B____.
    (a) red marrow
    (b) yellow marrow
    (c) the matrix of bone tissue
    (d) the ground substance

17. The two types of osseous tissue are ____A____.
    (a) compact bone and spongy bone
    (b) dense bone and compact bone
    (c) spongy bone and cartilage
    (d) a, b, and c are correct

18. The cells that maintain mature compact bone are ____C____.
    (a) lacunae   (b) osteocytes
    (c) osteoblasts   (d) osteoclasts

19. The axial skeleton consists of the bones of the ____D____.
    (a) pectoral and pelvic girdles
    (b) skull, thorax, and vertebral column
    (c) arm, legs, hand, and feet
    (d) limbs, pectoral girdle, and pelvic girdle

20. The appendicular skeleton consists of the bones of the ____B____.
    (a) pectoral and pelvic girdles
    (b) skull, thorax, and vertebral column
    (c) arm, legs, hands, and feet
    (d) limbs, pectoral girdle, and pelvic girdle

21. Of the following sets of bones, _____ A _____ lists only bones of the cranium.
    (a) mandible, parietal, occipital, sphenoid
    (b) frontal, occipital, zygomatic, parietal
    (c) occipital, sphenoid, temporal, parietal
    (d) mandible, maxillary, nasal, zygomatic

22. Of the following bones, the _____ A _____ is unpaired.
    (a) vomer   (b) maxillary bone
    (c) palatine bone (d) nasal bone

23. At the glenoid cavity, the scapula articulates with the proximal end of the _____ C _____.
    (a) humerus   (b) radius
    (c) ulna   (d) femur

24. Each coxa of the pelvic girdle consists of three fused bones, the _____ C _____.
    (a) ulna, radius, humerus
    (b) hamate, capitate, trapezium
    (c) femur, tibia, fibula
    (d) ilium, ischium, pubis

25. The function of the synovial fluid is _____ B _____.
    (a) to nourish chondrocytes
    (b) to provide lubrication
    (c) to absorb shock
    (d) a, b, and c are correct

26. Standing on tiptoe is an example of a movement called _____ D _____.
    (a) elevation   (b) dorsiflexion
    (c) plantar flexion (d) retraction

TRUE/FALSE

F   27. In anatomical position, the ulna lies medial to the radius.
T   28. The red marrow is the site of production of red blood cells and other blood elements.
T   29. Joints typically found at the end of long bones are amphiarthroses.
T   30. Abduction and adduction always refer to movements of the appendicular skeleton.
F   31. Both the scapula and clavicle form joints with the axial skeleton.

SHORT ESSAY

32. What are the five primary functions of the skeletal system?

33. During the growth of a long bone, how is the epiphysis forced farther from the shaft?

34. What two primary functions are performed by the thoracic cage?

35. What is the difference between the *pelvic girdle* and the *pelvis*?

36. While working at an excavation, an archaeologist finds several small skull bones. She examines the frontal, parietal, and occipital bones and concludes that the skulls are those of children not yet 1 year old. How can she tell their ages from examining the bones?

✔ Answers to Concept Check Questions

(p. 92)   **1.** Concentric layers of bone around a central canal indicate a *Haversian system* that makes up compact bone. Since the ends (epiphyses) of long bones are mostly spongy bone, this sample most likely came from the shaft (diaphysis). **2.** Because osteoclasts break down, or demineralize, bone, the bone would have less mineral content and be weaker.

(p. 94)   **1.** Long bones of the body, like the femur, have a plate of cartilage (the *epiphyseal plate*) that separates the epiphysis from the diaphysis as long as the bone is growing in length. An X-ray would reveal whether the epiphyseal plate was still present. If it was, then growth was still occurring; if not, the bone had reached its adult length. **2.** The increase in the male sex hormone, testosterone, that occurs at puberty contributes to an increased rate of bone growth and the closure of the epiphyseal plates. Since the source of testosterone, the testes, is removed in castration, the boys would be expected to have a longer, though slower, growth period and be taller than if they had not been castrated. **3.** The larger arm muscles of the weight lifter apply more mechanical stress to the bones of the arm. In response to the stress, the bones will grow thicker. We would expect the jogger to have heavier thigh bones for similar reasons.

(p. 100)   **1.** The *frontal bone* of the cranium lies under the forehead. **2.** The opening in the occipital bone is called the *occipital foramen*. It provides a passage for the spinal cord that connects to the brain. **3.** The paranasal sinuses function to make some of the heavier skull bones lighter, and their epithelial linings produce mucus.

(p. 103)   **1.** An intervertebral disc between the first and second vertebrae would not allow the head to rotate, or turn, to the right and left. **2.** In adults, the five sacral vertebrae fuse to form a single sacrum. **3.** The *thoracic cage* is made up of the thoracic vertebrae, the ribs, and the sternum.

(p. 107)   **1.** The only direct connection between the pectoral girdle and the axial skeleton occurs between the clavicle and the *manubrium* of the sternum. **2.** Only the *radius* of the forearm is involved in forming the wrist joint.

(p. 109)   **1.** The three bones that make up the coxa are the ilium, ischium, and pubis. **2.** Although the fibula is not part of the knee joint nor does it bear weight, it is an important point of attachment for many leg muscles. When the fibula is fractured, these muscles cannot function properly to move the leg and walking is difficult and painful. **3.** Joey has most likely fractured the *calcaneus* (heel bone).

(p. 115)   **1.** At first, the joint is a type of amphiarthrotic joint. Later, when the bones interlock, they form sutural (synarthrotic) joints. **2.** (a) abduction; (b) supination; (c) flexion.

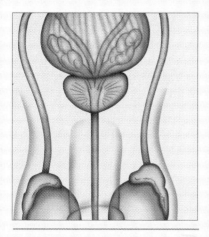

5

MEDICAL TERMINOLOGY OF THE MALE REPRODUCTIVE SYSTEM

OBJECTIVES

On completion of this chapter, you should be able to:

- Describe the male's external organs of reproduction.

- Describe and state the functions of the testes, epididymis, ductus deferens, seminal vesicles, prostate gland, bulbourethral glands, and urethra.

- Analyze, build, spell, and pronounce medical words that relate to surgical procedures and pathology.

- Identify and give the meaning of selected vocabulary words.

- Identify and define selected abbreviations.

- Review Drug Highlights presented in this chapter.

- Provide the description of diagnostic and laboratory tests related to the male reproductive system.

- Successfully complete the study and review section.

▶ ANATOMY AND PHYSIOLOGY OVERVIEW

The male reproductive system consists of the *testes, various ducts,* the *urethra,* and the following accessory glands: *bulbourethral, prostate,* and the *seminal vesicles.* The supporting structures and accessory sex organs are the *scrotum* and the *penis* (Fig. 5–1). The vital function of the male reproductive system is to provide the sperm cells necessary to fertilize the ovum thereby perpetuating the species. The following is a general overview of the organs and functions of this system.

▶ EXTERNAL ORGANS

In the male, the scrotum and the penis are the external organs of reproduction.

THE SCROTUM

The *scrotum* is a pouch-like structure located behind the penis. It is suspended from the perineal region and is divided by a septum into two sacs, each containing one of the testes along with its connecting tube called the *epididymis.* Within the tissues of the scrotum are fibers of smooth muscle that contract in the absence of sufficient heat, giving the scrotum a wrinkled appearance. This contractile action brings the testes closer to the perineum where they can absorb sufficient body heat to maintain the viability of the *spermatozoa.* Under normal conditions, the walls of the scrotum are generally free of wrinkles, and it hangs loosely between the thighs (Fig. 5–1).

THE PENIS

The *penis* is the external male sex organ and is composed of erectile tissue covered with skin. The size and shape of the penis varies, with an average erect penis being 15 to 20 cm in length. The penis has three longitudinal columns of erectile tissue that are capable of significant enlargement when engorged with blood, as is the case during sexual stimulation. Two of these columns, located

THE MALE REPRODUCTIVE SYSTEM

ORGAN/STRUCTURE	PRIMARY FUNCTIONS
The Scrotum	Contains testes and connecting tubes; contractile action brings the testes closer to the perineum, where they can absorb sufficient body heat to maintain the viability of the spermatozoa
The Penis	Male organ of copulation; site of the orifice for the elimination of urine and semen from the body
The Testes	Contains seminiferous tubules that are the site of the development of spermatozoa; cells within the testes also produce the male sex hormone, testosterone
The Epididymis	Storage site for the maturation of sperm
The Ductus Deferens or Vas Deferens	Excretory duct of the testis
The Seminal Vesicles	Produce a slightly alkaline fluid that becomes a part of the seminal fluid or semen
The Prostate Gland	Secretes an alkaline fluid that aids in maintaining the viability of spermatozoa
The Bulbourethral or Cowper's Glands	Produce a mucous secretion before ejaculation, which becomes a part of the semen
The Urethra	Transmits urine and semen out of the body

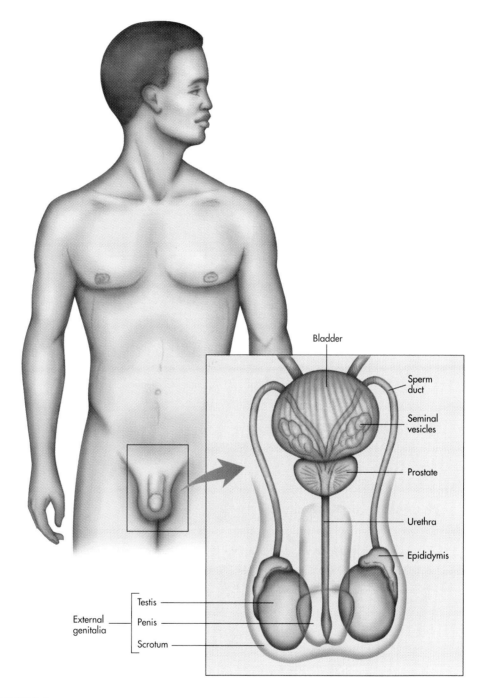

FIGURE 5–1

The male reproductive system: seminal vesicles, prostate, urethra, sperm duct, epididymis, and external genitalia.

side by side, form the greater part of the penis. These columns are known as the *corpora cavernosa penis.* The third longitudinal column, the *corpus spongiosum,* has the same function as the first two columns but is transversed by the penile portion of the urethra and tends to be more elastic when in an erectile state. The *corpus spongiosum,* at its distal end, expands to form the *glans penis.* The glans penis is the cone-shaped head of the penis and is the site of the urethral orifice. It is covered with loose skin folds called the *foreskin* or prepuce. See Figure 5–2. The foreskin contains glands that secrete a lubricating fluid called *smegma*. The foreskin may be removed by a surgical procedure known as *circumcision.*

The erectile state in the penis results when sexual stimulation causes large quantities of blood from dilated arteries supplying the penis to fill the cavernous spaces in the erectile tissue. When the arteries constrict, the pressure on the veins in the area is reduced, thus allowing more blood to leave the penis than enters, and the penis returns to its normal state. The functions of the penis are to serve as the male organ of *copulation* and as the site of the orifice for the elimination of urine and semen from the body.

▶ THE TESTES

The male has two ovoid-shaped organs, the *testes,* located in the scrotum. Each testis is about 4 cm long and 2.5 cm wide. The interior of each testis is divided into about 250 wedge-shaped lobes by fibrous tissues. Coiled within each lobe are one to three small tubes called the *seminiferous tubules.* These tubules are the site of the development of male reproductive cells, the *spermatozoa.* Cells within the testes also produce the male sex hormone, *testosterone,* which is responsible for the development of secondary male characteristics during puberty. Testosterone is essential for normal growth and development of the male accessory sex organs. It plays a vital role in the erection process of the penis, and thus, is necessary for the reproductive act, copulation. Additionally, it affects the growth of hair on the face, muscular development, and vocal timbre. The *seminiferous tubules* form a plexus or network called the rete testis from which 15 to 20 small ducts, the efferent ductules, leave the testis and open into the epididymis (Figs. 5–1 and 5–2).

▶ THE EPIDIDYMIS

Each testis is connected by efferent ductules to an *epididymis,* which is a coiled tube lying on the posterior aspect of the testis. The epididymis is between 13 and 20 feet in length but is coiled into a space less than 2 inches (5 cm) long and ends in the ductus deferens. Each epididymis functions as a storage site for the maturation of *sperm* (Fig. 5–3) and as the first part of the duct system through which sperm pass on their journey to the urethra (see Figs. 5–1 and 5–2).

▶ THE DUCTUS DEFERENS OR VAS DEFERENS

The *ductus deferens* is a slim muscular tube, about 45 cm in length, and is a continuation of the epididymis. It has been described as the *excretory duct* of the testis and extends from a point adjacent to the testis to enter the abdomen through the inguinal canal. It is later joined by the duct from the seminal vesicle. Between the testis and the part of the abdomen known as the internal inguinal ring, the ductus deferens is contained within a structure known as the *spermatic cord.* The spermatic cord also contains arteries, veins, lymphatic vessels, and nerves (see Fig. 5–4).

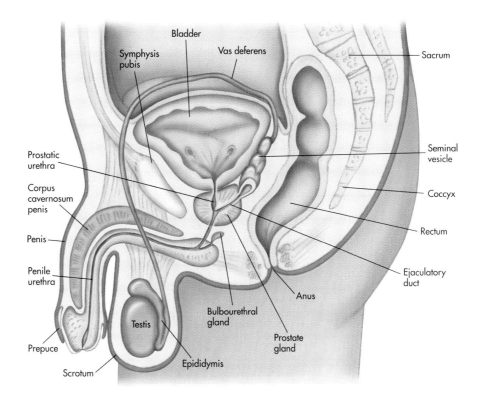

FIGURE 5–2

Sagittal section of the male pelvis, showing the organs of the reproductive system.

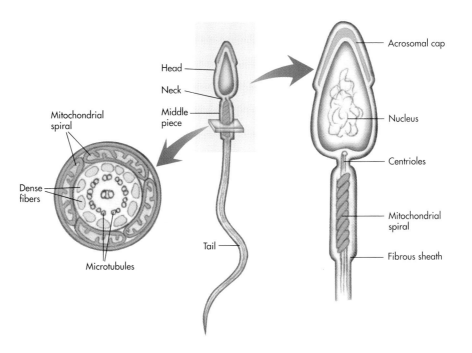

FIGURE 5–3

The basic structure of a spermatozoon (sperm).

▶ THE SEMINAL VESICLES

There are *two seminal vesicles,* each connected by a narrow duct to a ductus deferens, which then forms a short tube, the *ejaculatory duct,* that penetrates the base of the prostate gland and opens into the prostatic portion of the urethra. The seminal vesicles produce a slightly alkaline fluid that becomes a part of the seminal fluid or semen (see Fig. 5–4).

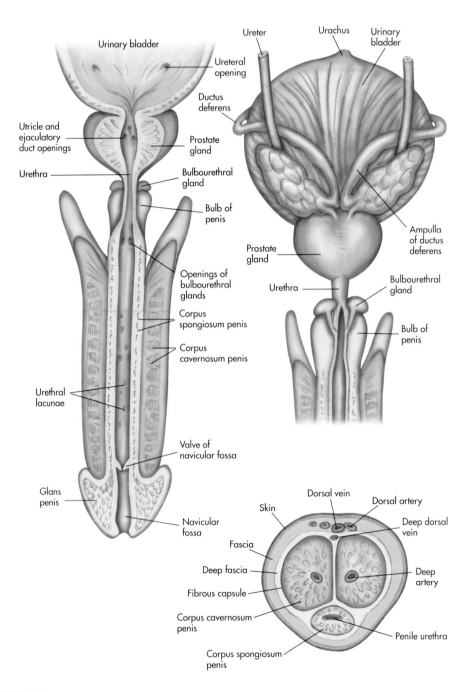

FIGURE 5–4

The structures of the bladder, prostate gland, and penis.

▶ THE PROSTATE GLAND

The *prostate gland* is about 4 cm wide and weighs about 20 g. It is composed of glandular, connective, and muscular tissue and lies behind the urinary bladder. It surrounds the first 2.5 cm of the urethra and secretes an alkaline fluid that aids in maintaining the viability of spermatozoa. Enlargement of the prostate *(benign prostatic hyperplasia)* is a condition that sometimes occurs in older men. In this condition, the prostate obstructs the urethra and causes interference with the normal passage of urine. When this occurs, a *prostatectomy* may be performed to remove a part of the gland. The prostate gland may also be a site for cancer in older men (see Fig. 5–4).

▶ THE BULBOURETHRAL OR COWPER'S GLANDS

The *bulbourethral glands* are two small pea-sized glands located below the prostate and on either side of the urethra. A duct about 2.5 cm long connects them with the wall of the urethra. The bulbourethral glands produce a mucous secretion before ejaculation, which becomes a part of the semen (see Fig. 5–4).

▶ THE URETHRA

The male *urethra* is approximately 20 cm long and is divided into three sections: prostatic, membranous, and penile. It extends from the urinary bladder to the external urethral orifice at the head of the penis. It serves the function of transmitting urine and semen out of the body (see Fig. 5–4).

Life Span Considerations

▶ THE CHILD

In the newborn, the **testicles** may appear large at birth. They may fail to descend into the scrotum, causing a condition, **cryptorchism.** The foreskin of the penis may be tight at birth, causing **phimosis,** a condition of narrowing of the opening of the prepuce wherein the foreskin cannot be drawn back over the glans penis.

Puberty is defined as a period of rapid change in the lives of boys and girls during which time the reproductive systems mature and become functionally capable of reproduction. In the male, puberty begins around 12 years of age, when the genitals start to increase in size and the shoulders broaden and become muscular. As testosterone is released, secondary sexual characteristics develop, such as pubic and axillary hair, increase in size of the penis and testes, voice changes, facial hair, erections, and noctural emissions.

▶ THE OLDER ADULT

With aging, the **prostate gland** enlarges and its glandular secretions decrease, the **testes** become smaller and more firm, there is a gradual decrease in the production of **testosterone,** and pubic hair becomes sparser and stiffer. This period of change in the male has been referred to as the "male climacteric" and may be associated with symptoms such as hot flashes, feelings of suffocation, insomnia, irritability, and emotional instability. Testosterone replacement therapy may be recommended for the "male climacteric."

In a healthy, normal male **spermatogenesis** and the ability to have erections lasts a lifetime. However, sexual arousal may be slowed with a longer refractory period between erections. In men, a "refractory period" is a time after one orgasm during which they are not physically able to have another one.

According to the National Institutes of Health (NIH) **erectile dysfunction** *(impotence)* affects as many as 20 million men in the United States. It was once thought to be an unavoidable result of aging, but now, erectile dysfunction is understood to be caused by a variety of factors. Erectile dysfunction is defined as the inability to achieve or maintain an erection sufficient for sexual intercourse. It occurs when not enough blood is supplied to the penis, when the smooth muscle in the penis fails to relax, or when the penis does not retain the blood that flows into it. According to studies by the NIH, 5% of men have some degree of erectile dysfunction at age 40 and approximately 15 to 25% at age 65 or older. Although the likelihood of erectile dysfunction increases with age, it is not an inevitable part of aging. About 80% of erectile dysfunction has a physical cause. See Table 5–1 for physical causes of erectile dysfunction.

TABLE 5–1   Some Physical Causes of Erectile Dysfunction

Vascular Diseases	Arteriosclerosis, hypertension, high cholesterol, and other medical conditions can obstruct blood flow and cause erectile dysfunction
Diabetes	Can alter nerve function and blood flow to the penis and cause erectile dysfunction
Prescription Drugs	Certain antihypertensive and cardiac medications, antihistamines, psychiatric medications, and other prescription drugs can cause erectile dysfunction
Substance Abuse	Excessive smoking, alcohol, and illegal drugs constrict blood vessels and can cause erectile dysfunction
Neurologic Diseases	Multiple sclerosis, Parkinson's disease, and other diseases can interrupt nerve impulses to the penis and cause erectile dysfunction
Surgery	Prostate, colon, bladder, and other types of pelvic surgery may damage nerves and blood vessels and cause erectile dysfunction
Spinal Injury	Interruptions of nerve impulses from the spinal cord to the penis can cause erectile dysfunction
Other	Hormonal imbalance, kidney failure, dialysis, and reduced testosterone levels can cause erectile dysfunction

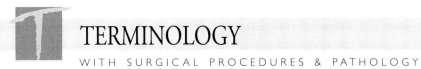

TERMINOLOGY

WITH SURGICAL PROCEDURES & PATHOLOGY

TERM	WORD PARTS			DEFINITION
anorchism (ăn-ōr′ kĭzm)	an orch ism	P R S	lack of testicle condition of	A condition in which there is a lack of one or both testes
aspermatism (ă-spĕr′ mă-tĭzm)	a spermat ism	P R S	lack of seed condition of	A condition in which there is a lack of secretion of the male seed
azoospermia (ă-zō″ ō-spĕr′ mē-ă)	a zoo sperm ia	P CF R S	lack of animal seed condition	A condition in which there is a lack of spermatozoa in the semen
balanitis (băl″ ă-nī′ tĭs)	balan itis	R S	glans inflammation	Inflammation of the glans penis
circumcision (sĕr″ kŭm-sĭ′ shŭn)	circum cis ion	P R S	around to cut process	The surgical process of removing the foreskin of the penis
cryptorchism (krĭpt-ōr′ kĭzm)	crypt orch ism	R R S	hidden testicle condition of	A condition in which the testes fail to descend into the scrotum
epididymectomy (ĕp″ ĭ-dĭd″ ĭ-mĕk′ tō-mē)	epi didym ectomy	P R S	upon testis excision	Surgical excision of the epididymis
epididymitis (ĕp″ ĭ-dĭd″ ĭ-mī′ tĭs)	epi didym itis	P R S	upon testis inflammation	Inflammation of the epididymis
epispadias (ĕp″ ĭ-spā′ dĭ-ăs)	epi spadias	P R	upon a rent, an opening	A congenital defect in which the urethra opens on the dorsum of the penis
hydrocele (hī′ drō-sēl)	hydro cele	P S	water hernia	A collection of serous fluid in a sac-like cavity; specifically the tunica vaginalis testis
hypospadias (hī″ pō-spā′ dĭ-ăs)	hypo spadias	P R	under a rent, an opening	A congenital defect in which the urethra opens on the underside of the penis

continued

Terminology - continued

TERM	WORD PARTS			DEFINITION
oligospermia (ŏl″ ĭ-gō-spĕr′ -mĭ-ă)	oligo sperm ia	P R S	scanty seed condition	A condition in which there is a scanty amount of spermatozoa in the semen
orchidectomy (or″ kĭ-dĕk′ tō-mē)	orchid ectomy	R S	testicle excision	Surgical excision of a testicle
orchidopexy (or′ kĭd-ō-pēk ″ sē)	orchido pexy	CF S	testicle fixation	Surgical fixation of a testicle
orchidoplasty (or′ kĭd-ō-plăs″ tē)	orchido plasty	CF S	testicle surgical repair	Surgical repair of a testicle
orchidotomy (or″ kĭd-ŏt′ ō-mē)	orchido tomy	CF S	testicle incision	Incision into a testicle
orchitis (or-kī′ tĭs)	orch itis	R S	testicle inflammation	Inflammation of a testicle
parenchyma (păr-ĕn′ kĭ-mă)	par enchyma	P R	beside to pour	The essential cells of a gland or organ that are concerned with its function
penitis (pē-nī′ tĭs)	pen itis	R S	penis inflammation	Inflammation of the penis
phimosis (fī-mō′ sĭs)	phim osis	R S	a muzzle condition of	A condition of narrowing of the opening of the prepuce wherein the foreskin cannot be drawn back over the glans penis
prostatalgia (prŏs″ tă-tăl′ jĭ-ă)	prostat algia	R S	prostate pain	Pain in the prostate
prostatectomy (prŏs″ tă-tĕk′ tō-mē)	prostat ectomy	R S	prostate excision	Surgical excision of the prostate
prostatitis (prŏs″ tă-tī′ tĭs)	prostat itis	R S	prostate inflammation	Inflammation of the prostate
prostatocystitis (prŏs″ tă-tō-sĭs-tī′ tĭs)	prostato cyst itis	CF R S	prostate bladder inflammation	Inflammation of the prostate and bladder
prostatomegaly (prŏs″ tă-tō-mĕg′ ă-lē)	prostato megaly	CF S	prostate enlargement	Enlargement of the prostate

Terminology - continued

TERM	WORD PARTS			DEFINITION

TERMINOLOGY SPOTLIGHT

Prostatomegaly is defined as enlargement of the prostate. Enlargement of the prostate gland may occur in men who are 50 years of age and older and is referred to as **benign prostatic hyperplasia** (BPH). By age 60, four out of five men may have an enlarged prostate. As the prostate enlarges, it compresses the **urethra,** thereby restricting the normal flow of urine. This restriction generally causes a number of symptoms and can be referred to as **prostatism.** Prostatism is any condition of the prostate gland that interferes with the flow of urine from the bladder. Symptoms usually include:

- A weak or hard-to-start urine stream
- A feeling that the bladder is not empty
- A need to urinate often, especially at night
- A feeling of urgency (a sudden need to urinate)
- Abdominal straining; a decrease in size and force of the urinary stream
- Interruption of the stream
- Acute urinary retention
- Recurrent urinary infections

Treatment for benign prostatic hyperplasia may include surgery, medication, and/or balloon dilation of the urethra.

Surgery. Transurethral resection of the prostate (TURP or TUR). During this procedure, an endoscopic instrument that has ocular and surgical capabilities is introduced directly through the urethra to the prostate and small pieces of the prostate gland are removed by using an electrical cutting loop.

Medication. Proscar (finasteride), an oral medication, may be prescribed by a physician to help relieve the symptoms of BPH. It lowers the levels of dihydrotestosterone (DHT), which is a major factor in enlargement of the prostate. Lowering of DHT leads to shrinkage of the enlarged prostate gland in most men. Although this can lead to gradual improvement in urine flow and symptoms, it does not work for all cases. Side effects may include impotence and less desire for sex. Proscar can alter the prostate-specific antigen test (PSA) that is used to screen for prostate cancer.

Balloon dilation. During this procedure, a balloon catheter is placed in the distal urethra and inflated by injecting a dilute contrast media at high pressure. The balloon is left in place for approximately 10 minutes and then the pressure is released.

TERM	WORD PARTS			DEFINITION
spermatoblast (spĕr-măt′ ō-blăst)	spermato blast	CF S	seed, sperm immature cell, germ cell	The sperm germ cell
spermatocyst (spĕr-măt′ ō-sĭst)	spermato cyst	CF R	seed, sperm sac, bladder	A cyst of the epididymis that contains spermatozoa
spermatogenesis (spĕr″ măt-ō-jĕn′ ĕ-sĭs)	spermato genesis	CF S	seed, sperm formation, produce	Formation of spermatozoa
spermatozoon (spĕr″ măt-ō-zō′ ŏn)	spermato zoon	CF R	seed, sperm life	The male sex cell. *The plural form is spermatozoa*

continued

TERM	WORD PARTS			DEFINITION
spermaturia (spĕr″ mă-tū′ rĭ-ă)	spermat uria	R S	seed, sperm urine	Discharge of semen with the urine
spermicide (spĕr′ mĭ-sīd)	spermi cide	CF S	sperm to kill	An agent that kills sperm
testicular (tĕs-tĭk′ ū-lar)	testicul ar	R S	testicle pertaining to	Pertaining to a testicle
varicocele (văr′ ĭ-kō-sēl)	varico cele	CF S	twisted vein hernia	An enlargement and twisting of the veins of the spermatic cord
vasectomy (văs-ĕk′ tō-mē)	vas ectomy	R S	vessel excision	Surgical excision of the vas deferens
vesiculitis (vĕ-sĭk″ ū-lī′ tĭs)	vesicul itis	R S	vesicle inflammation	Inflammation of a vesicle; in particular, the seminal vesicle

VOCABULARY WORDS

Vocabulary words are terms that have not been divided into component parts. They are common words or specialized terms associated with the subject of this chapter. These words are provided to enhance your medical vocabulary.

WORD	DEFINITION
artificial insemination (ăr″ tĭ-fĭsh′ ăl ĭn-sĕm″ ĭn-ā′ shŭn)	The process of artificial placement of semen into the vagina so that conception may take place
capacitation (kăh-păs″ ĭ-tā′ shŭn)	The process by which spermatozoa are conditioned to fertilize an ovum in the female genital tract
castrate (kăs′ trāt)	To remove the testicles or ovaries; *to geld, to spay*
cloning (klōn′ ing)	The process of creating a genetic duplicate of an individual organism through asexual reproduction

Vocabulary - continued

WORD	DEFINITION
coitus (kō′ ĭ-tŭs)	Sexual intercourse between a man and a woman
condom (kŏn′ dŭm)	A thin, flexible protective sheath, usually rubber, worn over the penis during copulation to help prevent impregnation or venereal disease
condyloma (kŏn″ dĭ-lō′ mă)	A wart-like growth of the skin, most often seen on the external genitalia; is either viral or syphilitic in origin
ejaculation (ē-jăk″ ū-lā′ shŭn)	The process of expulsion of seminal fluid from the male urethra
Ericsson sperm separation method (er′ ik-son sperm sĕp″ă-rā′ shŭn mĕth′ od)	A process of separating the Y-chromosome sperm from the X-chromosome sperm. A sperm sample is taken and placed in a tube of albumin. Those that survive are Y-chromosome sperm, which make male babies. Women inseminated with these sperm have a 75 to 80% chance of producing a male child.
eugenics (ū-jĕn′ ĭks)	The study and control of the bringing forth of offspring as a means of improving genetic characteristics of future generations
eunuch (ū′ nŭk)	A male who has been castrated, ie, had his testicles removed
gamete (găm′ ēt)	A mature reproductive cell of the male or female; *a spermatozoon or ovum*
gonorrhea (gŏn″ŏ-rē′ ă)	A highly contagious venereal disease of the genital mucous membrane of either sex; the infection transmitted by the gonococcus *Neisseria gonorrhoeae*
gossypol (gŏs′ sĕ-pŏl)	An extract of cottonseed oil that acts as a spermicide and may inhibit or prevent herpes simplex virus infection
gynecomastia (ji″ nĕ-kō-măs′ tĭ-ă)	A condition of excessive development of the mammary glands in the male
herpes genitalis (hĕr′ pēz jĕn-ĭ-tăl′ ĭs)	A highly contagious venereal disease of the genitalia of either sex; caused by herpes simplex virus-2 (HSV-2)
heterosexual (hĕt″ ĕr-ō-sĕk′ shū-ăl)	Pertaining to the opposite sex; refers to an individual who has a sexual preference for the opposite sex
homosexual (hō″ mō-sĕks′ ū-ăl)	Pertaining to the same sex; refers to an individual who has a sexual preference for the same sex

continued

Vocabulary - continued

WORD	DEFINITION
infertility (ĭn″ fĕr-tĭl′ ĭ-tē)	The inability to produce a viable offspring
mitosis (mī-tō′ sĭs)	The ordinary condition of cell division
prepuce (prē′ pūs)	The foreskin over the glans penis in the male
puberty (pū′ ber-tē)	The stage of development in the male and female when secondary sex characteristics begin to develop and become functionally capable of reproduction
semen (sē′ mĕn)	The fluid-transporting medium for spermatozoa discharged during ejaculation
syphilis (sĭf′ ĭ-lĭs)	A chronic infectious venereal disease caused by *Treponema pallidum,* which is transmitted sexually
trisomy (trī′ sōm-ē)	A genetic condition of having three chromosomes instead of two. The condition causes various birth defects.

ABBREVIATIONS

AIH	artificial insemination homologous	**SPP**	suprapubic prostatectomy
BPH	benign prostatic hyperplasia	**STDs**	sexually transmitted diseases
FTA-ABS	fluorescent treponemal antibody absorption	**STS**	serologic test for syphilis
		TPA	*Treponema pallidum* agglutination
Gc	gonorrhea	**TUR**	transurethral resection
HLA	human leukocyte antigen	**UG**	urogenital
HPV	human papilloma virus	**VD**	venereal disease
HSV-2	herpes simplex virus-2	**VDRL**	venereal disease research laboratory
NPT	nocturnal penile tumescence	**WR**	Wassermann reaction
PSA	prostate-specific antigen		

DRUG HIGHLIGHTS

Drugs that are generally used for the male reproductive system include androgenic hormones. Testosterone is the most important androgen and adequate secretions of this hormone are necessary to maintain normal male sex characteristics, the male libido, and sexual potency.

Testosterone	Is responsible for growth, development, and maintenance of the male reproductive system, and secondary sex characteristics.
Therapeutic use	As replacement therapy in primary hypogonadism, and to stimulate puberty in carefully selected males. It may be used to relieve male menopause symptoms due to androgen deficiency. It may also be used to help stimulate sperm production in oligospermia and in impotence due to androgen deficiency. It may be used when there is advanced inoperable metastatic breast cancer in women who are 1 to 5 years postmenopausal and to prevent postpartum breast pain and engorgement in the non-nursing mother. *Examples: Halotestin (fluoxymesterone), Metandren (methyltestosterone), Andro (testosterone enanthate in oil), and Testex (testosterone propionate in oil).*
Patient teaching	Educate the patient to be aware of possible adverse reactions and report any of the following to the physician. *All patients:* nausea, vomiting, jaundice, edema. *Males:* frequent or persistent erection of the penis. Adolescent males: signs of premature epiphyseal closure. Should have bone development checked every 6 months. *Females:* hoarseness, acne, changes in menstrual periods, growth of hair on face and/or body.
Special Considerations	In diabetic patients, the effects of testosterone may decrease blood glucose and insulin requirements.
	Testosterone may decrease the anticoagulant requirements of patients receiving oral anticoagulants. These patients require close monitoring when testosterone therapy is begun and then when it is stopped.
	Anabolic steroids (testosterone) may be abused by individuals who seek to increase muscle mass, strength, and overall athletic ability. This form of use is illegal and signs of abuse may include flu-like symptoms, headaches, muscle aches, dizziness, bruises, needle marks, increased bleeding (nosebleeds, petechiae, gums, conjunctiva), enlarged spleen, liver, and/or prostate, edema, and in the female increased facial hair, menstrual irregularities, and enlarged clitoris.

DIAGNOSTIC AND LABORATORY TESTS

Test	Description
fluorescent treponemal antibody absorption (floo-ō-rĕs′ ĕnt trĕp″ ō-nē′ măl ăn′ tĭ-bŏd″ ē ab-sorp′ shŭn)	A test performed on blood serum to determine the presence of *Treponema pallidum.* Used to detect syphilis.
paternity (pă-tĕr′ nĭ-tē)	A test to determine whether a certain man could be the father of a specific child. The test can indicate only who is not the father. Types of tests that may be used are blood type, human leukocyte antigen (HLA), white blood cell, enzyme and protein, and genetic. The blood type of the child and accused father are analyzed for compatibility. For example, a parent with type O blood cannot be the parent of a child with type AB blood. The HLA looks at the body's tissue compatibility system, and the white blood cell test looks at chemical markers (antigens) on the surface of the white blood cells. Enzyme and protein looks at red blood cell enzymes, and a new genetic test is being developed that uses molecular and protein biology to look at family-related patterns among genes.
prostate-specific antigen (PSA) immunoassay (prŏs′ tāt-spĕ-sĭf′ ĭk ăn′ tĭ-jĕn ĭm″ ū-nō-ăs′ sā)	A blood test that measures concentrations of a special type of protein known as prostate-specific antigen. Increased level indicates prostate disease or possibly prostate cancer.
semen (sē′ mĕn)	A test performed on semen that looks at the volume, pH, sperm count, sperm motility, and morphology. Used to evaluate infertility in men.
testosterone toxicology (tĕs-tŏs′ tĕr-ōn tŏks″ ĭ-kŏl′ ō-jē)	A test performed on blood serum to identify the level of testosterone. Increased level may indicate benign prostatic hyperplasia. Decreased level may indicate hypogonadism, testicular hypofunction, hypopituitarism, and/or orchidectomy.
venereal disease research laboratory (vē- nē′ rē- ăl dĭ-zēz rē′ sĕrch lăb′ ră-tor″ ē)	A test performed on blood serum to determine the presence of *Treponema pallidum.* Used to detect syphilis.

SEXUALLY TRANSMITTED DISEASES (STDS)

Sexually transmitted diseases can occur in men, women, and children. They are passed from person to person through sexual contact or from mother to child. The following is a summary of the most common sexually transmitted diseases:

Disease	Cause	Symptoms	Treatment
Chlamydia (klă-mĭd′ ē-ă)	*Chlamydia trachomatis* (bacterium)	**MAY BE ASYMPTOMATIC OR** **MALE:** Mucopurulent discharge from penis, burning, itching in genital area, dysuria, swollen testes. Can lead to sterility **FEMALE:** Mucopurulent discharge from vagina, cystitis, pelvic pain, cervicitis. Can lead to pelvic inflammatory disease (PID) and sterility **NEWBORN:** Eye infection, pneumonia. Can cause death	Antibiotics—tetracycline or erythromycin
Genital warts (jĕn′ ĭ-tăl wŏrts)	Human papilloma virus (HPV)	**MALE:** Cauliflower-like growths on the penis and perianal area **FEMALE:** Cauliflower-like growths around vagina and perianal area	Laser surgery, chemotherapy, cryosurgery, cauterization
Gonorrhea (gŏn″ ŏ-rē′ ā)	*Neisseria gonorrhoeae* (bacterium)	**MALE:** Purulent urethral discharge, dysuria, urinary frequency **FEMALE:** Purulent vaginal discharge, dysuria, urinary frequency, abnormal menstrual bleeding, abdominal tenderness. Can lead to PID and sterility **NEWBORN:** Gonorrheal ophthalmia neonatorum, purulent eye discharge. Can cause blindness	Antibiotics—penicillin or tetracycline
Herpes genitalis (hĕr′ pēz jĕn-ĭ-tāl′ ĭs)	Herpes simplex virus-2 (HSV-2)	**ACTIVE PHASE MALE:** Fluid-filled vesicles (blisters) on penis. Rupture causes acute pain and itching **FEMALE:** Blisters in and around vagina **NEWBORN:** Can be infected during vaginal delivery. Severe infection, physical and mental damage **GENERALIZED:** "Flu-like" symptoms, fever, headache, malaise, anorexia, muscle pain	**NO CURE:** Antiviral drug acyclovir (Zovirax) may be used to relieve symptoms during acute phase
Syphilis (sĭf′ ĭ-lĭs)	*Treponema pallidum* (bacterium)	**PRIMARY**—1st stage Chancre at point of infection. See Figures 5–5 and 5–6. **Male**—penis, anus, rectum. **Female**—vagina, cervix. **Both**—lips, tongue, fingers, or nipples **SECONDARY**—2nd stage "Flu-like" symptoms with a skin rash over moist, fatty areas of the body. See Figure 5–7. Alopecia	Antibiotics—penicillin, tetracycline, or erythromycin

Disease	Cause	Symptoms	Treatment
		TERTIARY—latent-3rd stage No symptoms —damage to internal organs **NEWBORN:** Congenital syphilis—may have a heart defect, bone deformity, or other deformities	
Trichomoniasis (trĭk″ ō-mō-nī′ ă-sĭs)	*Trichomonas* (parasitic protozoa)	**MALE:** Usually asymptomatic. Can lead to cystitis, urethritis, prostatitis **FEMALE:** White frothy vaginal discharge, burning and itching of vulva. Can lead to cystitis, urethritis, vaginitis	Metronidazole (Flagyl)

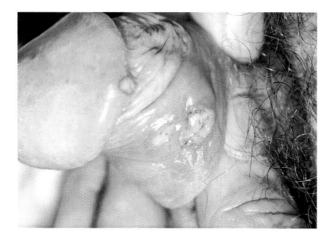

FIGURE 5–5

Chancre. *(Courtesy of Jason L. Smith, MD.)*

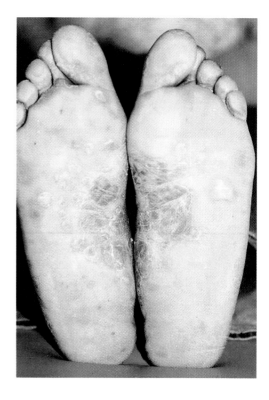

FIGURE 5–7

Secondary syphilis. *(Courtesy of Jason L. Smith, MD.)*

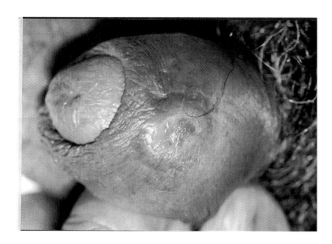

FIGURE 5–6

Chancre. *(Courtesy of Jason L. Smith, MD.)*

COMMUNICATION ENRICHMENT

This segment is provided for those who wish to enhance their ability to communicate in either English or Spanish.

▶ **Related Terms**

English	Spanish	English	Spanish
AIDS (Acquired Immune Deficiency Syndrome)	SIDA (Síndrome de Immune Deficiencia Adquirida) (sĭ-*dă* [sĭn-*drō*-mĕ dĕ ĭmm-*mū*-n-dĕ-f ĭ-cĭ-ĕn-cĭ-ă *ăd*-kĭ-rĭ-dă])	homosexual	homosexual (ō-mō-sĕx-sū-ăl)
		impotence	impotencia (ĭm-pō-*tĕn*-sĭ-ă)
		masturbate	masturbarse (*măs*-tūr-băr-sĕ)
bisexual	bisexual (bĭ-*sĕx*-sū-ăl)	masturbation	masturbación (*măs*-tūr-bă-sĭ-ōn)
chlamydia	chlamydia (klă-*mĭ*-dī-ă)	penis	pene (*pĕ*-nĕ)
circumcision	circuncisión (sĭr-*cūn*-sĭ-ōn)	prostate	prostático; prostata (prōs-*ta*-tĭ-kō; prōs-*tă*-tă)
condom	condon (*cōn*-dōn)		
ejaculation	eyaculación (ĕ-yă-kū-lă-sĭ-*ōn*)	prostatectomy	prostatectomia (prōs-*tă*-tĕk-tō-mĭ-ă)
ejaculate	eyacular (ĕ-yă-kū-*lăr*)	prostate gland	glándula prostática (*glăn*-dū-lă prōs-*tă*-tĭ-ka)
erection	erección (ĕ-rĕk-sĭ-*ōn*)	reproduction	reproducción (rĕ-prō-dūk-sĭ-*ōn*)
genitals	genitales (hĕ-nĭ-*tă*-lĕs)	reproductive system	sistema reproductivo (sĭs-*tĕ*-mă rĕ-prō-*dūk*-tĭ-vō)
gonorrhea	gonorrea (gō-*nō*-rĕ-ă)		
herpes	herpe (*ĕr*-pĕ)	semen	semen (*sĕ*-mĕn)
heterosexual	heterosexual (ĕ-tĕ-rō-sĕx-sū-ăl)	sexual desires	deseos sexual (dĕ-*sĕ*-ōs *sĕx*-sū-ăl)

English	Spanish	English	Spanish
sexual relations	relaciones sexual (re-*lă*-sĭ-ō-něs *sĕx*-sū-ăl)	underwear	ropa interior (*rŏ*-pă ĭn-*tĕ*-rĭ-ōr)
sterile	estéril (ĕs-*tĕ*-rĭl)	venereal	venéreo (vĕ-*nĕ*-rĕ-ō)
syphilis	sífilis (*sĭ*-fĭ-lĭs)	veneral infection	enfermedad venérea (ĕn-*fĕr*-mĕ-dăd vĕ-*nĕ*-rĕ-ă)
testicle	testículo (tĕs-*tĭ*-kū-lō)		

CHAPTER REVIEW SECTION

LEARNING EXERCISES

▶ **Anatomy and Physiology**

Write your answers to the following questions. Do not refer back to the text.

1. List the primary and accessory glands of the male reproductive system.

   a. _____   b. _____

   c. _____   d. _____

   e. _____   f. _____

2. Name the supporting structure and accessory sex organs of the male reproductive system.

   a. _____   b. _____

3. State the vital function of the male reproductive system. _____

   _____

4. Describe the scrotum. _____

   _____

5. The _____ _____ _____ and the

   _____ _____ are names of the three longitudinal

   columns of erectile tissue in the penis.

6. The average erect penis measures _____ to _____ cm in length.

7. The _____ _____ is the cone-shaped head of the penis.

8. Define prepuce. _____

_____

9. Define smegma. _____

10. State two functions of the penis.

    a. _____   b. _____

11. Describe the testes. _____

    _____

    _____

12. _____ _____ are the site of the development of spermatozoa.

13. List five effects of testosterone regarding male development.

    a. _____   b. _____

    c. _____   d. _____

    e. _____

14. Name the plexus that the seminiferous tubules form. _____

15. Describe the epididymis. _____

    _____

16. State two functions of the epididymis.

    a. _____   b. _____

17. The excretory duct of the testes is known by two names, _____

    _____ or _____ _____.

18. The spermatic cord contains five types of structures and connects the testes with organs in the abdomen. Name these five structures.

    a. _____   b. _____

    c. _____   d. _____

    e. _____

19. State the function of the seminal vesicles. _____

    _____

20. Describe the prostate gland. _____

_____

21. Define the condition known as benign prostatic hyperplasia. _____

_____

22. The two small pea-sized glands located below the prostate and on either side of the urethra
    are known as the _____ glands or as _____ glands.

23. Name the three sections of the male urethra.

    a. _____   b. _____

    c. _____

24. State a function of the male urethra. _____

25. The male urethra is approximately _____ cm long.

▶ **Word Parts**

1. In the spaces provided, write the definitions of these prefixes, roots, combining forms, and
   suffixes. Do not refer to the listings of terminology words. Leave blank those terms you cannot
   define.

2. After completing as many as you can, refer back to the terminology word listings to check your
   work. For each word missed or left blank, write the term and its definition several times on the
   margins of these pages or on a separate sheet of paper.

3. To maximize the learning process, it is to your advantage to do the following exercises as
   directed. To refer to the terminology listings before completing these exercises invalidates the
   learning process.

Prefixes
Give the definitions of the following prefixes:

1. a- _____   2. an- _____

3. circum- _____   4. epi- _____

5. hydro- _____   6. hypo- _____

7. oligo- _____   8. par- _____

Roots and Combining Forms
Give the definitions of the following roots and combining forms:

1. balan _____   2. cis _____

3. crypt _____

4. cyst _____

5. didym _____

6. enchyma _____

7. orch _____

8. orchid _____

9. orchido _____

10. pen _____

11. phim _____

12. prostat _____

13. prostato _____

14. spadias _____

15. sperm _____

16. spermat _____

17. spermato _____

18. spermi _____

19. testicul _____

20. varico _____

21. vas _____

22. vesicul _____

23. zoo _____

24. zoon _____

Suffixes

Give the definitions of the following suffixes:

1. -algia _____

2. -ar _____

3. -blast _____

4. -cele _____

5. -cide _____

6. -ectomy _____

7. -genesis _____

8. -ia _____

9. -ion _____

10. -ism _____

11. -itis _____

12. -megaly _____

13. -osis _____

14. -pexy _____

15. -plasty _____

16. -tomy _____

17. -uria _____

▶ **Identifying Medical Terms**

In the spaces provided, write the medical terms for the following meanings:

1. _____   Inflammation of the glans penis

2. _____   Surgical excision of the epididymis

3. _____   Surgical excision of a testicle

4. _____   Surgical repair of a testicle

5. _____ Pain in the prostate

6. _____ Inflammation of the prostate and bladder

7. _____ The sperm germ cell

8. _____ The male sex cell

9. _____ An agent that kills sperm

10. _____ Pertaining to a testicle

▶ **Spelling**

In the spaces provided, write the correct spelling of these misspelled terms:

1. crptorchism Cryptorchism

2. hyospadias Hypospadias

3. orchdotomy orchidotomy

4. prostatmegaly Prostatomegaly

5. spermauria Spermaturia

WORD PARTS STUDY SHEET

Word Parts	Give the Meaning
circum-	around
epi-	upon
hydro-	water
hypo-	under
oligo-	scanty
balan-	glans
cis-	cut
crypt-	hidden
cyst-	bladder
didym-	testis
orch-, orchid-, orchido-	testicle
pen-	penis
phim-	muzzle
prostat-, prostato-	prostat

spadias-	rent, an opening
sperm-, spermat-, spermi-, spermato-	seed
testicul-	testicul
varico-	twisted vein
vas-	vessel
vesicul-	vesicle
zoo-	animal
zoon-	life
-algia	pain
-blast	Immature cell
-cele	hernia
-cide	to kill
-ectomy	excision
-genesis	formation
-ia, -ism, -osis	condition
-ion	process
-itis	Inflammation
-megaly	Inflammation
-pexy	fixation
-plasty	surgical repair
-tomy	Incision
-uria	urine

REVIEW QUESTIONS

▶ Matching

Select the appropriate lettered meaning for each numbered line.

___E___ 1. circumcision

___C___ 2. coitus

___F___ 3. condom

a. Caused by the bacterium *Treponema pallidum*

b. A mature reproductive cell of the male or female

c. Sexual intercourse between a man and a woman

_____ **B** 4. gamete

_____ **J** 5. genital warts

_____ **G** 6. gonorrhea

_____ **H** 7. infertility

_____ **K** 8. prepuce

_____ **A** 9. syphilis

_____ **D** 10. trichomoniasis

d. Caused by a parasitic protozoa

e. The surgical process of removing the foreskin of the penis

f. A thin, flexible protective sheath worn over the penis during copulation to help prevent impregnation or venereal disease

g. Caused by the human papilloma virus

h. The inability to produce a viable offspring

i. Causes purulent urethral discharge in the male and purulent vaginal discharge in the female

j. Caused by the bacterium *Chlamydia trachomatis*

k. The foreskin over the glans penis in the male

▶ **Abbreviations**

Place the correct word, phrase, or abbreviation in the space provided.

1. benign prostatic hyperplasia __BPH__

2. Gc __gonorrhea__

3. human papilloma virus __HPV__

4. HSV-2 __herpes simplex virus-2__

5. STDs __Sexually Transmited Disease__

6. *Treponema pallidum* agglutination __TPA__

7. TUR __Transurethal resection__

8. UG __urogenital__

9. venereal disease __VD__

10. Wassermann reaction __WR__

▶ **Diagnostic and Laboratory Tests**

Select the best answer to each multiple choice question. Circle the letter of your choice.

1. A test performed on blood serum to detect syphilis.
   a. paternity
   b. semen
   c. FTA-ABS
   d. HSV-2

2. A test to determine whether a certain man could be the father of a specific child.
   a. paternity
   b. semen
   c. FTA-ABS
   d. HSV-2

3. An increased level indicates prostate disease or possibly prostate cancer.
   a. fluorescent treponemal antibody
   b. prostate-specific antigen
   c. semen
   d. testosterone toxicology

4. Used to determine infertility in men.
   a. paternity
   b. prostate-specific antigen
   c. semen
   d. testosterone toxicology

5. An increased level may indicate benign prostatic hyperplasia.
   a. fluorescent treponemal antibody
   b. prostate-specific antigen
   c. testosterone toxicology
   d. venereal disease research

CRITICAL THINKING ACTIVITY

▶ **Case Study**

Benign Prostatic Hyperplasia

Please read the following case study and then answer the questions that follow.

A 58-year-old male was seen by a physician, and the following is a synopsis of the visit.

Present History: The patient states that he is having difficulty with urination. He is having a need to urinate often, especially at night, urgency, and a decrease in size and force of the urinary stream.

Signs and Symptoms: Chief complaint: frequency, urgency, and decrease in size and force of the urinary stream.

Diagnosis: Benign prostatic hyperplasia

Treatment: Proscar (finasteride) was ordered by the physician to help relieve the symptoms of benign prostatic hyperplasia. It lowers the levels of dihydrotestosterone (DHT), which is a major factor in enlargement of the prostate. Lowering of DHT leads to shrinkage of the enlarged prostate gland in most men. It may take 6 months or more to determine if it is working for an individual. The patient was scheduled for a follow-up visit in 6 months and informed that side effects of Proscar may include impotence and less desire for sex, and that this medication can alter the prostate-specific antigen test (PSA) that is used to screen for prostate cancer.

Critical Thinking Questions

1. Signs and symptoms of benign prostatic hyperplasia include frequency, _____, and decrease in size and force of the urinary stream.

2. Treatment included _____ (finasteride).

3. Side effects of this medication may include _____ and less desire for sex.

4. This medication can alter the _____-specific antigen test that is used to screen for prostate cancer.

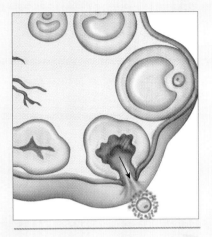

6

MEDICAL TERMINOLOGY OF THE FEMALE REPRODUCTIVE SYSTEM

OBJECTIVES

On completion of this chapter, you should be able to:

- Describe the uterus and state its functions.
- Describe the fallopian tubes and state their functions.
- Describe the ovaries and state their functions.
- Describe the vagina and state its functions.
- Describe the breast.
- Describe the menstrual cycle.
- Analyze, build, spell, and pronounce medical words that relate to surgical procedures and pathology.
- Identify and give the meaning of selected vocabulary words.
- Identify and define selected abbreviations.
- Review Drug Highlights presented in this chapter.
- Provide the description of diagnostic and laboratory tests related to the female reproductive system.
- Successfully complete the study and review section.

► ANATOMY AND PHYSIOLOGY OVERVIEW

The female reproductive system consists of the left and right *ovaries,* which are the female's primary sex organs, and the following accessory sex organs: two *fallopian tubes,* the *uterus,* the *vagina,* the *vulva,* and two *breasts.* The vital function of the female reproductive system is to perpetuate the species through sexual or germ cell reproduction.

► THE UTERUS

The *uterus* is a muscular, hollow, pear-shaped organ having three identifiable areas: the *body* or upper portion, the *isthmus* or central area, and the *cervix,* which is the lower cylindrical portion or neck. The *fundus* is the bulging surface of the body of the uterus extending from the internal os *(mouth)* of the cervix upward above the fallopian tubes. The uterus is suspended in the anterior part of the pelvic cavity, halfway between the sacrum and the symphysis pubis, above the bladder, and in front of the rectum. A number of ligaments support the uterus and hold it in position. These are two broad ligaments, two round ligaments, two uterosacral ligaments, and the ligaments that are attached to the bladder. The normal position of the uterus is with the cervix pointing toward the lower end of the sacrum and the fundus toward the suprapubic region. An average, normal uterus is about 8 cm long, 5 cm wide, and 2.5 cm thick (Figs. 6–1 and 6–2).

THE UTERINE WALL

The wall of the uterus consists of three layers: the *peritoneum* or outer layer, the *myometrium* or muscular middle layer, and the *endometrium,* which is the mucous membrane lining the inner surface of the uterus. The endometrium is composed of columnar epithelium and connective tissue and is supplied with blood by both straight and spiral arteries. It undergoes marked changes in

THE FEMALE REPRODUCTIVE SYSTEM

ORGAN/STRUCTURE	PRIMARY FUNCTIONS
The Uterus	Organ of the cyclic discharge of menses; provides place for the nourishment and development of the fetus; contracts during labor to help expel the fetus
The Fallopian Tubes	Serve as a duct for the conveyance of the ovum from the ovary to the uterus; serve as ducts for the conveyance of spermatozoa from the uterus toward the ovary
The Ovaries	Production of ova and hormones
The Vagina	Female organ of copulation; serves as a passageway for the discharge of menstruation; serves as a passageway for the birth of the fetus
The Vulva	External female genitalia
Mons pubis	Provides pad of fatty tissue
Labia majora	Provides two folds of adipose tissue
Labia minora	Lies within the labia majora and encloses the vestibule
Vestibule	Opening for the urethra, the vagina, and two excretory ducts of Bartholin's glands
Clitoris	Erectile tissue that is homologous to the penis of the male; produces pleasurable sensations during the sexual act
The Breast	Following childbirth, mammary glands produce milk

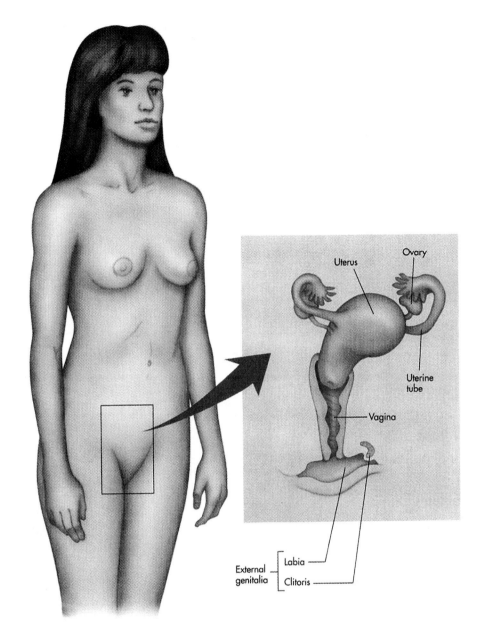

FIGURE 6–1

The female reproductive system.

response to hormonal stimulation during the menstrual cycle. These changes are discussed in the last section of this overview.

FUNCTIONS OF THE UTERUS

There are three primary functions associated with the uterus:

- It is the organ of the cyclic discharge of a bloody fluid from the uterus and the changes that occur to its endometrium.

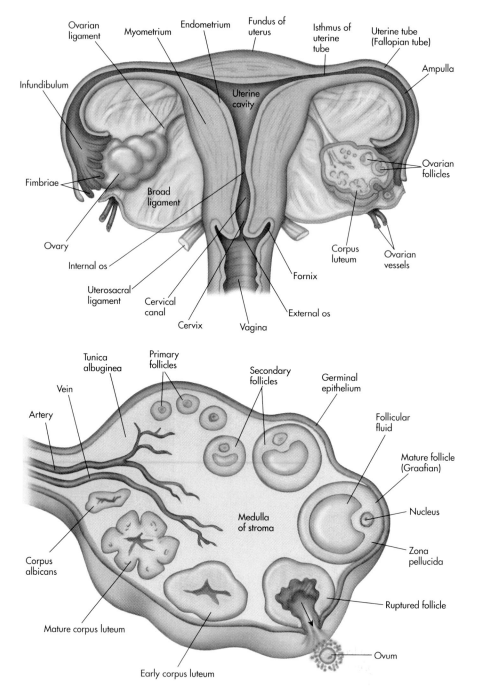

FIGURE 6–2

The uterus, ovaries, and associated structures with an expanded view of a mammalian ovary showing stages of graafian follicle and ovum development.

- It functions as a place for the protection and nourishment of the fetus during pregnancy.
- During labor, the muscular uterine wall contracts rhythmically and powerfully to expel the fetus from the uterus.

ABNORMAL POSITIONS OF THE UTERUS

The uterus may become malpositioned because of weakness of any of its supporting ligaments. Trauma, disease processes of the uterus, or multiple pregnancies may contribute to the weakening of the supporting ligaments. The following terms describe some of the abnormal positions of the uterus:

Anteflexion. The process of bending forward of the uterus at its body and neck

Retroflexion. The process of bending the body of the uterus backward at an angle with the cervix usually unchanged from its normal position

Anteversion. The process of turning the fundus forward toward the pubis, with the cervix tilted up toward the sacrum

Retroversion. The process of turning the uterus backward, with the cervix pointing forward toward the symphysis pubis

Prolapse. The downward displacement of the uterus so that the cervix is within the vaginal orifice, the cervix is outside the orifice, or the entire uterus is outside the orifice

▶ THE FALLOPIAN TUBES

Also called the *uterine tubes* or *oviducts,* the *fallopian tubes* extend laterally from either side of the uterus and end near each ovary. An average, normal fallopian tube is about 11.5 cm long and 6 mm wide. Its wall is composed of three layers: the *serosa* or outermost layer, composed of connective tissue; the *muscular layer,* containing inner circular and outer longitudinal layers of smooth muscle; and the *mucosa* or inner layer, consisting of simple columnar epithelium.

ANATOMICAL FEATURES OF THE FALLOPIAN TUBES

The *isthmus* is the constricted portion of the tube nearest the uterus (see Fig. 6–2). From the isthmus, the tube continues laterally and widens to form a section called the *ampulla.* Beyond the ampulla, the tube continues to expand and ends as a funnel-shaped opening. This end of the tube is called the *infundibulum,* and its opening is the *ostium.* Surrounding each ostium are *fimbriae* or *finger-like processes* that work to propel the discharged ovum into the tube, where ciliary action aids in moving it toward the uterus. Should the ovum become impregnated by a spermatozoon while in the tube, the process of *fertilization* occurs.

FUNCTIONS OF THE FALLOPIAN TUBES

The two basic functions of the fallopian tubes are as follows:

- Each tube serves as a duct for the conveyance of the ovum from the ovary to the uterus.
- The tubes serve as ducts for the conveyance of spermatozoa from the uterus toward each ovary.

▶ THE OVARIES

Located on either side of the uterus, the *ovaries* are almond-shaped organs attached to the uterus by the ovarian ligament and lie close to the fimbriae of the fallopian tubes. The anterior border of each ovary is connected to the posterior layer of the broad ligament by the *mesovarium.* Each ovary is attached to the side of the pelvis by the *suspensory ligaments.* An average, normal ovary is about 4 cm long, 2 cm wide, and 1.5 cm thick.

MICROSCOPIC ANATOMY

Each ovary consists of two distinct areas: the *cortex* or outer layer and the *medulla* or inner portion. The cortex contains small secretory sacs or follicles in three stages of development. These stages are known as *primary, growing,* and *graafian,* which is the follicles' mature stage (see Fig. 6–2). The ovarian medulla contains connective tissue, nerves, blood and lymphatic vessels, and some smooth muscle tissue in the region of the hilus.

FUNCTION OF THE OVARIES

The functional activity of the ovary is primarily controlled by the anterior lobe of the pituitary gland, which produces the *gonadotropic hormones* FSH and LH. These abbreviations are for follicle-stimulating hormone, instrumental in the development of the ovarian follicles, and luteinizing horome, which stimulates the development of the *corpus luteum,* a small yellow mass of cells that develops within a ruptured ovarian follicle.

Two functions have been identified for the ovary: the production of ova or female reproductive cells and the production of hormones.

The Production of Ova

Each month a *graafian follicle* ruptures on the ovarian cortex, and an *ovum* (singular of ova) discharges into the pelvic cavity, where it enters the fallopian tube. This process is known as *ovulation.* In an average, normal woman more than 400 ova may be produced during her reproductive years (see Fig. 6–2).

The Production of Hormones

The ovary is also an endocrine gland, producing *estrogen* and *progesterone.* Estrogen is the female sex hormone secreted by the follicles. Progesterone is a steroid hormone secreted by the corpus luteum. These hormones are essential in promoting growth, development, and maintenance of the female secondary sex organs and characteristics. They also prepare the uterus for pregnancy, promote development of the mammary glands, and play a vital role in a woman's emotional well-being and sexual drive.

▶ THE VAGINA

The *vagina* is a musculomembranous tube extending from the vestibule to the uterus (Fig. 6–2). It is 10 to 15 cm in length and is situated between the bladder and the rectum. It is lined by mucous membrane made up of *squamous epithelium.* A fold of mucous membrane, the *hymen,* partially covers the external opening of the vagina.

FUNCTIONS OF THE VAGINA

The vagina has three basic functions:

- It is the female organ of copulation. The vagina receives the seminal fluid from the male penis.

- It serves as a passageway for the discharge of menstruation.
- It serves as a passageway for the birth of the fetus.

▶ THE VULVA

The *vulva* consists of the following five organs that comprise the external female genitalia (Fig. 6–3):

Mons pubis. A pad of fatty tissue of triangular shape and, after puberty, covered with pubic hair. It may be referred to as the mons veneris or "mound of Venus," and is the rounded area over the symphysis pubis.

Labia majora. The two folds of adipose tissue, which are large lip-like structures, lying on either side of the vaginal opening.

Labia minora. Two thin folds of skin that lie within the labia majora and enclose the vestibule.

Vestibule. The cleft between the labia minora. It is approximately 4 to 5 cm long and 2 cm wide. Four major structures open into it: the urethra, the vagina, and two excretory ducts of the Bartholin glands.

Clitoris. A small organ consisting of sensitive erectile tissue that is homologous to the penis of the male.

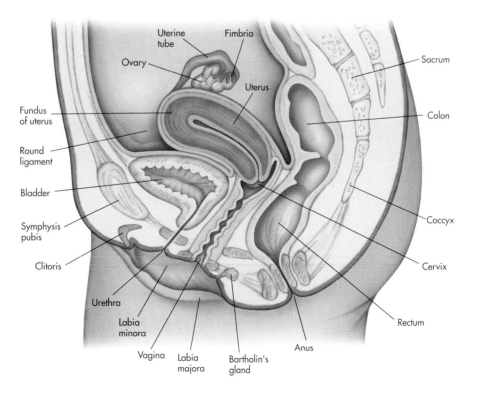

FIGURE 6–3

Sagittal section of the female pelvis, showing organs of the reproductive system.

Between the vulva and the anus is an external region known as the *perineum*. It is composed of muscle covered with skin. During the second stage of labor, a decision is made by the attending physician as to the need to perform an *episiotomy*, a surgical procedure to prevent tearing of the perineum and to facilitate delivery of the fetus.

▶ THE BREAST

The *breasts* or mammary glands are compound *alveolar structures* consisting of 15 to 20 glandular tissue lobes separated by septa of connective tissue. Most women have two breasts that lie anterior to the pectoral muscles and curve outward from the lateral margins of the sternum to the anterior border of the axilla. The size of the breast may greatly vary according to age, heredity, and adipose *(fatty)* tissue present. The *areola* is the dark, pigmented area found in the skin over each breast, and the nipple is the elevated area in the center of the areola. During pregnancy, the areola changes from its pinkish color to a dark brown or reddish color. The areola is supplied with a row of small sebaceous glands that secrete an oily substance to keep it resilient. The *lactiferous glands* consist of 20 to 24 glands in the areola of the nipple and, during lactation, secrete and convey milk to a suck-

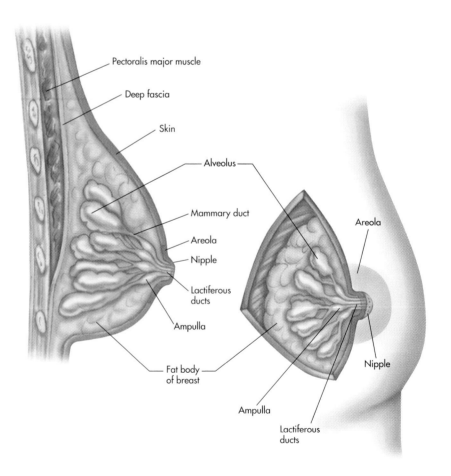

FIGURE 6–4

The breast.

ling infant (Fig. 6–4). The hormone *prolactin,* which is produced by the anterior lobe of the pituitary, stimulates the mammary glands to produce milk after childbirth. Other hormones playing a role in milk production are insulin and glucocorticoids. *Colostrum,* a thin yellowish secretion, is the "first milk" and contains mainly serum and white blood cells. Suckling stimulates the production of oxytocin by the posterior lobe of the pituitary gland. It acts on the mammary glands to stimulate the release of milk and stimulates the uterus to contract during parturition.

BREAST-FEEDING

Among the natural advantages of breast-feeding are the following:

- It provides an ideal food for most newborn babies.
- The milk provides essential nutrients for growth and development.
- The milk is virtually free from harmful bacteria.

After the first 2 weeks, the nursing mother may produce 1 or more pints of milk per day. Milk production may be affected by emotions, food, fluids, physical health, and medications. The nursing mother will usually have a supply of milk for her suckling infant for a period of 6 to 9 months. The nursing process is usually a satisfying experience for both mother and infant. For the mother, the nursing causes contractions of the muscles of the uterus, which aid in its rapid return to normal size. For the infant, breast milk is a natural substance that provides almost everything needed for the first months of life.

► THE MENSTRUAL CYCLE

The onset of the *menstrual cycle,* menarche, occurs at the age of *puberty* and its cessation is at *menopause.* It is a periodic recurrent series of changes occurring in the uterus, ovaries, vagina, and breasts approximately every 28 days. The menstrual cycle is divided into four phases, each of which is described for you.

MENSTRUATION PHASE

The *menstruation phase* is characterized by the discharge of a bloody fluid from the uterus accompanied by a shedding of the endometrium. This phase averages 4 to 5 days and is considered to be the first to the fifth days of the cycle.

PROLIFERATION PHASE

The *proliferation phase* is characterized by the stimulation of estrogen, the thickening and vascularization of the endometrium, along with the maturing of the ovarian follicle. This phase begins about the fifth day and ends at the time of rupture of the graafian follicle—about 14 days before the onset of menstruation.

LUTEAL OR SECRETORY PHASE

The *luteal phase is* characterized by continued thickening of the endometrium, by the glands within the endometrium becoming tortuous, and by the appearance of coiled arteries in its tissues. The endometrium becomes edematous, and the stroma becomes compact. During this phase, the corpus luteum in the ovary is developing and secreting progesterone. The progesterone level is highest during this phase as the estrogen level decreases. This phase lasts about 10 to 14 days.

PREMENSTRUAL OR ISCHEMIC PHASE

During the *premenstrual phase,* the coiled arteries become constricted, the endometrium becomes anemic and begins to shrink, and the corpus luteum decreases in functional activity. This phase lasts about 2 days and ends with the occurrence of menstruation.

Premenstrual syndrome is a condition that affects certain women and may cause distressful symptoms such as constipation, diarrhea, nausea, anorexia, appetite cravings, headache, backache, muscular aches, edema, insomnia, clumsiness, malaise, irritability, indecisiveness, mental confusion, and depression. These symptoms may begin 2 weeks before the onset of *menstruation.* Although the exact cause of this syndrome has not been determined, it may be due to the amount of prostaglandin produced, a deficient or excessive amount of estrogen or progesterone, or an inter-relationship between these factors.

▶ THE CHILD

The sex of the child is determined at the time of **fertilization.** When a spermatozoon carrying the X sex chromosome fertilizes the X-bearing ovum, the result is a female child (X + X = female). When the X-bearing ovum is fertilized by the Y-bearing spermatozoon, a male child is produced (X + Y = male). Sex differentiation occurs early in the embryo. At 16 weeks the external **genitals** of the fetus are recognizably male or female. This difference may be seen during ultrasonography. See Figure 6–5.

The genitals of the newborn are not fully developed at birth. They may be slightly swollen, and in the female infant, blood-tinged mucus may be discharged from the vagina. This is due to hormones transmitted from the mother to the infant. The labia minora may protrude beyond the labia majora.

The sex organs do not mature until the onset of **puberty.** At puberty the female experiences breast development, vaginal secretions, and menarche. A study published in the *Journal of Pediatrics,* April 1997, revealed that many girls begin to develop sexually by age 8. This study involved 17,000 American girls ages 3 to 12, who were seen in 65 pediatric practices nationwide. At age 8, 48.3% of African-American girls and 14.7% of white girls had begun developing breasts, pubic hair, or both. Among African-American girls, menstruation began on average at 12.16 years; among white girls, the average was 12.88 years. The study raised questions about whether environmental estrogens, chemicals that mimic the female hormone estrogen, are bringing on puberty at an earlier age. The study also suggested that sex education should begin sooner than it often does.

▶ THE OLDER ADULT

At about 50 years of age, men and women begin experiencing bodily changes that are directly related to **hormonal** production. In women, the ovaries cease to produce estrogen and progesterone. With decreased production of the female hormones, estrogen and progesterone, women enter the phase of life known as **menopause.** Natural menopause will occur in 25% of women by age 47, in 50% by age 50, 75% by age 52, and in 95% by age 55.

The symptoms of menopause vary from being hardly noticeable to being severe. Symptoms may include irregular periods, hot flashes, vaginal dryness, insomnia, joint pain, headache, emotional instability, irritability, and depression. Breast tissue may lose its firmness, and pubic and axillary hair becomes sparse. Without estrogen, the uterus becomes smaller, the vagina shortens and vaginal tissues become drier. There may be loss of bone mass leading to **osteoporosis.**

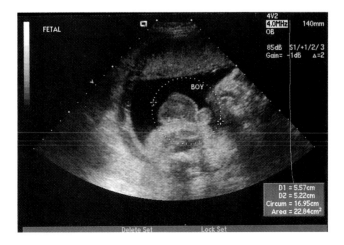

FIGURE 6–5

Ultrasonogram showing a male fetus. *(Courtesy of Nancy West.)*

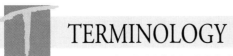

TERMINOLOGY

WITH SURGICAL PROCEDURES & PATHOLOGY

TERM	WORD PARTS			DEFINITION
abortion (ă-bōr′ shŭn)	abort ion	R S	to miscarry process	The process of miscarrying
amenorrhea (ă-mĕn″ ō-rē′ ă)	a meno rrhea	P CF S	lack of month flow	A lack of the monthly flow or menstruation
amniocentesis (ăm″ nĭ-ō-sĕn-tē′ sĭs)	amnio centesis	CF S	lamb surgical puncture	Surgical puncture of the amniotic sac to obtain a sample of amniotic fluid
amniotome (ăm′ nĭ-ō-tōm)	amnio tome	CF S	lamb instrument to cut	An instrument used to cut fetal membranes
anovular (ăn-ŏv′ ū-lăr)	an ovul ar	P R S	lack of ovary pertaining to	Pertaining to the lack of production and discharge of an ovum
antenatal (ăn″ tē- nā′ tal)	ante nat al	P R S	before birth pertaining to	Pertaining to before birth
ante partum (ăn′ tē pär′ tŭm)	ante partum	P R	before labor	The time before the onset of labor
bartholinitis (bar″ tō-lĭn-ī′ tĭs)	bartholin itis	R S	Bartholin's glands inflammation	Inflammation of Bartholin's glands
catamenia (kăt ă-mē′ nĭ-ă)	cata men ia	P R S	down month condition	The condition of monthly discharge of blood from the uterus
cervicitis (sĕr-vĭ-sī′ tĭs)	cervic itis	R S	cervix inflammation	Inflammation of the uterine cervix
colpoperineo-plasty (kŏl″ pō-pĕr″ĭn-ē′ ō-plăs″ tē)	colpo perineo plasty	CF CF S	vagina perineum surgical repair	Surgical repair of the vagina and perineum
colporrhaphy (kŏl-pōr′ ă-fē)	colpo rrhaphy	CF S	vagina suture	Suture of the vagina

Terminology - continued

TERM	WORD PARTS			DEFINITION
colposcope (kŏl′ pō-skōp)	colpo scope	CF S	vagina instrument	An instrument used to examine the vagina and cervix by means of a magnifying lens
conception (kŏn-sĕp′ shŭn)	con cept ion	P R S	together receive process	Process of the union of the male's sperm and the female's ovum; *fertilization*
contraception (kŏn″ tră-sĕp′ shŭn)	contra cept ion	P R S	against receive process	Process of preventing conception

TERMINOLOGY SPOTLIGHT

Contraception is the process of preventing conception. According to the Association of Reproductive Health Professional's survey, 4 out of 5 American women ages 18 to 50 are sexually active. Of these, 9 out of 10, were interested in becoming more educated about various methods of birth control.

In the United States, there are numerous methods that may be used for contraception; some of these are birth control pills, condoms, a diaphragm, foams, jellies, suppositories, natural planning (rhythm method), an intrauterine device (IUD), a cervical cap, a contraceptive sponge, a vasectomy, female sterilization, the Norplant system, Depo-Provera contraceptive injection, and the female condom (Reality).

The most frequently used contraceptives cited by 4000 women ages 18 to 50 were:

Pill	86%
Barrier method (condom, diaphragm, etc.)	76%
Sterilization	34%
Natural planning	25%
IUD	14%
Depo-Provera	2%
Norplant system	1%
None	5%

TERM	WORD PARTS			DEFINITION
culdocentesis (kŭl″ dō-sĕn-tē′ sĭs)	culdo centesis	CF S	cul-de-sac surgical puncture	Surgical puncture of the cul-de-sac for removal of fluid
cystocele (sĭs′ tō-sēl)	cysto cele	CF S	bladder hernia	A hernia of the bladder that protrudes into the vagina
dysmenorrhea (dĭs″ mĕn-ō-rē′ ă)	dys meno rrhea	P CF S	difficult, painful month flow	Difficult or painful monthly flow

continued

Terminology - continued

TERM	WORD PARTS			DEFINITION
dyspareunia (dĭs′ pă-rū′ nĭ-ă)	dys	P	difficult, painful	Difficult or painful sexual intercourse
	par	P	beside	
	eunia	R	a bed	
dystocia (dĭs-tō′ sĭ-ă)	dys	P	difficult, painful	The condition of a difficult and painful childbirth
	toc	R	birth	
	ia	S	condition	
endometriosis (ĕn″ dō-mĕ″ trĭ-ō′ sĭs)	endo	P	within	A condition in which endometrial tissue occurs in various sites in the abdominal or pelvic cavity
	metri	CF	uterus	
	osis	S	condition of	
episiotomy (ĕ-pĭs″ ĭ-ŏt′ ō-mē)	episio	CF	vulva, pudenda	Incision of the perineum to prevent tearing of the perineum and to facilitate delivery
	tomy	S	incision	
eutocia (ū-tō′ sĭ-ă)	eu	P	good, normal	The condition of a good, normal childbirth
	toc	R	birth	
	ia	S	condition	
fibroma (fī-brō′ mă)	fibr	R	fibrous tissue	A fibrous tissue tumor
	oma	S	tumor	
genitalia (jĕn-ĭ-tăl′ ĭ-ă)	genital	R	belonging to birth	The male or female reproductive organs
	ia	S	condition	
gynecologist (gī″ nĕ-kōl′ ō-jĭst)	gyneco	CF	female	One who specializes in the study of the female
	log	R	study of	
	ist	S	one who specializes	
gynecology (gī″ nĕ-kōl′ ō-jē)	gyneco	CF	female	The study of the female
	logy	S	study of	
hematosalpinx (hē″ mă-tō-săl′ pĭnks)	hemato	CF	blood	A collection of blood in the fallopian tube that may be associated with tubal pregnancy
	salpinx	R	tube	
hymenectomy (hī″ mĕn-ĕk′ tō-mē)	hymen	R	hymen	Surgical excision of the hymen
	ectomy	S	excision	
hysterectomy (hĭs″ tĕr-ĕk′ tō-mē)	hyster	R	womb, uterus	Surgical excision of the uterus
	ectomy	S	excision	

Terminology - continued

TERM	WORD PARTS			DEFINITION
hysterotomy (hĭs″tĕr-ŏt′ō-mē)	hystero tomy	CF S	womb, uterus incision	Incision into the uterus; also called a cesarean section
intrauterine (ĭn′tră-ū′tĕr-ĭn)	intra uter ine	P R S	within uterus pertaining to	Pertaining to within the uterus
mammography (măm-ŏg′ră-fē)	mammo graphy	CF S	breast recording	Process of obtaining pictures of the breast by the use of x-rays
mammoplasty (măm′ō-plăs″tē)	mammo plasty	CF S	breast surgical repair	Surgical repair of the breast
mastectomy (măs-tĕk′tō-mē)	mast ectomy	R S	breast excision	Surgical excision of the breast
mastitis (măs-tī′tĭs)	mast itis	R S	breast inflammation	Inflammation of the breast
menopause (mĕn′ō-pawz)	meno pause	CF R	month cessation	Cessation of the monthly flow; *also called climacteric*
menorrhagia (mĕn″ō-rā′jĭ-ă)	meno rrhagia	CF S	month to burst forth	Excessive bursting forth of blood at the time of the monthly flow
menorrhea (mĕn″ō-rē′ă)	meno rrhea	CF S	month flow	A normal monthly flow
multipara (mŭl-tĭp′ă-ră)	multi para	P R	many to bear	A woman who has borne more than one child
myometritis (mī″ō-mē-trī′tĭs)	myo metr itis	CF R S	muscle womb, uterus inflammation	Inflammation of the muscular wall of the uterus
neonatal (nē″ō-nā′tăl)	neo nat al	P R S	new birth pertaining to	Pertaining to the first 4 weeks after birth
nullipara (nŭl-ĭp′ă-ră)	nulli para	P R	none to bear	A woman who has borne no offspring
oligomenorrhea (ŏl″ĭ-gō-mĕn″ō-rē′ă)	oligo meno rrhea	P CF S	scanty month flow	A scanty monthly flow

continued

Terminology - continued

TERM	WORD PARTS			DEFINITION
oogenesis (ō″ō-jĕn′ĕ-sĭs)	oo genesis	CF S	ovum, egg formation, produce	Formation of the ovum
oophorectomy (ō″ŏf-ō-rĕk′tō-mē)	oophor ectomy	R S	ovary excision	Surgical excision of an ovary
oophoritis (ō″ŏf-ō-rī′tĭs)	oophor itis	R S	ovary inflammation	Inflammation of an ovary
panhysterectomy (păn″hĭs-tĕr-ĕk′ tō-mē)	pan hyster ectomy	P R S	all womb, uterus excision	Surgical excision of the entire uterus
pelvimetry (pĕl-vĭm′ĕt-rē)	pelvi metry	CF S	pelvis measurement	Measurement of the pelvis to determine its capacity and diameter
perinatalogy (pĕr″ĭ-nă-tŏl′ō-jē)	peri nata logy	P CF S	around birth study of	Study of the fetus and infant from 20 to 29 weeks of gestation to 1 to 4 weeks after birth
postcoital (pōst-kō′ĭt-ăl)	post coit al	P R S	after a coming together pertaining to	Pertaining to after sexual intercourse
postpartum (pōst păr′tŭm)	post partum	P R	after labor	Pertaining to after childbirth
prenatal (prē-nā′tl)	pre nat al	P R S	before birth pertaining to	Pertaining to before birth
primipara (prī-mĭp′ă-ră)	primi para	P R	first to bear	A woman who is bearing her first child
pseudocyesis (sū″dō-sī-ē′sĭs)	pseudo cyesis	P S	false pregnancy	A false pregnancy
pyometritis (pī″ō-mē-trī′tĭs)	pyo metr itis	CF R S	pus womb, uterus inflammation	Purulent (pus) inflammation of the uterus
pyosalpinx (pī″ō-săl′pĭnks)	pyo salpinx	CF R	pus tube	Accumulation of pus in the fallopian tube

Terminology - continued

TERM	WORD PARTS			DEFINITION
rectovaginal (rĕk″ tō-văj′ ĭ-năl)	recto vagin al	CF R S	rectum vagina pertaining to	Pertaining to the rectum and vagina
retroversion (rĕt″ rō-vur′ shŭn)	retro vers ion	P R S	backward turning process	The process of being turned backward, such as the displacement of the uterus with the cervix pointed forward
salpingectomy (săl″ pĭn-jĕk′ tō-mē)	salping ectomy	R S	tube excision	Surgical excision of a fallopian tube
salpingitis (săl″ pĭn-jī′ tĭs)	salping itis	R S	tube inflammation	Inflammation of a fallopian tube
salpingo-oophor-ectomy (săl′ pĭng″ gō-ō″ ŏf-ō-rĕk′ tō-mē)	salpingo oophor ectomy	CF R S	tube ovary excision	Surgical excision of an ovary and a fallopian tube
trimester (trī-mĕs′ tĕr)	tri mester	P R	three month	A period of 3 months
vaginitis (văj″ ĭn-ī′ tĭs)	vagin itis	R S	vagina inflammation	Inflammation of the vagina
venereal (vē- nē′ rē-ăl)	venere al	R S	sexual intercourse pertaining to	Pertaining to or resulting from sexual intercourse

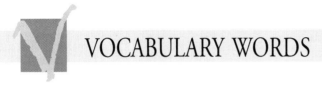

VOCABULARY WORDS

Vocabulary words are terms that have not been divided into component parts. They are common words or specialized terms associated with the subject of this chapter. These words are provided to enhance your medical vocabulary.

WORD	DEFINITION
amniocentesis (ăm″ nĭ-ō-sĕn-tē′ sĭs)	A surgical puncture of the amniotic sac to obtain amniotic fluid from which it can be determined if the fetus has Down syndrome, neural tube defects, Tay-Sachs disease, or other genetic defects
biotics (bī-ŏt′ ĭks)	The science of living organisms and the sum of knowledge regarding the life process
blastocyst (blăs′ tō-sĭst)	An embryonic cell mass that attaches to the uterus wall and is a stage in the development of a mammalian embryo
decidua (dē- sĭd′ ū-ă)	The endometrium or mucous membrane of the pregnant uterus that envelops the impregnated ovum
diagnostic ultrasound (dī″ ăg-nŏs′ tĭk ŭl′ tră-sŏund)	The use of extremely high-frequency sound waves for the purpose of diagnosing genetic defects and hydrocephalic conditions in the unborn fetus
Doppler ultrasound (dăp′ lər ŭl′ trăh-sŏund)	A procedure using an audio transformation of high-frequency sounds to monitor the fetal heartbeat
fetus (fē′ tŭs)	The developing young in the uterus from the third month to birth
gamete intrafallopian transfer (GIFT) (găm′ ēt ĭn″ tră-fă-lō′ pē-ăn)	A procedure that places the sperm *(spermatozoa)* and eggs *(oocytes)* directly in the fimbriated end of the fallopian tube via a laparoscope
genetics (jĕn-ĕt′ ĭks)	The science of biology that studies the phenomenon of heredity and the laws governing it
hysteroscope (hĭs′ tĕr-ō-skōp)	An instrument used in the biopsy of uterine tissue before 12 weeks of gestation. This tissue is then analyzed for chromosome arrangement, DNA sequence, and genetic defects.

Vocabulary - continued

WORD	DEFINITION
laser ablation (lā′ zĕr ăb-lā′ shŭn)	A procedure that uses a laser to destroy the uterine lining. A biopsy is performed before the procedure to make sure no cancer is present. This procedure may be used for disabling menstrual bleeding. *It does cause sterility.*
laser laparoscopy (lā′ zĕr lăp-ăr-ŏs′ kō-pē)	A procedure that uses a long, telescope-like instrument equipped with a laser, lights, and a tiny video camera. It may be used to explore the abdominal area and to treat ectopic pregnancy.
laser lumpectomy (lā-zĕr lŭm-pĕk′ tō-mē)	The use of a contact Yag laser to remove a tumor from the breast. It appears to cause less pain for the patient and discharge time from the hospital is sooner.
lumpectomy (lŭm-pĕk′ tō-mē)	The surgical removal of a tumor from the breast. In this procedure, no other tissue or lymph nodes are removed, only the tumor; usually not considered for large tumors, although the latest strategy involves shrinking large tumors with chemotherapy so that they become small enough to be removed by this method
menarche (mĕn-ar′ kē)	The beginning of the monthly flow; *menses*
mittelschmerz (mĭt′ ĕl-shmārts)	Abdominal pain that occurs midway between the menstrual periods at ovulation
morula (mor′ ū-lă)	A solid mass of cells resulting from cell division after fertilization of an ovum
nonstress test (nŏn′ strĕs tĕst)	A diagnostic procedure, often done in a physician's office, wherein a monitor is placed on the mother's abdomen and fetal heartbeats are recorded. The fetal heartbeats should accelerate if the fetus moves.
ovulation (ŏv″ ū-lā′ shăn)	The process in which an ovum is discharged from the cortex of the ovary
ovum transfer (ō′ vum trăns′ fer)	A method of fertilization for women who cannot conceive children. A donor ovum is impregnated within the donor's body by artificial insemination and later transferred to the recipient female.
"parking" (părk′ ĭng)	A surgical procedure in which the fallopian tube is detached from the ovary. An incision is made into the peritoneum and the tube is sewn into it. This is a reversible sterilization procedure.
parturition (par″ tū-rĭsh′ ŭn)	The act of giving birth; *also known as childbirth or delivery*
pudendal (pū-dĕn′ dăl)	Pertaining to the external female genitalia

continued

Vocabulary - continued

WORD	DEFINITION
puerperium (pū″ ĕr-pē′ rĭ-ŭm)	The 4 to 6 weeks after childbirth when the female generative organs usually return to a normal state
quickening (kwĭk′ ĕn-ĭng)	The first movement of the fetus felt in the uterus, occurring during the 16th to 20th week of pregnancy
secundines (sĕk′ ŭn-dīnz)	The afterbirth consisting of the placenta, umbilical cord, and fetal membranes
sonogram (sō′ nŏ-grăm)	A procedure using high-frequency sound waves to display a visual echo image of the fetus; used to determine size of the fetus and to diagnose genetic defects
surrogate mother (sur′ ō-gāt mŭth′ ēr)	A female who contracts to bear a child for another. Pregnancy may occur as a result of artificial insemination
"test-tube baby" (tĕs′ tūb bā′ bē)	An in vitro fertilization technique whereby the ovum is fertilized outside the body and later implanted in the host female
toxic shock syndrome (tŏk′ sĭk shŏk sĭn′ drōm)	A poisonous *Staphylococcus aureus* infection that may strike young, menstruating women
uterine adnexa (ū′ tĕr-ĭn ăd-nĕk′ sah)	The ovaries and fallopian tubes
zygote (zī′ gōt)	The fertilized ovum. The zygote is produced by the union of two gametes.

ABBREVIATIONS

AB	abortion	**CS**	cesarean section
AFP	alpha-fetoprotein	**CVS**	chorionic villus sampling
AH	abdominal hysterectomy	**D&C**	dilation (dilatation) and curettage
Ascus	atypical squamous cells of undetermined significance	**DES**	diethylstilbestrol
BBT	basal body temperature	**DUB**	dysfunctional uterine bleeding
C-section	cesarean section	**EDC**	expected date of confinement
CIN	cervical intraepithelial neoplasia	**FSH**	follicle-stimulating hormone
CIS	carcinoma-in-situ	**GIFT**	gamete intrafallopian transfer
		grav I	pregnancy one

Gyn	gynecology	**OB**	obstetrics
HCG	human chorionic gonadotropin	**Pap**	Papanicolaou (smear)
HPV	human papillomavirus	**PID**	pelvic inflammatory disease
HRT	hormone replacement therapy	**PMP**	previous menstrual period
HSG	hysterosalpingography	**PMS**	premenstrual syndrome
IUD	intrauterine device	**TSS**	toxic shock syndrome
LH	luteinizing hormone	**UC**	uterine contractions
LMP	last menstrual period	**WNL**	within normal limits
MH	marital history		

DRUG HIGHLIGHTS

Drugs that are generally used for the female reproductive system include hormones, contraceptives, and those used during labor and delivery.

Female Hormones

Estrogens
Are used for a variety of conditions. They may be used in the treatment of amenorrhea, dysfunctional bleeding, and hirsutism and in palliative therapy for breast cancer in women and prostatic cancer in men. They are also used as replacement therapy in the treatment of uncomfortable symptoms that are related to menopause. In this instance, it is believed that estrogen replacement therapy is useful in preventing osteoporosis and possibly heart disease.
Examples: TACE (chlorotrianisene), Premarin (conjugated estrogens, USP), DES (diethylstilbestrol), Estrace (estradiol), Theelin (estrone), and Estraderm (estradiol) transdermal system.

Progestogens/
progestins
Synthetic preparations of progesterone. They are used to prevent uterine bleeding and are combined with estrogen for treatment of amenorrhea. They may be used in cases of infertility and threatened or habitual miscarriage. Progesterone is responsible for changes in the uterine endometrium during the second half of the menstrual cycle, development of maternal placenta after implantation, and development of mammary glands.
Examples: Provera (medroxyprogesterone acetate), Norlutin (norethindrone), Norlutate (norethindrone acetate), and Gesterol (progesterone).

Contraceptives

Oral
Nearly 100% effective when used as directed. These pills contain mixtures of estrogen and progestin in various levels of strength. The estrogen in the pill inhibits ovulation and the progestin inhibits pituitary secretion of luteinizing hormone (LH), causes changes in the cervical mucus that renders it unfavorable to penetration by sperm, and alters the nature of the endometrium.
Examples: Ortho-Novum 10/11-21, Triphasil-21, Micronor, Enovid-E 21, Ovulen-28, Brevicon 21-day, Demulen 1/50-21, and Lo/Ovral-21.

The Norplant
system
Consists of six thin capsules that contain levonorgestrel (a progestin). The capsules are made of a soft flexible material and are placed in a fan-like pattern just under the skin on the inside surface of the upper arm. They have a 99% effective contraceptive action that begins within hours after placement and lasts up to 5 years.

Uterine Stimulants	Oxytocic agents (uterine stimulants) may be used in obstetrics to induce labor at term. They are also used to control postpartum hemorrhage and to induce therapeutic abortion. *Examples: Ergotate Maleate (ergonovine maleate) and Pitocin (oxytocin).*
Uterine Relaxants	May be administered to delay labor until the fetus has gained sufficient maturity as to be likely to survive outside the uterus. *Examples: Ethanol (ethyl alcohol) and Yutopar (ritodrine HCl).*

DIAGNOSTIC AND LABORATORY TESTS

Test	Description
amniotic fluid analysis (ăm-nē-ŏt′ ĭk floo′ ĭd ă-năl′ ĭ-sĭs)	A procedure that involves the removal of amniotic fluid via a large needle. Ultrasound is used to give the location of the fetus, and then the needle is inserted into a suprapubic site of the mother. Abnormal results can indicate spina bifida, Down syndrome, hemophilia, hemolytic disease, and/or poor fetal maturity.
breast examination (brest ĕks-ăm″ ĭ-nā′ shŭn)	Visual inspection and manual examination of the breast for changes in contour, symmetry, "dimpling" of skin, retraction of the nipple(s), and for the presence of lumps.
chorionic villus sampling (CVS) (kō-rē-ŏn′ ĭk vĭl′ ŭs sam′ plĭng)	A procedure that involves the insertion of a catheter into the cervix and into the outer portion of the membranes surrounding the fetus. A sample of the chorionic villi can be examined for the chromosomal abnormalities and biochemical disorders. This procedure can be done 8 weeks into pregnancy.
colposcopy (kŏl-pŏs′ kō-pē)	Visual examination of the vagina and cervix via a colposcope. Abnormal results may indicate cervical or vaginal erosion, tumors, and dysplasia.
culdoscopy (kŭl-dŏs′ kō-pē)	Visual examination of the viscera of the female pelvis via a culdoscope. May be used in suspected ectopic pregnancy and unexplained pelvic pain, and to check for pelvic masses.
estrogens (es′ trō-jĕns)	A urine test or blood serum test to determine the level of estrone, estradiol, and estriol.
human chorionic gonadotropin (HCG) (hū′ măn kō-rē-ŏn′ ĭk gŏn″ ă-dō- trō′ pĭn)	A urine test or blood serum test to determine the presence of HCG. A positive result may indicate pregnancy.

hysterosalpingography
(hĭs″ tĕr-ō-săl″ pĭn-gŏg′ ră-fē)

X-ray of the uterus and fallopian tubes after the injection of a radiopaque substance. Size and structure of the uterus and fallopian tubes can be evaluated. Uterine tumors, fibroids, tubal pregnancy, and tubal occlusion may be observed. Also used for treatment of an occluded fallopian tube.

laparoscopy
(lăp-ăr-ŏs′ kō-pē)

Visual examination of the abdominal cavity via a laparoscope. Used to examine the ovaries and fallopian tubes.

mammography
(măm-ŏg′ ră-fē)

The process of obtaining pictures of the breast by use of x-rays. This procedure is able to locate breast tumors before they grow to 1 cm. It is the most effective means of detecting early breast cancers.

Papanicolaou (Pap smear)
(păp′ ăh-nĭk″ ō-lă′ oo)

A screening technique to aid in the detection of cervical/uterine cancer and cancer precursors. It is not a diagnostic procedure. Both false-positive and false-negative results have been experienced with Pap smears. Any lesion should be biopsied unless not indicated clinically. The Pap smear should not be used as a sole means to diagnose or exclude malignant and premalignant lesions. It is a screening procedure only.

Pap smear results are generally reported as: within normal limits (WNL); abnormal squamous cells of undetermined significance (Ascus); mild dysplasia (CIN I); moderate dysplasia (CIN II); and severe dysplasia and/or carcinoma-in-situ (CIN III).

pregnanediol
(prĕg″ nān-dī-ŏl)

A urine test that determines menstrual disorders or possible abortion.

wet mat or wet-prep
(wĕt măt or wĕt-prĕp)

Examination of vaginal discharge for the presence of bacteria and yeast. A vaginal smear is placed on a microscopic slide, wet with normal saline, and then viewed under a microscope by the physician.

COMMUNICATION ENRICHMENT

This segment is provided for those who wish to enhance their ability to communicate in either English or Spanish.

▶ Related Terms

English	Spanish
abortion	aborto (ă-*bōr*-tō)
breast examination	examen de pecho (ex-*să*-mĕn dĕ *pĕ*-chō)
breasts	pechos; senos (*pe*-chōs; *sĕ*-nōs)
cesarean	cesarea (sĕ-*să*-rĕ-ă)
contraception	contracepción (cōn-tră-*cĕp*-sĭ-ōn)
Do you use?	¿usa? (¿ū-să?)
the pill	la píldora (lă pĭl-*dō*-ră)
the diaphragm	el diafragma (ĕl *dĭ*-ă-frăg-mă)
an IUD	un dispositivo ultra intrauterino (ūn dĭs-*pō*-sĭ-*tĭ*-vō *ūl*-tră *ū*-tĕ-rĭ-nō)
foam	espuma (ĕs-*pū*-mă)
condoms	preservativos (condones) (*prĕ*-sĕr-vă-tĭ-vōs; cōn-*dō*-nĕs)
the rhythm method	el método de ritmo (ĕl *mĕ*-tō-dō dĕ *rĭt*-mō)
the method of withdrawal	el método de retirar (ĕl *mĕ*-tō-dō dĕ *rĕ*-tĭ-răr)
abstinence	abstinencia (ăbs-tĭ-*nĕn*-sĭ-ă)
injection	inyección (ĭn-jĕc-sĭ-*ōn*)

English	Spanish
cramps	calambres (că-*lăm*-brĕs)
delivery	parto (*pă*r-tō)
episiotomy	episiotomia (ĕ-*pĭ*-sĭ-ō-tō-mĭ-ă)
intercourse	acto sexual; cópula (ăk-*tō sĕx*-sū-ăl; *cō*-pū-lă)
lump	protuberancia (prō-tū-bĕ-*răn*-sĭ-ă)
marital status	estado civil (ĕs-*tă*-dō *sĭ*-vĭl)
menopause	menopausia (mĕ-nō-*pă*-ū-sĭ-ă)
menstrual history	historia menstrual (ĭs-*tō*-rĭ-ă *mĕns*-trū-ăl)
multiple births	nacimientos múltiples (*nă*-sĭ-mĭ-ĕn-tōs *mūl*-tĭ-plĕs)
nipple	pezón (pĕ-*zōn*)
ovary	ovario (ō-*vă*-rĭ-ō)
Pap smear	papanicolao (*pă*-pă-nĭ-kō-lă-ō)
pelvic examination	examen de la pelvis (ĕx-*să*-mĕn dĕ lă pĕlvĭs)
period	periódo (pĕ-rĭ-*ō*-dō)
placenta	placenta (plă-*cĕn*-tă)
pregnancy	embarazo; preñez (ĕm-bă-*ră*-zō; prĕn-*yĕz*)
pregnant	embarazada (ĕm-bă-ră-*să*-dă)
premature	prematuro (prĕ-mă-*tū*-rō)

English	Spanish
sanitary napkin	toalla sanitaria (tō-*ă*-jă săn-nĭ-*tă*-rĭ-ă)
uterus	útero (*ū*-tĕ-rō)
vagina	vagina (vă-*hĭ*-nă)
womb	matriz (*mă*-trĭz)

CHAPTER REVIEW SECTION

LEARNING EXERCISES

▶ **Anatomy and Physiology**

Write your answers to the following questions. Do not refer back to the text

1. List the primary and accessory sex organs of the female reproductive system.

    a. _____   b. _____

    c. _____   d. _____

    e. _____   f. _____

2. State the vital function of the female reproductive system. _____

    _____

3. Name the three identifiable areas of the uterus.

    a. _____   b. _____

    c. _____

4. Define fundus. _____

    _____

5. Name the ligaments that support the uterus and hold it in position.

    a. _____   b. _____

    c. _____   d. _____

6. Name the three layers of the uterine wall.

    a. _____   b. _____

    c. _____

7. State the three primary functions associated with the uterus.

    a. _____

    b. _____

    c. _____

8. Define the following terms:

    a. Anteflexion_____

    _____

    b. Retroflexion _____

    _____

    c. Anteversion _____

    _____

    d. Retroversion _____

    _____

9. The fallopian tubes are also called the _____ _____

    or _____.

10. Name the three layers of the fallopian tubes.

    a. _____   b. _____

    c. _____

11. Define fimbriae. _____

    _____

12. Should the ovum become impregnated by a spermatozoon while in the fallopian tube,

    the process of _____ occurs.

13. State two functions of the fallopian tubes.

    a. _____   b. _____

    c. _____

14. Describe the ovaries. _____

    _____

15. Name the three stages of an ovarian follicle.

   a. _____   b. _____

   c. _____

16. The functional activity of the ovary is controlled by the _____.

17. State the two functions of the ovary.

   a. _____   b. _____

18. The vagina is a _____ tube extending from the _____ to the uterus.

19. State the three functions of the vagina.

   a. _____   b. _____

   c. _____

20. Name the organs that comprise the external female genitalia.

   a. _____   b. _____

   c. _____   d. _____

   e. _____

21. Between the vulva and the anus is an external region known as the _____

   _____.

22. Define episiotomy. _____

   _____

23. The breasts or _____ _____ are compound alveolar structures.

24. The _____ is the dark pigmented area found in the skin over each

   breast and the _____ is the elevated area in its center.

25. Name the three hormones that play a role in milk production.

   a. _____   b. _____

   c. _____

26. Define colostrum. _____

   _____

27. Name the four phases of the menstrual cycle.

   a. _____   b. _____

   c. _____   d. _____

28. Define premenstrual syndrome. _____

_____

_____

▷ **Word Parts**

1. In the spaces provided, write the definitions of these prefixes, roots, combining forms, and suffixes. Do not refer to the listings of terminology words. Leave blank those terms you cannot define.

2. After completing as many as you can, refer back to the terminology word listings to check your work. For each word missed or left blank, write the term and its definition several times on the margins of these pages or on a separate sheet of paper.

3. To maximize the learning process, it is to your advantage to do the following exercises as directed. To refer to the terminology listings before completing these exercises invalidates the learning process.

Prefixes

Give the definitions of the following prefixes:

1. a- _____   2. an- _____

3. ante- _____   4. cata- _____

5. con- _____   6. contra- _____

7. dys- _____   8. endo- _____

9. eu- _____   10. intra- _____

11. multi- _____   12. neo- _____

13. nulli- _____   14. oligo- _____

15. pan- _____   16. par- _____

17. peri- _____   18. post- _____

19. pre- _____   20. primi- _____

21. pseudo- _____   22. retro- _____

23. tri- _____

Roots and Combining Forms

Give the definition of the following roots and combining forms:

1. abort _____
2. amnio _____
3. bartholin _____
4. cept _____
5. cervic _____
6. coit _____
7. colpo _____
8. culdo _____
9. cysto _____
10. episio _____
11. eunia _____
12. fibr _____
13. genital _____
14. gyneco _____
15. hemato _____
16. hymen _____
17. hyster _____
18. hystero _____
19. log _____
20. mammo _____
21. mast _____
22. men _____
23. meno _____
24. mester _____
25. metr _____
26. metri _____
27. myo _____
28. nat _____
29. nata _____
30. oo _____
31. oophor _____
32. ovul _____
33. para _____
34. partum _____
35. pause _____
36. pelvi _____
37. perineo _____
38. pyo _____
39. recto _____
40. salping _____
41. salpingo _____
42. salpinx _____
43. toc _____
44. uter _____
45. vagin _____
46. venere _____
47. vers _____

Suffixes

Give the definitions of the following suffixes:

1. -al _____
2. -ar _____

3. -cele _____   4. -centesis _____

5. -cyesis _____   6. -ectomy _____

7. -genesis _____   8. -graphy _____

9. -ia _____   10. -ine _____

11. -ion _____   12. -ist _____

13. -itis _____   14. -logy _____

15. -metry _____   16. -oma _____

17. -osis _____   18. -plasty _____

19. -rrhagia _____   20. -rrhaphy _____

21. -rrhea _____   22. -scope _____

23. -tome _____   24. -tomy _____

▶ Identifying Medical Terms

In the spaces provided, write the medical terms for the following meanings:

1. _____   The process of miscarrying

2. _____   An instrument used to cut fetal membranes

3. _____   The time before the onset of labor

4. _____   Inflammation of the uterine cervix

5. _____   Suture of the vagina

6. _____   A difficult or painful monthly flow

7. _____   A good, normal childbirth

8. _____   A fibrous tissue tumor

9. _____   The study of the female

10. _____   Surgical excision of the hymen

11. _____   Surgical repair of the breast

12. _____   A normal monthly flow

13. _____   Pertaining to the first 4 weeks after birth

14. _____   Formation of the ovum

15. _____   Pertaining to after childbirth

▶   Spelling

In the spaces provided, write the correct spelling of these misspelled terms:

1. amiocentesis _____
2. bartolinitis _____
3. dytocia _____
4. epsiotomy _____
5. hystrotomy _____
6. menorhagia _____
7. oophritis _____
8. salpinitis _____
9. vajinitis _____
10. veneral _____

WORD PARTS STUDY SHEET

Word Parts	Give the Meaning
ante-	_____
contra-	_____
dys-	_____
multi-	_____
nulli-	_____
primi-	_____
tri-	_____
abort-	_____
amnio-	_____
bartholin-	_____
cervic-	_____
coit-	_____
colpo-	_____
genital-	_____
gyneco-	_____
hymen-	_____
hyster-, hystero-	_____
mammo-, mast-	_____

men-, meno- _____

metr-, metri-, metro- _____

oo- _____

oophor- _____

partum- _____

perineo- _____

salping-, salpingo- _____

uter- _____

vagin- _____

venere- _____

-cele _____

-centesis _____

-cyesis _____

-genesis _____

-ia, -osis _____

-oma _____

-plasty _____

-rrhagia _____

-rrhaphy _____

-rrhea _____

-scope _____

-tome _____

-tomy _____

REVIEW QUESTIONS

▶ **Matching**

Select the appropriate lettered meaning for each numbered line.

_____	1.	gamete intrafal-lopian transfer
_____	2.	laser ablation
_____	3.	lumpectomy
_____	4.	menarche
_____	5.	mittelschmerz
_____	6.	morula
_____	7.	ovulation
_____	8.	parturition
_____	9.	pudendal
_____	10.	quickening

a. A solid mass of cells resulting from cell division after fertilization of an ovum
b. Pertaining to the external female genitalia
c. The beginning of the monthly flow; menses
d. Surgical removal of a tumor from the breast
e. Abdominal pain that occurs midway between the menstrual periods at ovulation
f. A procedure that places the sperm and eggs directly in the fimbriated end of the fallopian tube
g. The process in which an ovum is discharged from the cortex of the ovary
h. The act of giving birth
i. The first movement of the fetus felt in the uterus, occurring during the 16th to 20th week of pregnancy
j. A procedure that uses a laser to destroy the uterine lining
k. The fertilized ovum

▶ **Abbreviations**

Place the correct word, phrase, or abbreviation in the space provided.

1. AB _____

2. alpha-fetoprotein _____

3. AH _____

4. cesarean section _____

5. DES _____

6. expected date of confinement _____

7. grav I _____

8. Gyn _____

9. intrauterine device _____

10. pelvic inflammatory disease _____

► **Diagnostic and Laboratory Tests**

Select the best answer to each multiple choice question. Circle the letter of your choice.

1. A procedure that involves the insertion of a catheter into the cervix and into the outer portion of the membranes surrounding the fetus.
    a. amniotic fluid analysis
    b. chorionic villus sampling
    c. colposcopy
    d. culdoscopy

2. A positive result may indicate pregnancy.
    a. colposcopy
    b. culdoscopy
    c. HCG
    d. laparoscopy

3. X-ray of the uterus and fallopian tubes after the injection of a radiopaque substance.
    a. hysterosalpingography
    b. laparoscopy
    c. culdoscopy
    d. mammography

4. Used to examine the ovaries and fallopian tubes.
    a. colposcopy
    b. culdoscopy
    c. laparoscopy
    d. mammography

5. The process of obtaining pictures of the breast by use of x-rays.
    a. colposcopy
    b. culdoscopy
    c. laparoscopy
    d. mammography

CRITICAL THINKING ACTIVITY

▶ **Case Study**

Menopause

Please read the following case study and then answer the questions that follow.

A 52-year-old female was seen by a physician and the following is a synopsis of the visit.

Present History: The patient states that her periods have become very irregular, that she has hot flashes and trouble sleeping, that sex with her husband has become uncomfortable, and that she is very moody.

Signs and Symptoms: Chief complaint: irregular periods, hot flashes, insomnia, dyspareunia, and emotional instability.

Diagnosis: Menopause. The diagnosis was determined by a complete gynecologic examination.

Treatment: Hormone replacement therapy (HRT) consisting of estrogens combined with progestin. The patient was placed on Prempro (conjugated estrogens/medroxyprogesterone acetate tablets) one tablet daily. Prempro is packaged in a special calendar blister pack that shows one instantly whether she has taken the pill for that day. The package is designed for 2 weeks, with directions for use: Begin either card with the tablet that is labeled for the day of the week on which your first day of therapy falls. Complete one card, then begin the second card the very next day. Complete second card.

Prevention: There are no known preventive measures.

Critical Thinking Questions

1. Symptoms of menopause include irregular periods, hot flashes, insomnia, _____, and emotional instability.

2. The diagnosis was determined by a complete _____ examination.

3. Treatment included hormone replacement therapy _____, a combination of estrogens and progestin.

4. The abbreviation for hormone replacement therapy is _____.

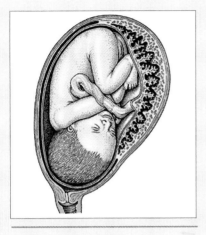

ANATOMY AND PHYSIOLOGY OF THE REPRODUCTIVE SYSTEM

OBJECTIVES

- Summarize the functions of the human reproductive system and its principal components.

- Describe the components of the male reproductive system.

- Describe the process of spermatogenesis.

- Describe the roles of the male reproductive tract and accessory glands in the maturation and transport of spermatozoa.

- Describe the hormones involved in sperm production.

- Describe the components of the female reproductive system.

- Describe the events of the ovarian and uterine cycles.

- Describe the hormonal regulation of the ovarian and uterine cycles.

- Describe the effects of age on the reproductive systems.

The reproductive system is the only one of our organ systems that is not essential for an individual's survival. It is indispensable, however, for the continuation of the human race.

Reproduction is the process that links one generation to the next in humans as well as in all other organisms. In simple, one-celled organisms reproduction occurs through the division of the organism itself. This type of reproduction is called *asexual*. Humans (and many familiar creatures) reproduce *sexually*, that is, they require two parents of opposite sexes for reproduction.

Human reproduction depends on the joining together of male and female reproductive cells, or **gametes** (GA-mēts), to form a new human being. The male and female gametes, a **sperm** from the father and an **ovum** (Ō-vum), or egg cell, from the mother, fuse in a process called **fertilization.** The resulting cell, called a **zygote** (ZĪ-gōt), divides repeatedly and gradually transforms into an individual with its own unique traits. This transformation process, called *development*, is the topic of the next chapter.

▶ SYSTEM BRIEF

Human reproductive systems are specialized to produce, store, nourish, and transport male and female gametes. In both sexes, the gametes result from a special form of cell division called **meiosis** (mī-Ō-sis) (Figure 7-1). The gametes produced through meiosis contain only half the number of chromosomes found in other cells. All other body cells contain 46 chromosomes, whereas gametes contain just 23. Thus the combination of a sperm and an egg produces a single cell with the normal complement of 46 chromosomes.

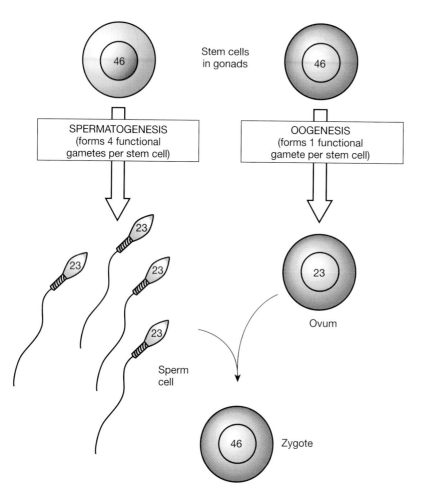

FIGURE 7-1

Meiosis and the Formation of Gametes.

Special stems cells within male and female gonads undergo meiosis, which results in the formation of sex cells that contain half the normal number of chromosomes.

Both male and female reproductive systems include reproductive organs, or **gonads** (GŌ-nads), that produce gametes and hormones; ducts that receive and transport the gametes; accessory glands and organs that secrete fluids into various ducts; and structures associated with the reproductive system, collectively known as the **external genitalia** (jen-i-TĀ-lē-a).

The roles of the male and female reproductive systems are quite different. In the adult male the gonads, or **testes** (TES-tēz; singular: *testis*), secrete male sex hormones (*androgens*), principally testosterone, and produce a half-billion sperm each day. The sperm then travel along a lengthy duct system where they are mixed with the secretions of accessory glands, creating **semen** (SĒ-men). During **ejaculation** (e-jak-ū-LĀ-shun) the semen is expelled from the body.

The gonads, or **ovaries**, of adult females typically release only one ovum each month. This gamete travels along short **uterine tubes**, also called *fallopian tubes* or *oviducts*, that terminate in a muscular chamber, the **uterus** (Ū-te-rus). A short passageway, the **vagina** (va-JĪ-na), connects the uterus with the exterior. During intercourse the male ejaculation introduces semen into the vagina, and the sperm move farther along the female reproductive tract. If a single sperm fuses with an egg, fertilization occurs. The resulting cell divides repeatedly, and the process of development begins. The uterus provides protection and support as the cluster of cells becomes an *embryo* (months 1–2) and then a *fetus* (months 3–9), until the time of delivery.

▶ STRUCTURE OF THE MALE REPRODUCTIVE SYSTEM

The principal structures of the male reproductive system are shown in Figure 7-2. Proceeding from the testes, the sperm cells, or **spermatozoa** (sper-ma-tō-ZŌ-a), travel along the **epididymis** (ep-i-DID-i-mus), the **ductus deferens** (DUK-tus DEF-e-renz), the **ejaculatory** (ē-JAK-ū-la-tō-rē) **duct**,

FIGURE 7-2

The Male Reproductive System.

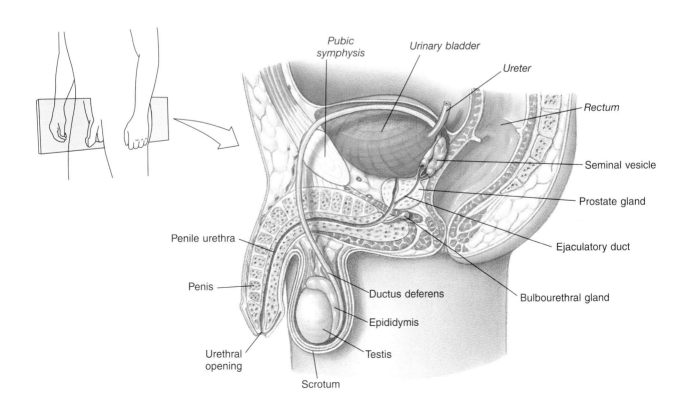

and the **urethra** before leaving the body. Accessory organs, notably the **seminal** (SEM-i-nal) **vesicles**, the **prostate** (PROS-tāt) **gland**, and the **bulbourethral** (bul-bō-ū-RĒ-thral) **glands**, empty their secretions into the ejaculatory ducts and urethra. Structures visible from the outside are the **scrotum** (SKRŌ-tum), which encloses the testes, and the **penis** (PĒ-nis). Together, the scrotum and penis constitute the external genitalia of the male.

THE TESTES

The *primary sex organs* of the male system are the testes. The testes hang within a fleshy pouch, the scrotum. The scrotum is subdivided into two chambers, each containing a testis. Each testis has the shape of an almond roughly 5 cm (2 in.) long and 2.5 cm (1 in.) wide.

The testes form in the abdominal cavity next to the kidneys. During fetal development the testes slowly descend from their original position and, in the seventh month, pass through openings (called *inguinal canals*) within the abdominal wall and into the scrotum. Each testis is attached to a **spermatic cord** made up of connective and muscle tissue surrounding a ductus deferens, blood vessels, lymphatic vessels, and nerves. The presence of the testes in the scrotum outside the body wall means that they are in an environment about 1.1°C (2°F) below normal body temperature. This cooler temperature is necessary for normal sperm development.

As Figure 7-3a shows, each testis is subdivided into compartments called *lobules*. Within the lobules, sperm production occurs in tightly coiled **seminiferous** (se-mi-NIF-e-rus) **tubules**. Each tubule averages around 80 cm (31 in.) in length, and a typical testis contains nearly half a mile of seminiferous tubules.

sperma, seed + *genesis*, origin
spermatogenesis: the process of sperm formation

Spermatozoa are produced by the process of **spermatogenesis** (sper-ma-tō-JEN-e-sis). This process begins with stem cells lying at the outermost layer of cells in the seminiferous tubules (Figure 7-3b). The descendants of the stem cells undergo a halving of their chromosome number (meiosis) as they proceed to the central opening, or *lumen*.

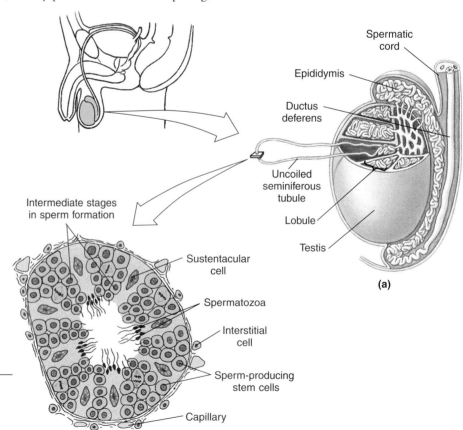

FIGURE 7-3

Structure of the Testes.

(a) Diagrammatic sketch and structural relationships of the testes. **(b)** A section through a coiled seminiferous tubule showing its organization of cells.

In addition, each seminiferous tubule also contains **sustentacular** (sus-ten-TAK-ū-lar) **cells** (*Sertoli cells*). These large "nurse cells" provide nutrients and chemical signals that promote the development of spermatozoa. The entire process of spermatogenesis takes approximately 9 weeks.

The spaces between the tubules contain large **interstitial cells** that produce the male sex hormone **testosterone** (Figure 7-3b).

The Sperm Cell

A sperm cell is quite small. For example, 1 ml of ejaculate can contain up to 100 million spermatozoa! Each sperm cell is made up of three regions: the *head*, the *middle piece*, and the *tail* (Figure 7-4). The **head** is a flattened oval filled with densely packed chromosomes. The top of the head is covered by an **acrosomal** (ak-rō-SŌ-mal) **cap**, or **acrosome**, which contains enzymes essential for fertilization. A very short **neck** attaches the head to the **middle piece**, which is filled with mitochondria providing the energy for moving the flagellum that forms the **tail**.

THE MALE REPRODUCTIVE TRACT

The testes produce physically mature spermatozoa that are, as yet, incapable of fertilizing an ovum. The other portions of the male reproductive system, sometimes called the accessory structures, are concerned with the functional maturation, nourishment, storage, and transport of spermatozoa.

The Epididymis

Late in their development the spermatozoa enter the central opening of the seminiferous tubule. Although they have most of the physical characteristics of mature sperm cells, they are still functionally immature and incapable of locomotion. At this point, fluid currents carry them into the **epididymis** (Figure 7-2). This tubule, almost 7 m (23 ft.) long, is so twisted and coiled that it actually

FIGURE 7-4

Structure of a Spermatozoon.

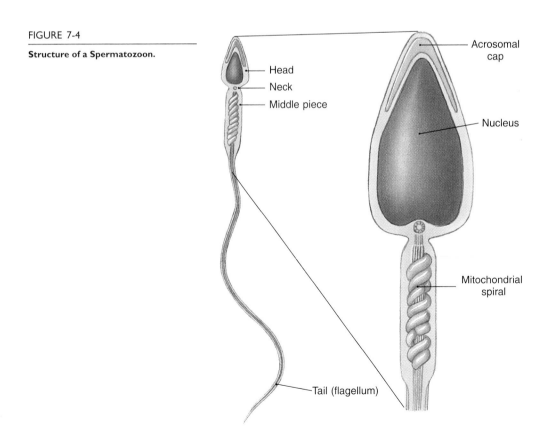

Head
Neck
Middle piece
Acrosomal cap
Nucleus
Mitochondrial spiral
Tail (flagellum)

takes up very little space. During the 2 weeks that a spermatozoon travels through the epididymis, it completes its physical maturation. The epididymis maintains suitable conditions for this process by absorbing cellular debris, providing organic nutrients, and recycling damaged or abnormal spermatozoa. Mature spermatozoa then arrive at the ductus deferens.

The Ductus Deferens

The **ductus deferens**, also known as the *vas deferens*, is 40 to 45 cm (16 to 18 in.) long. It extends toward the abdominal cavity within the spermatic cord. The ductus deferens curves downward alongside the urinary bladder toward the prostate gland (Figure 7-2).

Peristaltic contractions in the muscular walls of the ductus deferens propel spermatozoa and fluid along the length of the duct. The ductus deferens can also store spermatozoa in an inactive state for up to several months.

The junction of the ductus deferens with the duct draining the seminal vesicle creates the **ejaculatory duct**, a relatively short (2 cm, or less than 1 in.) passageway that penetrates the muscular wall of the prostate and fuses with the ejaculatory duct from the other side before emptying into the urethra.

The Urethra

The urethra of the male extends from the urinary bladder to the tip of the penis, a distance of 15 to 20 cm (6 to 8 in.). The urethra in the male is a passageway used by both the urinary and reproductive systems.

THE ACCESSORY GLANDS

A typical ejaculation releases 2 to 5 ml of semen. This volume of fluid, called an **ejaculate**, is made up of spermatozoa, seminal fluid, and various enzymes. A normal **sperm count** ranges from 20 million to 100 million spermatozoa per milliliter. Because of their small size, sperm make up only about 1 percent of semen volume. **Seminal fluid**, the fluid component of semen, is a mixture of the combined secretions of the seminiferous tubules, the epididymis, and the accessory glands.

The fluids contributed by the seminiferous tubules and the epididymis account for only about 5 percent of the final volume of semen. The major fraction of seminal fluid is composed of secretions from the *seminal vesicles*, the *prostate gland*, and the *bulbourethral glands*. Major functions of these glandular organs include (1) activating the spermatozoa, (2) providing the nutrients that spermatozoa need for their own movement, (3) pushing spermatozoa and fluids along the reproductive tract by peristaltic contractions, and (4) producing buffers that counteract the acids found in the vagina.

The Seminal Vesicles

Each seminal vesicle is a tubular gland with a total length of around 15 cm (6 in.) that is compactly folded into a 5 cm x 2.5 cm (2 in. x 1 in.) mass.

The seminal vesicles contribute about 60 percent of the volume of semen. In particular, their secretions contain relatively high concentrations of fructose, a six-carbon sugar easily broken down by spermatozoa. The secretions are also slightly alkaline, and this alkalinity helps neutralize acids in the prostatic secretions and within the vagina. When mixed with the secretions of the seminal vesicles, previously inactive but mature spermatozoa begin beating their flagella and become highly mobile.

The Prostate Gland

The **prostate gland** is a small, muscular, rounded organ with a diameter of about 4 cm (1.6 in.) that surrounds the urethra as it leaves the bladder. The prostate produces an acidic secretion that contributes about 30 percent of the volume of semen.

The Bulbourethral Glands

The paired **bulbourethral glands**, or *Cowper's glands*, are round, with diameters approaching 10 mm (less than 0.5 in.) (Figure 7-2). These glands secrete a thick, sticky, alkaline mucus that has lubricating properties.

THE PENIS

The **penis** is a tubular organ that surrounds the urethra (Figure 7-2). It conducts urine to the exterior and introduces semen into the female vagina during sexual intercourse. The penis (Figure 7-5a) is divided into three regions: (1) the **root**, the fixed portion that attaches the penis to the body wall; (2) the **body (shaft)**, the tubular portion that contains masses of *erectile tissue*; and (3) the **glans**, the expanded end that surrounds the external urethral opening.

The skin overlying the penis resembles that of the scrotum. A fold of skin, the **prepuce** (PRĒ-pūs), or *foreskin*, surrounds the tip of the penis. The prepuce attaches to the relatively narrow **neck** of the penis and continues over the glans. The surgical removal of the prepuce is called a *circumcision* (ser-kum-SIZH-un). In Western societies this procedure is usually performed soon after birth.

The body, or shaft, of the penis contains three columns, or bodies (singular: *corpus*; plural: *corpora*), of spongy, **erectile tissue** (Figure 7-5b). Erectile tissue consists of a maze of blood channels incompletely divided by sheets of elastic connective tissue and smooth muscle. The two cylindrical **corpora cavernosa** (KOR-po-ra ka-ver-NŌ-sa) lie side by side and above the relatively slender **corpus spongiosum** (spon-jē-Ō-sum) that surrounds the urethra.

In the resting state, there is little blood flow into the erectile tissues because their arterial branches are constricted. In response to involuntary nerve impulses during *arousal*, the walls of the arterial blood vessels to the erectile tissue open, blood flow increases, the penis becomes engorged with blood, and **erection** occurs.

FIGURE 7-5

The Penis.

(a) Anterior and lateral view of the penis, showing positions of the erectile tissues. **(b)** Sectional view through the penis.

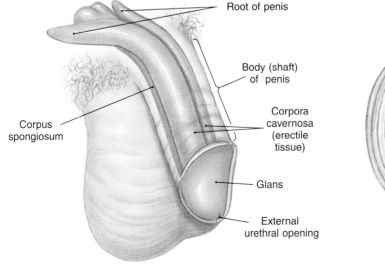

(a) Anterior and lateral view of penis

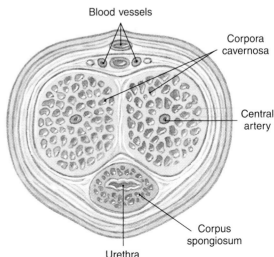

(b) Section through shaft of penis

► HORMONES AND MALE REPRODUCTIVE FUNCTION

The hormones that regulate the male reproductive system are produced by the pituitary gland, the hypothalamus, and the testes. The pituitary gland releases *follicle-stimulating hormone* (**FSH**) and *luteinizing hormone* (**LH**). The pituitary release of these hormones occurs in the presence of *gonadotropin-releasing hormone* (**GnRH**), a hormone released by the hypothalamus.

In the male, FSH stimulates the sustentacular cells of the seminiferous tubules. Under FSH stimulation, and in the presence of testosterone from the interstitial cells, sustentacular cells promote the production of sperm cells.

LH (formerly called *interstitial cell–stimulating hormone (ICSH)* in males) causes the secretion of testosterone by the interstitial cells of the testes. Testosterone levels and sperm production are both regulated by negative feedback. Low levels of testosterone stimulate the secretion of LH and FSH by the pituitary gland. The LH stimulates testosterone secretion, and testosterone and FSH stimulate sperm production. High levels of testosterone inhibit the secretion of LH and FSH, and the decline in LH inhibits testosterone secretion. The combination of reduced testosterone levels and reduced FSH levels slows the rate of sperm production.

Testosterone also has numerous functions in addition to promoting sperm production. It also determines the *secondary sexual characteristics* such as the distribution of facial hair, increased muscle mass and body size, and the quantity and location of fat deposits; stimulates protein synthesis and muscle growth; and influences brain development by stimulating sexual behaviors and sexual drive.

Testosterone production begins around the seventh week of embryonic development and reaches a peak after roughly 6 months of development. This early presence of testosterone stimulates the formation of the male duct system and accessory organs. Testosterone production then declines until it accelerates markedly at puberty, initiating sexual maturation and the appearance of secondary sexual characteristics.

Concept Questions

✔ How do you think the lack of an acrosomal cap would affect the ability of a sperm cell to fertilize an egg cell?

✔ What happens when the arteries serving the penis dilate (increase in diameter)?

✔ What effect would low levels of FSH have on sperm production?

► STRUCTURE OF THE FEMALE REPRODUCTIVE SYSTEM

A woman's reproductive system must produce sex hormones and gametes and also protect and support a developing embryo and nourish the newborn infant. The primary sex organs of the female reproductive system are the *ovaries*. The internal and external accessory organs include the *uterine tubes* (*fallopian tubes* or *oviducts*), the *uterus* (womb), the *vagina*, and the components of the external genitalia (Figure 7-6). As in the male, various accessory glands secrete into the reproductive tract. Physicians specializing in the female reproductive system are called **gynecologists** (gī-ne-KOL-o-jists).

THE OVARIES

A typical ovary measures approximately 5 cm x 2.5 cm (2 in. x 1 in.). It has a pale white or yellowish coloration and a nodular consistency that resembles cottage cheese or lumpy oatmeal. The production of gametes occurs in the outer layer of the ovary. Arteries, veins, lymphatics, and nerves within its interior link the ovary with other body systems.

The ovaries are responsible for the production of female gametes, eggs or **ova** (singular: **ovum**), and the secretion of female sex hormones, including *estrogens* and *progestins*.

Through the process of meiosis, ovum production, or **oogenesis** (ō-ō-JEN-e-sis), produces gametes with half the number of normal chromosomes. Oogenesis begins before birth, accelerates at puberty, and ends at *menopause*. During the years between puberty and menopause, oogenesis occurs on a monthly basis as part of the *ovarian cycle*.

oon, egg + *genesis*, origin
oogenesis: the process of ovum formation

The Ovarian Cycle

Ovum production occurs within specialized structures called **ovarian follicles** (ō-VAR-ē-an FOL-i-klz). Before puberty, each ovary contains some 200,000 immature egg cells. Each of these egg cells is enclosed by a layer of follicle cells. The combination is known as a **primordial** (prī-MOR-dē-al)

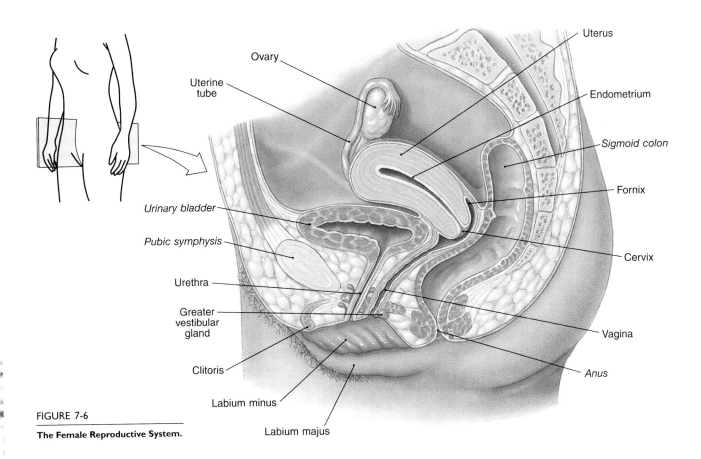

FIGURE 7-6

The Female Reproductive System.

follicle. At puberty, rising levels of FSH begin to activate a different group of primordial follicles each month. This monthly process, shown in Figure 7-7, is known as the **ovarian cycle**.

The cycle begins as the activated follicles develop into **primary follicles**. The follicle cells, which divide and form several layers around the immature ovum, provide nutrients to the growing ovum.

Although many primordial follicles develop into primary follicles, usually only a few will take the next step. The deeper follicular cells begin secreting a fluid that gradually accumulates and enlarges the entire follicle. At this stage the complex is known as a **secondary follicle**.

Eight to 10 days after the start of the ovarian cycle, the ovaries usually contain only a single secondary follicle. By days 10 to 14 of the cycle it has formed a mature **tertiary follicle**, or *Graafian* (GRAF-ē-an) *follicle*, roughly 15 mm (about 0.6 in.) in diameter. This complex is so large that it creates a prominent bulge in the surface of the ovary.

Ovulation, the release of the ovum, through the ovary wall, usually occurs at day 14 of a 28-day cycle. After ovulation, the ovum is drawn into the entrance of the uterine tube. The empty follicle collapses, and the remaining follicular cells multiply to create a hormone-producing structure known as the **corpus luteum** (LOO-tē-um). *Luteum* means "yellow," and the corpus luteum is also described as a "yellow body." Unless pregnancy occurs, after about 12 days the corpus luteum begins to degenerate. The disintegration marks the end of the ovarian cycle, but almost immediately the activation of another set of primordial follicles begins the next ovarian cycle.

THE UTERINE TUBES

Each **uterine tube** is about 13 cm (5 in.) long. The end closest to the ovary forms an expanded funnel, the *infundibulum*, with numerous fingerlike projections (Figure 7-8). The projections, called *fimbriae* (FIM-brē-ē), and the inner surfaces of the uterine tube are carpeted with cilia that produce a current that moves the ovum into the broad entrance to the uterine tube. Once inside the uterine

FIGURE 7-7

The Ovarian Cycle.

Follicular development
during the ovarian cycle.

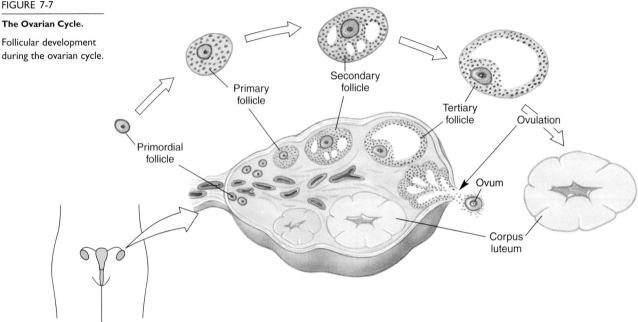

tube, the ciliary current and peristaltic contractions transport the ovum over 3 to 4 days to the uterine chamber. If fertilization is to occur, the ovum must encounter sperm during the first 12 to 24 hours of its passage down the uterine tube. Unfertilized ova disintegrate in the uterine tubes or uterus.

THE UTERUS

The **uterus** provides physical protection and nutritional support to the developing embryo and fetus (Figure 7-8). The typical uterus is a small, pear-shaped organ about 7.5 cm (3 in.) long with a maximum diameter of 5 cm (2 in.). It weighs 30 to 40 g and is held in place by various ligaments.

The uterus can be divided into two regions: the *body* and the *cervix*. The **body** is the largest division of the uterus. The *fundus* is the rounded portion of the body superior to the attachment of the uterine tubes. The **cervix** (SER-viks) is the inferior portion of the uterus and projects a short distance into the vagina. The cervical opening leads into the *cervical canal*, a narrow passageway that opens into the **uterine cavity**.

In section, the thick uterine wall can be divided into an inner **endometrium** (en-dō-MĒ-trē-um) and a muscular **myometrium** (mī-ō-MĒ-trē-um) covered by a layer of visceral peritoneum. The myometrium is made up of interwoven smooth muscle cells capable of stretching during the growth of the embryo and fetus. The endometrium of the uterus undergoes regular, cyclical changes in response to changing levels of sexual hormones. These alterations produce the characteristic features of the *uterine cycle*.

endo, inside + *metria*,
uterus
endometrium: the lining
of the uterus; the region
that supports a developing embryo and fetus

mys, muscle + *metria*,
uterus
myometrium: the muscular walls of the uterus

The Uterine Cycle

The **uterine cycle**, or **menstrual** (MEN-stroo-al) **cycle,** is a repeating series of changes in the structure of the endometrium. This cycle averages 28 days in length, but it can range from 21 to 35 days in normal individuals. It can be divided into three stages: the *menstrual period (menstruation)*, the *proliferative phase*, and the *secretory phase* (Figure 7-9).

The uterine cycle begins with **menstruation** (men-stroo-Ā-shun), a period of time marked by the breakdown and degeneration of the endometrium. The process is triggered by the decline in hormone concentrations as the corpus luteum disintegrates. Blood cells from broken blood vessels, and degenerating endometrial tissues and glands break away into the uterine chamber and then pass

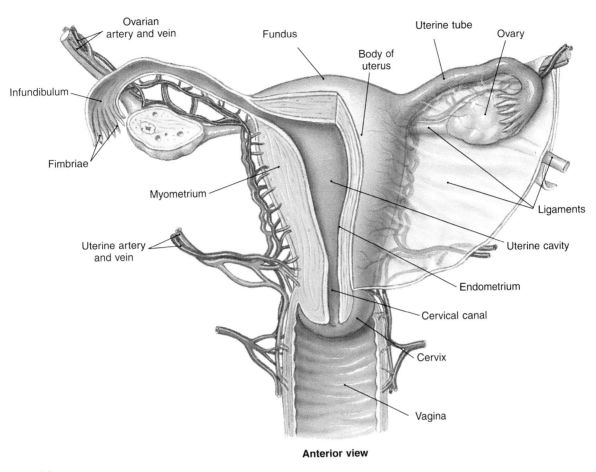

Anterior view

FIGURE 7-8

The Uterus and Associated Structures.

Anterior view with right portion of uterus, uterine tube, and ovary shown in section.

into the vagina. Menstruation usually lasts from 1 to 7 days, and over this period roughly 35 to 50 ml of blood is lost.

The *proliferative phase* begins in the days following the completion of menstruation as the surviving epithelial cells multiply and spread across the surface of the endometrium. This repair process is stimulated by the rising hormone levels that accompany the growth of another set of ovarian follicles. By the time ovulation occurs, the repaired endometrium is filled with small arteries, and endometrial (uterine) glands are secreting a glycogen-rich mucus. The proliferative phase ends with ovulation.

During the *secretory phase*, which begins at ovulation, the endometrial glands enlarge, steadily increasing their rates of secretion. This activity is stimulated by the hormones from the corpus luteum. The secretory phase persists as long as the corpus luteum remains intact. Secretions from the corpus luteum peak about 12 days after ovulation. Over the next day or two the glandular activity declines, and the menstrual cycle comes to a close. A new cycle then begins with the onset of menstruation and the disintegration of the endometrium.

The first menstrual period, called **menarche** (me-NAR-kē), occurs at puberty, typically at age 11 to 12. Uterine cycles continue until age 45 to 50, when **menopause** (ME-nō-paws), the last uterine cycle, occurs. At that time, few, if any, follicles are left in the ovaries. Over the intervening years some 500 ova will have been ovulated.

FIGURE 7-9

Phases of the Uterine (Menstrual) Cycle.

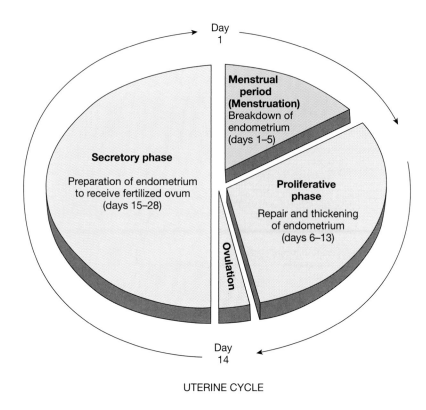

UTERINE CYCLE

THE VAGINA

The **vagina** is a muscular tube extending between the uterus and the external genitalia (Figures 7-6 and 7-8). It has an average length of 7.5 to 9 cm (3 to 3.5 in.), but because the vagina is highly distensible, its length and width are quite variable. The cervix of the uterus projects into the **vaginal canal**. The vagina lies parallel to the rectum, and the two are in close contact. After leaving the urinary bladder the urethra turns and travels along the superior wall of the vagina.

The vagina (1) serves as a passageway for the elimination of menstrual fluids, (2) receives the penis during sexual intercourse, and (3) in childbirth forms the birth canal through which the fetus passes on its way to an independent existence.

The vagina is lined by a mucous membrane thrown into folds called *rugae*. Its walls contain a network of blood vessels and layers of smooth muscle. An elastic epithelial fold, the **hymen** (HĪ-men), may partially or completely block the entrance to the vagina.

The vagina normally contains resident bacteria supported by the nutrients found in the mucus secreted by the cervix. As a result of the bacteria's metabolic activities the normal pH of the vagina ranges between 3.5 and 4.5, and this acid environment restricts the growth of many pathogenic organisms.

THE EXTERNAL GENITALIA

The region enclosing the female external genitalia is the **vulva** (VUL-va) (see Figure 7-10). The vagina opens into the **vestibule**, a central space bounded by the **labia minora** (LĀ-bē-a mi-NŌR-a; singular: *labium minus*). The labia minora are covered with a smooth, hairless skin. The urethra opens into the vestibule just anterior to the vaginal entrance. Anterior to the urethral opening, the **clitoris** (KLI-to-ris) projects into the vestibule. The clitoris is the female equivalent of the penis, derived from the same embryonic structures. Internally it contains erectile tissues that become engorged with blood during arousal.

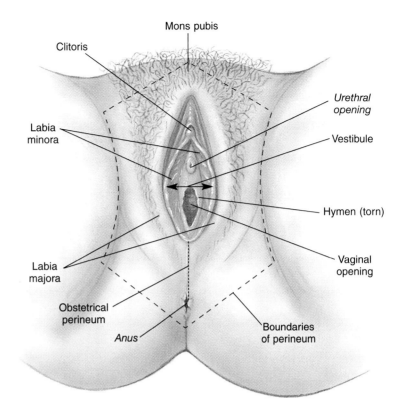

FIGURE 7-10

The Female External Genitalia.

An external view of the female perineum (outlined by dashed lines).

Mons pubis

Clitoris

Urethral opening

Labia minora

Vestibule

Hymen (torn)

Labia majora

Vaginal opening

Obstetrical perineum

Anus

Boundaries of perineum

During sexual arousal a pair of ducts discharges the lubricating secretions of the **greater vestibular glands** (refer to Figure 7-6) into the vestibule near the vaginal entrance. These mucous glands resemble the bulbourethral glands of the male.

The outer limits of the vulva are established by the *mons pubis* and the *labia majora*. The prominent bulge of the **mons pubis** is created by fat tissue beneath the skin anterior to the pubic symphysis. The fleshy **labia majora** (singular: *labium majus*) encircle and partially conceal the labia minora and underlying vestibular structures.

In both sexes, the **perineum** refers to the muscular pelvic floor that includes the external genitalia and anus. In the pregnant female, this term is also used more specifically for the region between the vaginal opening and the anus (the *obstetrical perineum*).

THE MAMMARY GLANDS

After its birth the newborn infant gains nourishment from the milk secreted by the mother's **mammary glands**. Milk production, or **lactation** (lak-TĀ-shun), occurs in the mammary glands of the breasts, specialized accessory organs of the female reproductive system (Figure 7-11).

The mammary glands lie within fatty tissue beneath the skin of the chest. Each breast bears a small conical projection, the **nipple**, where the ducts of underlying mammary glands open onto the body surface. The skin surrounding each nipple has a reddish brown coloration, and this region is known as the **areola** (a-RĒ-ō-la).

The glandular tissue of the breast consists of a number of separate lobes, each containing several secretory lobules. Within each lobe the ducts leaving the lobules converge, giving rise to a single **lactiferous** (lak-TIF-e-rus) **duct**. Near the nipple, the lactiferous duct expands, forming an expanded chamber called a **lactiferous sinus**. There are usually 15 to 20 lactiferous sinuses opening onto the surface of each nipple. Bands of connective tissue, the *suspensory ligaments of the breast*, surround the duct system and help support the breasts. A layer of loose connective tissue separates the mammary complex from the underlying muscles, and the two can move relatively independently.

Concept Questions

✔ As the result of infections such as gonorrhea, scar tissue can block the opening of each uterine tube. How would this blockage affect a woman's ability to conceive?

✔ What tissue breaks away and is lost during menstruation?

✔ Would blockage of a single lac-tiferous sinus interfere with delivery of milk to the nipple? Explain.

FIGURE 7-11
_____

The Mammary Glands of the Female Breast.

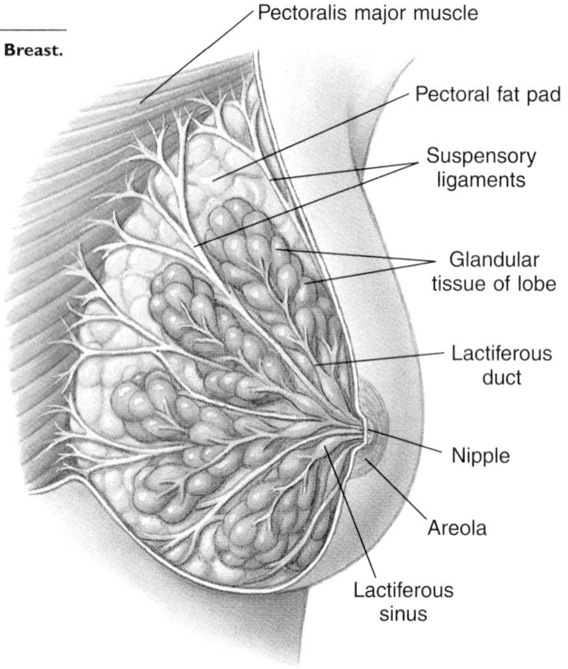

Pectoralis major muscle

Pectoral fat pad

Suspensory
ligaments

Glandular
tissue of lobe

Lactiferous
duct

Nipple

Areola

Lactiferous
sinus

► HORMONES AND THE FEMALE REPRODUCTIVE CYCLE

As in the male, the activity of the female reproductive tract is controlled by both pituitary and gonadal hormones. But the regulatory pattern is much more complicated, for a woman's reproductive system does not just produce gametes; it must also coordinate the ovarian and uterine cycles. Circulating hormones, especially estrogen, regulate the **female reproductive cycle** to ensure proper reproductive function.

THE OVARIAN CYCLE

Hormonal regulation of the ovarian cycle differs between the *preovulatory period* and *postovulatory period*.

Hormones and the Preovulatory Period

Each month some of the follicles begin their development into primary follicles under the stimulation of FSH. As the follicular cells enlarge and multiply, they release steroid hormones collectively known as *estrogens*, the most important being **estradiol** (es-tra-DĪ-ol). Estrogens have multiple functions, including (1) stimulating bone and muscle growth, (2) maintaining female secondary sex characteristics such as body hair distribution and the location of adipose tissue deposits, (3) affecting CNS activity, including sex-related behaviors and drives, (4) maintaining functional accessory reproductive glands and organs, and (5) initiating repair and growth of the endometrium.

The upper portion of Figure 7-12 summarizes the hormonal events associated with the ovarian cycle. As in the male, the primary hormones involved are produced by the anterior pituitary gland, under the control of the hypothalamus. As estrogen levels rise, they cause a decrease in the rate of FSH secretion. Estrogen also affects the rate of LH secretion—the rate of LH release increases as estrogen concentrations rise. Thus as the follicles develop and estrogen concentrations rise, the pituitary output of LH increases. The combination of estrogens, FSH, and LH continues to support follicular development and maturation.

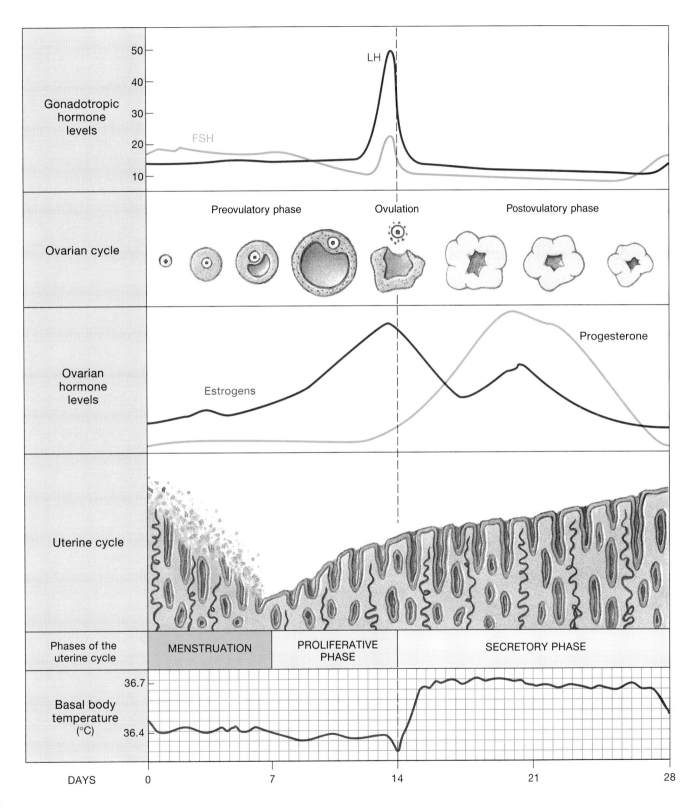

FIGURE 7-12

Hormonal Regulation of the Female Reproductive Cycle.

Estrogen concentrations take a sharp upturn in the second week of the ovarian cycle, as one tertiary follicle enlarges in preparation for ovulation. At about day 14 estrogen levels peak, accompanying the maturation of that follicle. The high estrogen concentration then triggers a massive outpouring of LH from the anterior pituitary, which triggers ovulation.

Hormones and the Postovulatory Period

LH levels remain elevated for only 2 days, but that is long enough to cause the empty follicle to change into a functional corpus luteum. In addition to estrogen, the corpus luteum begins to manufacture steroid hormones known as **progestins** (prō-JES-tinz), in particular, **progesterone** (prō-JES-ter-ōn). Progesterone is the principal hormone of the postovulatory period. It prepares the uterus for pregnancy by stimulating the growth of the endometrium. It also stimulates metabolic activity, leading to a rise in basal body temperature.

Progesterone secretion continues at relatively high levels for the following week, but unless pregnancy occurs, the corpus luteum then begins to degenerate. Roughly 12 days after ovulation, the corpus luteum becomes nonfunctional, and progesterone and estrogen levels fall markedly. This decline leads to an increase in FSH and LH production in the anterior pituitary, and the entire cycle begins again.

THE UTERINE CYCLE

The hormonal changes that regulate the ovarian cycle also affect the uterus. The lower portion of Figure 7-12 follows changes in the endometrium during a single uterine cycle. The sudden declines in progesterone and estrogen levels that accompany the breakdown of the corpus luteum result in menstruation. The loss of endometrial tissue continues for several days until rising estrogen levels stimulate the regeneration of the endometrium. The preovulatory phase continues until rising progesterone levels mark the arrival of the postovulatory phase. The combination of estrogen and progesterone then causes a further thickening of the endometrium that prepares it for the arrival of an embryo.

Concept Questions

✔ What changes would you expect to observe in the ovulatory cycle if the LH surge did not occur?

✔ What event occurs in the menstrual cycle when the levels of estrogen and progesterone decline?

HORMONES AND BODY TEMPERATURE

The changing levels of hormones also cause physiological changes that affect body temperature. During the preovulatory period, when estrogen is the dominant hormone, the resting, or "basal," body temperature measured upon awakening in the morning is about 0.3°C (or 0.5°F) lower than it is during the postovulatory period, when progesterone dominates. At the time of ovulation, basal temperature declines sharply, making the temperature rise over the following day even more noticeable (Figure 7-12). By keeping records of body temperature over a few menstrual cycles a woman can often determine the precise day of ovulation. This information can be important for those wishing to avoid or promote a pregnancy, for this can occur only if an ovum becomes fertilized within a day of its ovulation.

▶ AGING AND THE REPRODUCTIVE SYSTEM

The aging process affects the reproductive systems of men and women. The most striking age-related changes in the female reproductive system occur at menopause, whereas changes in the male reproductive system occur more gradually and over a longer period of time.

MENOPAUSE

Menopause is usually defined as the time that ovulation and menstruation cease. It typically occurs between the ages of 45 and 55, but in the years preceding it the ovarian and uterine cycles become irregular. A shortage of primordial follicles is the underlying cause of these developments; by age 50 there are often no primordial follicles left to respond to FSH.

Menopause is accompanied by a sharp and sustained rise in the production of FSH and LH and a decline in circulating concentrations of estrogen and progesterone. The decline in estrogen levels leads to reductions in the size of the uterus and breasts, accompanied by a thinning of the urethral and vaginal walls. The reduced estrogen concentrations have also been linked to the development of *osteoporosis*, presumably because bone deposition proceeds at a slower rate. A variety of nervous system effects are also reported, including "hot flashes," anxiety, and depression, but the hormonal mechanisms involved are not well understood. In addition, the risk of atherosclerosis and other forms of cardiovascular disease increase after menopause.

The symptoms accompanying and following menopause are sufficiently unpleasant that about 40 percent of menopausal women eventually seek medical assistance. Hormone replacement therapies involving a combination of estrogens and progestins can often prevent osteoporosis and the nervous and circulatory system changes associated with menopause.

Concept Question

✔ Why does the level of FSH rise and remain high during menopause?

THE MALE CLIMACTERIC

Changes in the male reproductive system occur more gradually, over a period known as the *male climacteric*. Circulating testosterone levels begin to decline between ages 50 and 60, coupled with increases in circulating levels of FSH and LH. Although sperm production continues (men well into their eighties can father children), there is a gradual reduction in sexual activity in older men.

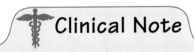

Clinical Note

Birth Control Strategies

Most adults practice some form of **contraception**, or birth control, during some part of their reproductive years. There are many different methods of preventing pregnancy. Fewer methods exist for the termination of a pregnancy.

CONCEPTION PREVENTION

Surgical Methods. *Sterilization* makes one unable to provide functional gametes for fertilization. Either sexual partner may be sterilized with the same net result. In a **vasectomy** (vaz-EK-to-mē) a segment of the ductus deferens is removed, making it impossible for spermatozoa to pass through the reproductive tract (see Figure 7-13a). The surgery can be performed in a physician's office in a matter of minutes. With the section removed, the cut ends do not reconnect; in time, scar tissue forms a permanent seal. After a vasectomy the man experiences normal sexual function, for the epididymal and testicular secretions normally account for only around 5 percent of the volume of the semen. Spermatozoa continue to develop, but they remain within the epididymis until they degenerate. The failure rate for this procedure is 0.08 percent (a failure is defined as a resulting pregnancy).

In the female the uterine tubes can be blocked through a surgical procedure known as a tubal ligation (see Figure 7-13b). Since the surgery involves entering the abdominopelvic cavity, complications are more likely than with vasectomy. The failure rate for this procedure is estimated at 0.45 percent. As in a vasectomy, attempts may be made to restore fertility after a tubal ligation.

Hormonal Methods. Oral contraceptives manipulate the female hormonal cycle so that ovulation does not occur. Contraceptive pills contain a combination of progestins and estrogens. These hormones suppress pituitary production of GnRH, so FSH is not released and ovulation does not occur. The hormones are administered in a cyclic fashion, beginning 5 days after the start of menstruation and continuing for the next 3 weeks. Over the fourth week the woman takes placebo pills or no pills at all. There are now at least 20 different brands of combination oral contraceptives available, and over 200 million women are using them worldwide. In the United States, 25 percent of women under age 45 use the combination pill to prevent conception. The failure rate for the combination oral contraceptives, when used as prescribed, is 0.24 percent over a 2-year period. Birth control pills are not without their risks, however. For example, women with severe hypertension, diabetes mellitus, epilepsy, gallbladder disease, heart trouble, or acne may find that their problems worsen when taking the combination pills. Women taking oral contraceptives are also at increased risk for venous thrombosis, strokes, pulmonary embolism, and (for women over 35) heart disease.

Two progesterone-only forms of birth control are now available. *Depo-provera*™ is injected every 3 months. The silastic tubes of the Norplant™ system are saturated with progesterone and inserted under the skin. This method provides birth control for a period of approximately 5 years. Both Depo-provera™ and the Norplant™ system can interrupt or cause irregular menstruation, but they are easy to use and extremely convenient. *(continued on next page)*

Barrier Methods. The **condom**, also called a *prophylactic* or "rubber," covers the body of the penis during intercourse and keeps spermatozoa from reaching the female reproductive tract. Condoms are also used to prevent transmission of sexually transmitted diseases, such as syphilis, gonorrhea, and AIDS. The condom failure rate has been estimated at over 6 percent. **Vaginal barriers** such as the *diaphragm, cervical cap,* or *vaginal sponge* rely on similar principles. A diaphragm, the most popular form of vaginal barrier in use at the moment, consists of a dome of latex rubber with a small metal hoop supporting the rim. Because vaginas vary in size, women choosing this method must be individually fitted. Before intercourse the diaphragm is inserted so that it covers the cervical opening. It is usually coated with a small amount of spermicidal jelly or cream, adding to the effectiveness of the barrier. The failure rate for a properly fitted diaphragm is estimated at 5 to 6 percent. The cervical cap is smaller and lacks the metal rim. It, too, must be fitted carefully, but unlike the diaphragm it may be left in place for several days. The failure rate (8 percent) is higher than that for a diaphragm. The vaginal sponge consists of a small synthetic sponge saturated with a *spermicide*—a sperm-killing foam or jelly. The failure rate for a contraceptive sponge is estimated at 6 to 10 percent.

Other Methods. An **intrauterine device (IUD)** consists of a small plastic loop or a T that can be inserted into the uterine chamber. The mechanism of action remains uncertain, but it is known that IUDs can change the intrauterine environment and lower the chances for fertilization and subsequent implantation of a fertilized ovum. IUDs are in limited use in the United States but they remain popular in many other countries. The failure rate is estimated at 5 to 6 percent.

The **rhythm method** involves abstaining from sexual activity on the days ovulation might be occurring. The timing is estimated based on previous patterns of menstruation and sometimes by following changes in basal body temperature. The failure rate for the rhythm method is very high, approaching 25 percent.

POST-CONCEPTION METHODS

If contraceptive methods fail, options exist to either prevent implantation or terminate the pregnancy.

Oral Methods. The "morning-after pills" contain estrogens or progestins. They may be taken within 72 hours of intercourse, and they appear to act by altering the transport of the zygote (fertilized egg) or preventing its attachment to the uterine wall. The drug known as *RU-486 (Mifepristone)* blocks the action of progesterone at the endometrial lining. The result is a normal menstrual period with degeneration of the endometrium whether or not fertilization has occurred.

Surgical Methods. **Abortion** refers to the termination of a pregnancy. Three classes of abortions are recognized. *Spontaneous abortions,* or *miscarriages,* occur naturally due to some developmental or physiological problem. *Therapeutic abortions* are performed when continuing the pregnancy represents a threat to the life and health of the mother. *Induced abortions* (elective abortions) are performed at the request of the individual. Induced abortions are currently legal during the first 3 months after conception, and many states permit abortions, sometimes with restrictions, until the fifth or sixth developmental month.

FIGURE 7-13

Surgical Sterilization.

(a) In a male **vasectomy**, the removal of a 1-cm, (1/2in.) section of the ductus deferens prevents the passage of sperm cells. **(b)** In a female **tubal ligation**, the removal of a section of the oviduct prevents both the passage of sperm and the movement of the ovum or embryo into the uterus.

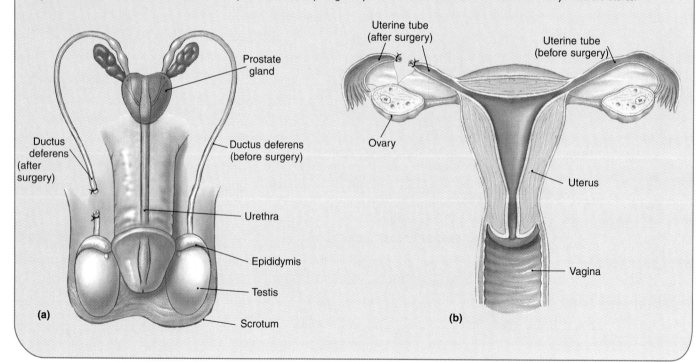

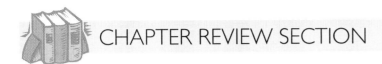

CHAPTER REVIEW SECTION

KEY WORDS

areola (a-RĒ-ō-la):

Pigmented area that surrounds the nipple of the breast.

estrogens (ES-trō-jenz):

Female sex hormones, notably estradiol; primary hormones regulating the female reproductive cycle.

genitalia:

External organs of the reproductive system.

lactation (lak-TĀ-shun):

The production of milk by the mammary glands.

meiosis (mī-Ō-sis):

Cell division that produces gametes with half the normal chromosome number.

menarche:

The first menstrual period that normally occurs at puberty.

menstruation (men-stroo-Ā-shun):

The monthly flow of blood that signifies the start of the uterine cycle.

oogenesis (ō-ō-JEN-e-sis):

Ovum production.

ovary:

Female reproductive gland; site of gamete production and hormone secretion.

ovulation (ov-ū-LĀ-shun):

The release of an ovum, following the rupture of the follicle wall.

progesterone (prō-JES-ter-ōn):

The most important progestin secreted by the corpus luteum following ovulation; prepares the uterus for pregnancy.

semen (SĒ-men):

Fluid ejaculate containing spermatozoa and the secretions of accessory glands of the male reproductive tract.

seminiferous tubules (se-mi-NIF-e-rus):

Coiled tubules where sperm production occurs in the testis.

spermatogenesis:

Sperm production.

spermatozoa (sper-ma-tō-ZŌ-a):

Sperm cells; singular: spermatozoon.

testes (TES-tēz):

The male gonads; sites of sperm production and hormone secretion.

testosterone (tes-TOS-te-rōn):

The principal androgen produced by the interstitial cells of the testes.

STUDY OUTLINE

INTRODUCTION

1. Human reproduction is *sexual*. It requires male and female **gametes** (reproductive cells). **Fertilization** is the fusion of a **sperm** from the father and an **ovum** from the mother to create a **zygote** (fertilized egg).

SYSTEM BRIEF

1. The reproductive system includes **gonads**, ducts, accessory glands and organs, and the **external genitalia**.

2. Gametes are produced through **meiosis**. Meiosis produces reproductive cells with half the normal chromosome number. *(Figure 7-1)*

3. In the male the **testes** produce sperm, which are expelled from the body in **semen** during **ejaculation**. Each month, the **ovaries** (gonads) of a sexually mature female produce an egg that travels along **uterine tubes** to reach the **uterus**. The **vagina** connects the uterus with the exterior.

STRUCTURE OF THE MALE REPRODUCTIVE SYSTEM

1. The **spermatozoa** travel along the **epididymis**, the **ductus deferens**, the **ejaculatory** duct, and the **urethra** before leaving the body. Accessory organs (notably the **seminal vesicles**, **prostate gland**, and **bulbourethral glands**) secrete fluids into the ejaculatory ducts and urethra. The **scrotum** encloses the testes, and the **penis** is an erectile organ. *(Figure 7-2)*

THE TESTES

2. Each testis is divided into a series of **lobules**. **Seminiferous tubules** within each lobule are the sites of sperm production. *(Figure 7-3a)*

3. Seminiferous tubules contain stem cells involved in **spermatogenesis**, and **sustentacular cells**, which nourish the developing spermatozoa. *(Figure 7-3b)*

4. Interstitial cells between the seminiferous tubules secrete sex hormones. *(Figure 7-3b)*

5. Each spermatozoon has a **head**, **middle piece**, and **tail**. *(Figure 7-4)*

THE MALE REPRODUCTIVE TRACT

6. From the testis the immature spermatozoa enter the **epididymis**, an elongate tubule. The epididymis aids their maturation and also serves as a recycling center for damaged spermatozoa. Spermatozoa leaving the epididymis are functionally mature, yet immobile.

7. The **ductus deferens,** or *vas deferens*, begins at the epididymis and passes through the inguinal canal as one component of the **spermatic cord**. The junction of the base of the seminal vesicle and the ductus deferens creates the **ejaculatory duct**, which empties into the urethra.

8. The urethra extends from the urinary bladder to the tip of the penis and carries products from both the urinary and reproductive systems.

THE ACCESSORY GLANDS

9. A typical ejaculation releases 2 to 5 ml of semen (an **ejaculate**), which contains 20 million to 100 million sperm per milliliter.

10. Each **seminal vesicle** is an active secretory gland that contributes about 60 percent of the volume of semen; its secretions contain fructose, which is easily metabolized by spermatozoa. These secretions also help neutralize the acids normally found in the urethra and vagina. The **prostate gland** secretes acidic fluids that make up about 30 percent of seminal fluid.

11. Alkaline mucus secreted by the **bulbourethral glands** has lubricating properties.

THE PENIS

12. The skin overlying the **penis** resembles that of the scrotum. Most of the body of the penis consists of three masses of **erectile tissue**. Beneath the superficial fascia there are two **corpora cavernosa** and a single **corpus spongiosum** that surrounds the urethra. Dilation of the erectile tissue with blood produces an **erection**. *(Figure 7-5)*

HORMONES AND MALE REPRODUCTIVE FUNCTION

1. Important regulatory hormones include **FSH** (follicle-stimulating hormone), **LH** (luteinizing hormone, formerly called *ICSH* or interstitial cell–stimulating hormone). Testosterone is the most important androgen.

2. FSH, along with testosterone, promotes spermatogenesis.

3. LH causes the secretion of testosterone by the interstitial cells of the testes.

STRUCTURE OF THE FEMALE REPRODUCTIVE SYSTEM

1. Principal organs of the female reproductive system include the *ovaries, uterine tubes, uterus, vagina,* and *external genitalia. (Figure 7-6)*

THE OVARIES

2. The ovaries are the site of ovum production, or **oogenesis**, which occurs monthly in **ovarian follicles** as part of the **ovarian cycle**.

3. As development proceeds **primordial, primary, secondary,** and **tertiary follicles** develop. At **ovulation**, an ovum is released at the ruptured wall of the ovary. *(Figure 7-7)*

THE UTERINE TUBES

4. Each **uterine tube** has an *infundibulum* with *fimbriae* (projections) that opens into the uterine cavity. For fertilization to occur, the ovum must encounter spermatozoa during the first 12 to 24 hours of its passage from the infundibulum to the uterus. *(Figure 7-8)*

THE UTERUS

5. The uterus provides protection and nutritional support to the developing embryo. Major anatomical landmarks of the uterus include the **body, cervix,** and **uterine cavity**. The uterine wall can be divided into an inner **endometrium** and a muscular **myometrium**. *(Figure 7-8)*

6. A typical 28-day **uterine cycle**, or **menstrual cycle**, begins with the onset of **menstruation** and the destruction of the endometrium. This process of menstruation continues from 1 to 7 days. *(Figure 7-9)*

7. After menstruation, the **proliferative phase** begins and the endometrium undergoes repair and thickens. Menstrual activity begins at **menarche** and continues until **menopause**. *(Figure 7-9)*

THE VAGINA

8. The **vagina** is a muscular tube extending between the uterus and external genitalia. A thin epithelial fold, the **hymen**, may partially block the entrance to the vagina.

THE EXTERNAL GENITALIA

9. The components of the **vulva** include the **vestibule**, **labia minora**, **clitoris**, **labia majora**, and the **lesser** and **greater vestibular glands**. *(Figure 7-10)*

THE MAMMARY GLANDS

10. At birth a newborn infant gains nourishment from milk secreted by maternal **mammary glands**. *(Figure 7-11)*

HORMONES AND THE FEMALE REPRODUCTIVE CYCLE

1. Hormonal regulation of the female reproductive system involves coordination of the ovarian and uterine cycles.

THE OVARIAN CYCLE

2. Estradiol, one of the *estrogens*, is the dominant hormone of the preovulatory period. Ovulation occurs in response to peak levels of estrogen and LH. *(Figure 7-12)*

3. Progesterone, one of the steroid hormones called *progestins*, is the principal hormone of the postovulatory period.

THE UTERINE CYCLE

4. Hormonal changes are responsible for the maintenance of the uterine cycle. *(Figure 7-12)*

HORMONES AND BODY TEMPERATURE

5. Body temperature is slightly lower during the preovulatory period than during the postovulatory period. *(Figure 7-12)*

AGING AND THE REPRODUCTIVE SYSTEM

MENOPAUSE

1. Menopause (the time that ovulation and menstruation cease in women) typically occurs around age 50. Production of FSH and LH rises, while circulating concentrations of estrogen and progesterone decline.

THE MALE CLIMACTERIC

2. During the **male climacteric**, between ages 50 and 60, circulating testosterone levels decline, while levels of FSH and LH rise.

REVIEW QUESTIONS

MATCHING

Match each item in Column A with the most closely related item in Column B. Use letters for answers in the spaces provided.

	Column A	Column B
K	1. gametes	a. production of androgens
J	2. gonads	b. muscular wall of uterus
G	3. interstitial cells	c. high concentration of fructose
A	4. seminal vesicles	d. reproductive organs
L	5. prostate gland	e. secretes thick, sticky, alkaline mucus
D	6. bulbourethral	f. female erectile tissue glands
H	7. prepuce	g. endocrine structure
B	8. corpus luteum	h. uterine lining
E	9. endometrium	i. reproductive cells
C	10. myometrium	j. ovum
F	11. female sex cell	k. milk production
M	12. lactation	l. secretes antibiotic
I	13. clitoris	m. foreskin of penis

MULTIPLE CHOICE

14. Chromosomes are carried within the _____ B _____ of a sperm cell.
    (a) acrosome   (b) head
    (c) middle piece   (d) tail

15. Spermatogenesis (sperm production) occurs in the _____ C _____ .
    (a) ductus deferens
    (b) epididymis
    (c) seminiferous tubules
    (d) prostate gland

16. The role of the epididymis is to _____ A _____ .
    (a) maintain an environment suitable for the maturation of spermatozoa
    (b) produce spermatozoa
    (c) transport spermatozoa to the urethra
    (d) secrete testosterone

17. The hormone that stimulates the growth of ovarian follicles is _____ B _____ .
    (a) estrogen
    (b) FSH
    (c) LH
    (d) progesterone

18. The female structure that corresponds to the male penis is the _____ D _____ .
    (a) vulva
    (b) labia minora
    (c) labia majora
    (d) clitoris

19. At the time of ovulation, the basal body temperature _____ B _____ .
    (a) is not affected
    (b) increases noticeably
    (c) declines sharply
    (d) may increase or decrease a few degrees

20. A sudden surge in LH concentration causes _____ A _____ .
    (a) the onset of menses
    (b) the end of the uterine cycle
    (c) menopause
    (d) breakdown of the follicular wall and ovulation

TRUE/FALSE

_F_ 21. The scrotum is an external sac that holds the testes.

_T_ 22. The inner lining of the uterus is the myometrium.

_T_ 23. Fertilization is the union of the egg and sperm.

_F_ 24. Circumcision is the surgical removal of the prepuce.

_F_ 25. Sperm production in the testes is stimulated by testosterone secreted by the pituitary gland.

_T_ 26. The principal hormone of the postovulatory period is progesterone.

SHORT ESSAY

27. What accessory organs and glands contribute to the composition of semen? What are the functions of each?

28. Using an average duration of 28 days, describe each of the three phases of the uterine cycle.

29. What are the three major functions of the vagina?

30. Diane has an inflammation of the peritoneum (peritonitis), which her doctor says resulted from a urinary tract infection. Why can this situation occur in females but not in males?

✔ ANSWERS TO CONCEPT CHECK QUESTIONS

(p. 168) **1.** The acrosomal cap contains enzymes necessary for fertilization of the ovum. Without these enzymes, fertilization would not occur. **2.** Dilation of the arteries serving the penis will result in erection. **3.** FSH is needed for maintaining a high level of testosterone, which supports the formation of spermatozoa. Low levels of FSH would lead to low levels of testosterone in the seminiferous tubules and thus a lower rate of sperm production and low sperm count.

(p. 173) **1.** Blockage of the uterine tube would cause sterility. **2.** The outer layer of the endometrium is sloughed off during menstruation. **3.** Blockage of a single lactiferous sinus would not interfere with the movement of milk to the nipple because each breast has between 15 and 20 lactiferous sinuses.

(p. 176) **1.** If the LH surge did not occur during an ovulatory cycle, ovulation and corpus luteum formation would not occur. **2.** A decline in the levels of estrogen and progesterone during the uterine, or menstrual cycle, signals the beginning of menstruation.

(p. 177) **1.** At menopause, circulating estrogen levels begin to drop. Estrogen has an inhibitory effect on GnRH and FSH, and as the level of estrogen declines, the levels of FSH and GnRH rise and remain elevated.

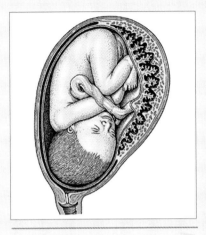

8

DEVELOPMENT AND INHERITANCE

OBJECTIVES

On completion of this chapter, you should be able to:

- Describe the process of fertilization

- List the three prenatal periods, and describe the major events of each period.

- List the three primary germ layers and their roles in forming major body systems.

- Describe the roles of the different membranes of the embryo.

- Describe the adjustments of the mother's organ systems in response to the presence of a developing embryo.

- Discuss the events that occur during labor and delivery.

- Describe the major stages of life after delivery.

- Describe the basic patterns of inheritance of human traits.

A human being develops in the womb for 9 months, grows to maturity in 15 to 20 years, and may live the better part of a century. During that whole time he or she will continue to change. Birth, growth, maturation, aging, and death are all parts of a single, continuous process. That process does not end with the individual, for human beings can pass at least some of their characteristics on to their offspring. Thus each generation gives rise to a new generation that will repeat the same cycle. In this chapter we examine **development**, the complex physical changes that occur from conception to maturity, and **inheritance**, the transfer of characteristics from parent to offspring.

▶ STAGES OF DEVELOPMENT

Development begins at fertilization, or **conception**. The period of **prenatal development** extends from conception to birth. **Postnatal development** begins at birth and continues to maturity. Prenatal development involves two stages. Over the first 2 months, the developing individual is called an **embryo. Embryology** (em-brē-OL-ō-jē) is the study of embryonic development. After 2 months, the developing individual is called a **fetus**. Fetal development begins at the start of the ninth week and continues up to the time of birth.

▶ FERTILIZATION

Fertilization involves the fusion of a sperm cell and an egg cell, each containing 23 chromosomes, to produce a single-celled *zygote* containing 46 chromosomes, the normal number of human chromosomes. As Figure 8-1a shows, normal fertilization occurs in the upper third of the uterine tube, usually within a day of ovulation.

Contractions of uterine muscles and ciliary currents in the uterine tubes aid the passage of sperm to the fertilization site. Of the 200 million spermatozoa introduced into the vagina in a typical ejaculate, only around 10,000 make it past the uterus, and fewer than 100 actually reach the egg. A male with a sperm count below 20 million per milliliter will usually be sterile because too few sperm survive to reach the egg.

Large numbers of sperm are needed for fertilization because when the egg leaves the ovary it is protected by a layer of follicle cells. Sperm cells release enzymes that separate these cells from one another to form an unobstructed passageway to the egg's cell membrane. One sperm cell cannot accomplish this—it takes the combined enzymes of many spermatozoa to clear the way to the egg. When one sperm does contact the egg surface, their cell membranes fuse, and the sperm nucleus is released into the cytoplasm of the egg. This event activates the egg and changes the cell membrane to prevent fertilization by other sperm.

▶ GESTATION

The time spent in prenatal development is known as **gestation** (jes-TĀ-shun). An average gestation period, that is, the length of a normal pregnancy, is 38 weeks or 266 days. For convenience, the gestation period is usually considered as three **trimesters**, each 3 months long.

The **first trimester** is the period of embryonic and early fetal development. During this period the basic components of all of the major organ systems appear.

In the **second trimester** the organs and organ systems complete most of their development. The body proportions change, and by the end of the second trimester the fetus looks distinctively human.

The **third trimester** is characterized by rapid fetal growth. Early in the third trimester most of the major organ systems become fully functional, and an infant born 1 month or even 2 months prematurely has a reasonable chance of survival.

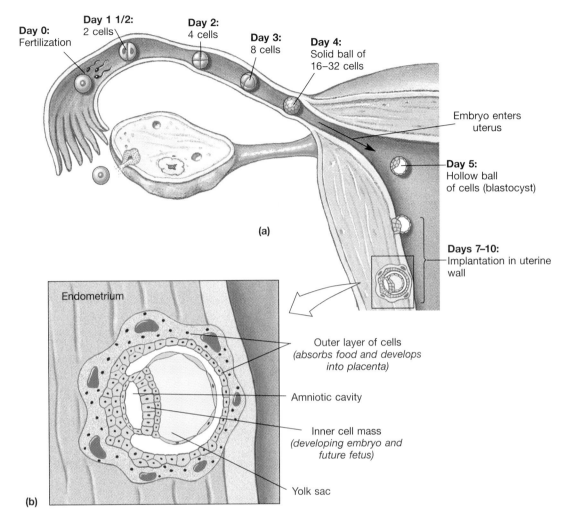

FIGURE 8-1

Fertilization and Implantation.

(a) Cleavage and formation of a blastocyst occurs within the oviduct over the first 5 days after fertilization. **(b)** After implantation, the outer cells absorb nutrients from the enclosing endometrium before forming the placenta. The inner mass of cells, which becomes the body, is separated from the outer cells by the formation of an amniotic cavity and yolk sac.

▶ THE FIRST TRIMESTER

The first trimester is the most dangerous period in prenatal or postnatal life. Only about 40 percent of the eggs that are fertilized produce embryos that survive the first trimester, and an additional number of fetuses enter the second trimester already doomed or deformed by some developmental mistake. Because the developmental events of the first trimester are easily disrupted, pregnant women are usually warned to take great care to avoid drugs or other physical or chemical stresses during this period. Major highlights of the first trimester include (1) embryo formation and the *implantation* of the embryo within the uterine wall, (2) formation of tissues and embryonic membranes, (3) formation of the placenta, and (4) the beginning of organ formation.

EMBRYO FORMATION

After fertilization, the newly formed zygote undergoes a period of rapid cell divisions called **cleavage** (KLĒ-vij). During cleavage, new cells form so rapidly that they do not have time to grow. The first division, resulting in two cells, is completed about 1.5 days after fertilization. This early stage is about the size of the period at the end of this sentence. As Figure 8-1a shows, by day 4, the embryo is a solid ball of cells, and it enters the chamber of the uterus. After 5 days of cleavage a hollow cavity appears, now forming an embryonic stage called a *blastocyst*. The cells making up this stage begin to form into outer and inner groups of cells. The outer layer of cells will be responsible for obtaining food for the *inner cell mass* that will form the developing embryo.

IMPLANTATION

Implantation begins on day 7 as the surface of the blastocyst touches and sticks to the uterine lining (Figure 8-1a). Within the next few days, the blastocyst becomes completely embedded within the uterine wall and loses contact with the uterine cavity; further development occurs entirely within the endometrium. Figure 8-1b shows the implanted blastocyst and the inner cell mass that will develop into the body. The breakdown of uterine gland cells within the endometrium releases glycogen and other nutrients. These nutrients provide the energy needed to support the early stages of embryo formation.

Implantation requires a functional endometrium. As implantation is occurring, some of the cells of the blastocyst begin secreting a hormone called **human chorionic** (kō-rē-ON-ik) **gonadotropin (hCG)**. Because of the hCG, the corpus luteum does not degenerate, and it maintains its production of estrogens and progesterone. As a result, the endometrial lining remains perfectly functional, and menstruation does not occur and terminate the pregnancy. The production of hCG is taken over by the placenta as it develops. The presence of hCG in blood or urine samples provides a reliable indication of pregnancy, and kits sold for the early detection of pregnancy are sensitive for the presence of this hormone.

TISSUE AND MEMBRANE FORMATION

Germ Layers

After implantation, the inner cell mass of the blastocyst becomes organized into three layers of cells. Each of these **germ layers** will form different body tissues. The outer layer is the **ectoderm**, the middle layer is the **mesoderm**, and innermost layer is the **endoderm**. Together, these layers form the body's organs and organ systems.

Briefly, ectoderm gives rise to tissues of the skin and nervous system, mesoderm gives rise to connective and muscle tissues, and the endoderm gives rise to the inner epithelium lining the digestive system. Table 8-1 lists the specific contributions each germ layer makes to the body systems described in earlier chapters.

Extraembryonic Membranes of the Embryo

Four **extraembryonic membranes** start forming outside the embryo after implantation. These are the *yolk sac*, the *amnion*, the *allantois*, and the *chorion*. Figure 8-2 shows these membranes at weeks 4 and 10.

The first of the extraembryonic membranes to appear is the **yolk sac** (see also Figure 8-1b). It aids in the transport of nutrients and is an important early site of blood cell formation. Its role is reduced after the first 6 weeks.

The **amnion** (AM-nē-on) encloses the *amniotic cavity*, which contains fluid that surrounds and cushions the developing embryo and fetus (see also Figure 8-1b). The amnion increases in size during development.

TABLE 8–1   Tissues and Organs Formed by the Primary Germ Layers

Primary Germ Layer	Developmental Contributions to the Body
Ectoderm	*Integumentary system:* epidermis, hair follicles and hairs, nails, and glands communicating with the skin (apocrine and merocrine sweat glands, mammary glands, and sebaceous glands)
	Skeletal system: pharyngeal cartilages of the embryo develop into portions of the sphenoid and hyoid bones, the auditory ossicles, and the styloid processes of the temporal bone
	Nervous system: all neural tissue, including brain and spinal cord
	Endocrine system: pituitary gland and the adrenal medullae
	Respiratory system: mucous epithelium of nasal passageways
	Digestive system: mucous epithelium of mouth and anus, salivary glands
Mesoderm	*Skeletal system:* all components except some ectodermal contributions
	Muscular system: all components
	Endocrine system: adrenal cortex, endocrine tissues of heart, kidneys, and gonads
	Cardiovascular system: all components, including bone marrow
	Lymphatic system: all components
	Urinary system: the kidneys, including the nephrons and the initial portions of the collecting system
	Reproductive system: the gonads and the adjacent portions of the duct systems
	Miscellaneous: the lining of the body cavities (pleural, pericardial, peritoneal) and the connective tissues that support all organ systems
Endoderm	*Endocrine system:* thymus, thyroid, and pancreas
	Respiratory system: respiratory epithelium (except nasal passageways) and associated mucous glands
	Digestive system: mucous epithelium (except mouth and anus), exocrine glands (except salivary glands), liver, and pancreas
	Urinary system: urinary bladder and distal portions of the duct system
	Reproductive system: distal portions of the duct system, stem cells that produce gametes

The **allantois** (a-LAN-tō-is) extends away from the embryo. The allantois accumulates some of the small amount of urine produced by the kidneys during embryonic development. The base of the allantois will form the urinary bladder. The remaining portion of the allantois will form much of the umbilical cord.

The **chorion** (KOR-ē-on) forms outside the amnion. Blood vessels that develop within the chorion provide the nutrients and oxygen needed for continued growth and development. The chorion develops into the *placenta*.

THE PLACENTA

The **placenta** begins its development as projections from the chorion, called *chorionic villi*, first come in contact with maternal tissues (Figure 8-2a). Embryonic blood vessels develop within each of the villi, and circulation through these chorionic blood vessels begins early in the third week of development, when the heart starts beating. These villi continue to enlarge and branch, forming an intricate network within the endometrium. Blood vessels break down and maternal blood flows slowly through these newly opened spaces. Chorionic blood vessels pass close by, and exchange between the embryonic and maternal circulations occurs by diffusion across the chorion.

FIGURE 8-2

Embryonic Membranes.

(a) The developing embryo and its external membranes at the fourth week of growth. **(b)** By week 10, the amnion has expanded greatly, filling the uterine cavity. The embryo, now making the transition to a fetus, is connected to the placenta (formed from the chorion) by the umbilical cord, which contains portions of the allantois and yolk sac membrane, and blood vessels.

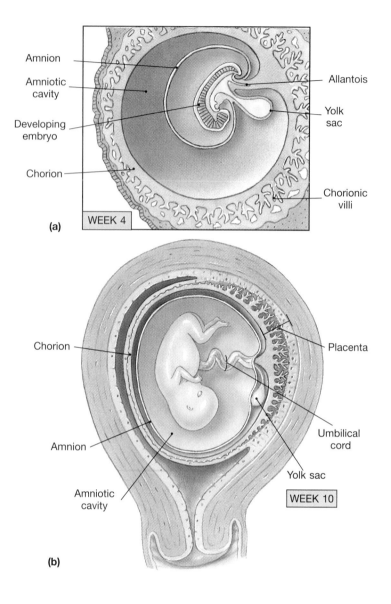

(a) WEEK 4

(b) WEEK 10

Placental Circulation

Figure 8-3 shows the fetal circulation at the placenta near the end of the first trimester. Blood flows to the placenta through the paired **umbilical arteries** and returns in a single **umbilical vein**. The chorionic villi provide the surface area for the exchange of gases, nutrients, and wastes between the fetal and maternal bloodstreams.

Placental Hormones

In addition to its role in the nutrition of the fetus, the placenta acts as an endocrine organ, releasing hormones. These hormones act to prevent menstruation during the pregnancy, prepare the mammary glands to produce milk, and prepare the body for labor and delivery.

Because of the human chorionic gonadotropin (hCG) secreted first by the blastocyst and then by the placenta, the corpus luteum persists for 3 to 4 months and maintains its production of progesterone, which helps keep the endometrium intact. The decline in the corpus luteum does not trigger menstruation because by the end of the first trimester the placenta is also secreting sufficient amounts of progesterone to maintain the endometrial lining and the pregnancy. As the end of the third trimester approaches, estrogen production by the placenta accelerates. The rising estrogen levels play a role in stimulating labor and delivery.

Concept Questions

✔ Why is it important that more than one spermatozoon contact the egg for fertilization to occur?

✔ What is the fate of the inner cell mass of the blastocyst?

✔ Which membrane encloses the fluid surrounding the developing embryo?

✔ What are two important functions of the placenta?

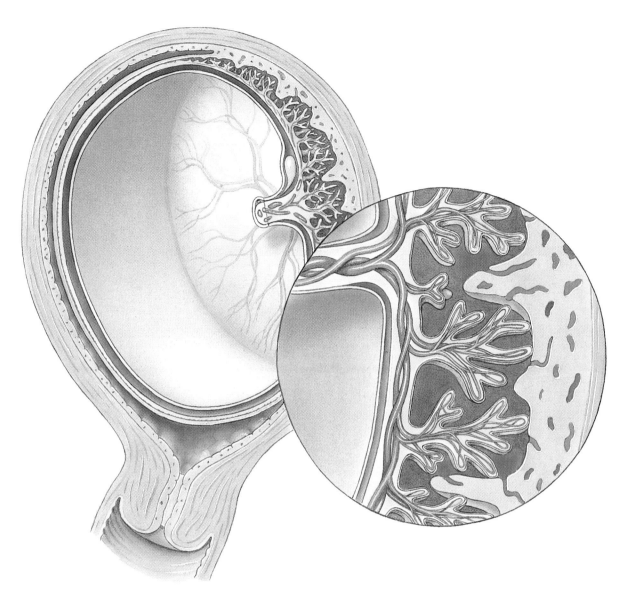

FIGURE 8-3

A Three-Dimensional View of the Placenta.

For clarity the uterus is shown after the embryo has been removed and the umbilical cord cut. Blood flows into the placenta through broken maternal blood arteries. It then flows around fingerlike projections of the chorion (chorionic villi), which contain fetal blood vessels. Fetal blood arrives over paired umbilical arteries and leaves over a single umbilical vein. Maternal blood reenters the venous system of the mother through the broken walls of small uterine veins. Actual mixing of maternal and fetal blood does not occur.

► THE SECOND AND THIRD TRIMESTERS

By the start of the second trimester the basic frameworks of all the major organ systems have formed. Over the next 4 months, the fetus grows from a weight of 0.026 kg (about 1 oz) to a weight of around 0.64 kg (1.4 lb). The changes in body form that occur during the first and second trimesters are shown in Figure 8-4.

During the third trimester, the basic structures of all the organ systems appear, and most become ready for their normal functions. The fetus also gains the most weight during this trimester. In 3 months the fetus puts on around 2.6 kg (5.7 lb), reaching a full-term weight of somewhere near 3.2 kg (7 lb).

FIGURE 8-4

FIGURE 8-4

Growth and Changes in Body Form.

These views of the embryos (4 and 8 weeks) and the fetus (16 weeks) are shown at actual size.

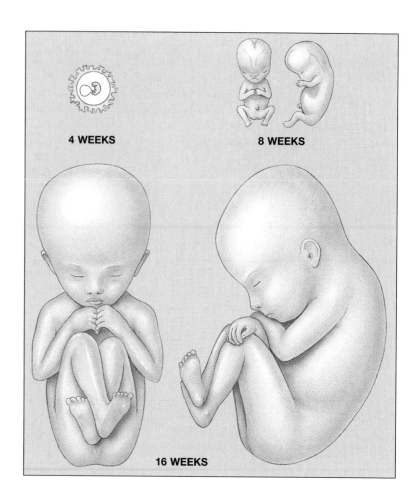

PREGNANCY AND THE MOTHER'S SYSTEMS

The developing fetus is totally dependent on the mother's organ systems for food, oxygen, and waste removal. This means that the mother must absorb enough oxygen, nutrients, and vitamins for herself *and* her fetus, and she must eliminate all the generated wastes. In practical terms, the mother must breathe, eat, and excrete for two. As the fetus grows, the demands on the mother increase, and her body systems must make major adjustments.

Maternal changes during pregnancy include increases in respiratory rate, blood volume, and appetite. Because of increased blood volume, the kidneys must increase their rate of filtration. As a result of increased urine production and the weight of the uterus pressing down on the urinary bladder, pregnant women need to urinate frequently. Changes in the reproductive organs include a tremendous increase in size of the uterus, and by the end of the sixth month of pregnancy, the mammary glands have increased in size and have begun producing and storing their secretions.

CHANGES IN THE UTERUS

At the end of gestation a typical uterus will have grown from 7.5 cm (3 in.) in length and 60 g (2 oz.) in weight to 30 cm (12 in.) in length and 1100 g (2.4 lbs.) in weight. It may then contain almost 5 L of fluid, giving the organ with its contained fetus a total weight of roughly 10 kg (22 lbs.). This remarkable expansion occurs through the enlargement and elongation of existing cells (especially smooth muscle cells) in the uterus.

The tremendous stretching of the uterine wall is associated with a gradual increase in the rates of spontaneous smooth muscle contractions. In the early stages of pregnancy the contractions are short, weak, and painless. The progesterone released by the placenta has an inhibitory, or calming, effect on the uterine smooth muscle, preventing more extensive and powerful contractions.

Three major factors oppose the calming action of progesterone:

1. **Rising estrogen levels**. Estrogens, also produced by the placenta, increase the sensitivity of the uterine smooth muscles and make contractions more likely. Throughout pregnancy the effects of progesterone are dominant, but as the time of delivery approaches, estrogen production accelerates, and the uterine muscles become more sensitive to stimulation.
2. Rising oxytocin levels. **Rising oxytocin levels stimulate an increase in the force and frequency of uterine contractions. Release of oxytocin by the pituitary gland is stimulated by high estrogen levels and by stretching of the uterine cervix.**
2. **Prostaglandin production**. In addition to estrogens and oxytocin, uterine tissues late in pregnancy produce prostaglandins that stimulate smooth muscle contractions.

After 9 months of gestation, **labor contractions** begin in the muscles of the uterine wall. Once begun, the contractions continue until delivery has been completed.

▶ LABOR AND DELIVERY

The goal of labor is the forcible expulsion of the fetus, a process known as **parturition** (par-tū-RISH-un), or **birth**. During labor, each contraction begins near the top of the uterus and sweeps in a wave toward the cervix. These contractions are strong and occur at regular intervals. As the birth nears, the contractions increase in force and frequency, changing the position of the fetus and moving it toward the cervical canal.

STAGES OF LABOR

Labor has traditionally been divided into three stages (Figure 8-5), the *dilation stage*, the *expulsion stage*, and the *placental stage*.

The Dilation Stage

The **dilation stage** begins with the onset of labor, as the cervix dilates completely and the fetus begins to slide down the cervical canal. This stage may last 8 or more hours, but during this period the labor contractions occur at intervals of once every 10 to 30 minutes. Late in the process the amnion usually ruptures, releasing the amniotic fluid. This event is sometimes referred to as having the "water break."

The Expulsion Stage

The **expulsion stage** begins after the cervix dilates completely, pushed open by the approaching fetus. Expulsion continues until the fetus has totally emerged from the vagina, a period usually lasting less than 2 hours. The arrival of the newborn infant into the outside world represents the birth, or **delivery**.

If the vaginal entrance is too small to permit the passage of the fetus and there is acute danger of perineal tearing, the entryway may be temporarily enlarged by making an incision through the perineal musculature between the vagina and anus. After delivery, this **episiotomy** (e-pē-zē-O-to-mē) can be repaired with sutures, a much simpler procedure than dealing with a potentially extensive perineal tear. If unexpected complications arise during the dilation or expulsion stages, the infant may be removed by **cesarean section,** or "C-section." In such cases an incision is made through the abdominal wall, and the uterus is opened just enough to allow passage of the infant's head, which is the widest part of its body.

FIGURE 8-5

The Stages of Labor.

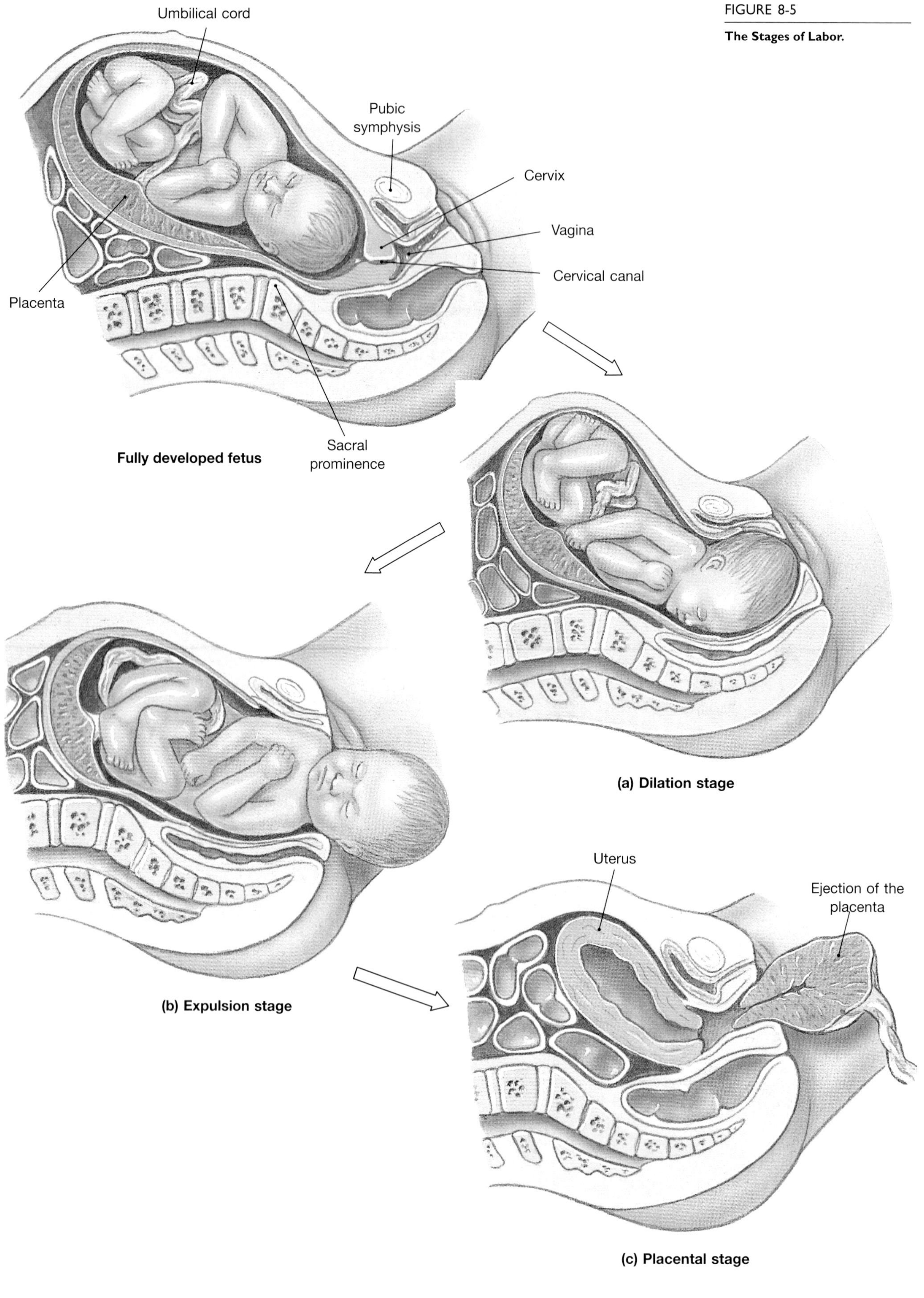

Umbilical cord

Pubic symphysis

Cervix

Vagina

Cervical canal

Placenta

Fully developed fetus

Sacral prominence

(a) Dilation stage

(b) Expulsion stage

Uterus

Ejection of the placenta

(c) Placental stage

The Placental Stage

During the third, or **placental**, stage of labor the muscle tension builds in the walls of the partially empty uterus, and the organ gradually decreases in size. This uterine contraction tears the connections between the endometrium and the placenta. Usually within an hour after delivery the placental stage ends with the ejection of the placenta, or "*afterbirth*." The disconnection of the placenta is accompanied by a loss of blood, perhaps as much as 500 to 600 ml, but because the maternal blood volume has increased during pregnancy the loss can be tolerated without difficulty.

Concept Questions

✔ Why does the rate of filtration at the mother's kidneys increase during pregnancy?

✔ By what process does the uterus increase in size during pregnancy?

✔ What effect would a decrease in progesterone have on the uterus during late pregnancy?

MULTIPLE BIRTHS

Multiple births (twins, triplets, quadruplets, and so forth) may occur for several reasons. The ratio of twin to single births in the U. S. population is 1:89. About 70 percent of all twins are **fraternal**, and the other 30 percent are **identical**. Fraternal twins are produced when two eggs are fertilized at the same time, forming two separate zygotes. Fraternal twins may be of the same or different genders. Identical twins result when cells from one zygote separate during an early stage of development. Such individuals have the same genetic makeup and are always the same gender (either both male or both female). Triplets and larger multiples can result from the same processes that produce twins.

▶ POSTNATAL DEVELOPMENT

Development does not stop at birth. In the course of postnatal development each individual passes through a number of **life stages**, that is, the neonatal period, *infancy, childhood, adolescence*, and *maturity*.

THE NEONATAL PERIOD, INFANCY, AND CHILDHOOD

The **neonatal period** extends from the moment of birth to 1 month thereafter. **Infancy** then continues to 2 years of age, and **childhood** lasts until puberty begins. Two major events are under way during these developmental stages.

1. The major organ systems other than those associated with reproduction become fully operational and gradually acquire the functional characteristics of adult structures.
2. The individual grows rapidly, and there are significant changes in body proportions.

Pediatrics is the medical specialty that focuses on the period of life from birth through childhood and adolescence.

The Neonatal Period

A variety of structural and functional changes occur as the fetus becomes a newborn infant, or **neonate**. Before delivery, the transfer of dissolved gases, nutrients, waste products, hormones, and antibodies occurred across the placenta. At birth the newborn infant must become relatively self-sufficient, with the processes of respiration, digestion, and excretion performed by its own organs and organ systems.

A newborn infant has little ability to control its body temperature, particularly in the first few days after delivery. For this reason newborn infants are usually kept bundled up in warm coverings. As the infant grows larger, it adds on fatty tissue which acts as an insulating blanket, its metabolic rate also rises, and its thermoregulatory abilities become better developed.

The nutritional needs of an infant are normally best met by the milk produced by the mammary glands. By the end of the sixth month of pregnancy the mammary glands are fully developed, and the gland cells begin producing a secretion known as **colostrum** (ko-LOS-trum). Colostrum, which is provided to the infant during the first 2 or 3 days of life, contains relatively more proteins and far less fat than milk. Many of the proteins are antibodies that help the infant fight off infections until its own immune system becomes functional.

FIGURE 8-6
_____

The Milk Let-down Reflex.

3. Stimulation of neurons
in the hypothalmus

Posterior
pituitary

4. Oxytocin released

5. Milk ejected

1. Receptors in
nipples stimulated

2. Impulses sent to
spinal cord

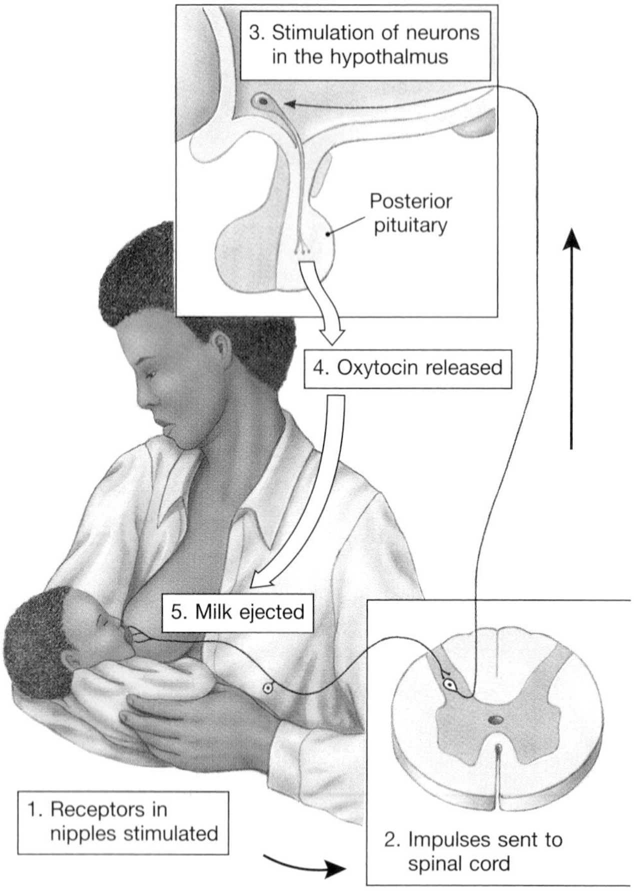

As colostrum production declines, milk production increases. Milk is a mixture of water, proteins, amino acids, lipids, sugars, and salts. It also contains large quantities of *lysozymes*, enzymes with antibiotic properties.

The actual secretion of the mammary glands is triggered when the newborn begins to suck on the nipple. Stimulation of touch receptors there leads to the release of oxytocin at the posterior pituitary. Oxytocin causes cells within the lactiferous ducts and sinuses to contract. This results in the ejection of milk, or *milk let-down* (Figure 8-6). The milk let-down reflex continues to function until *weaning* occurs, typically 1 to 2 years after birth.

Infancy and Childhood

The most rapid growth occurs during prenatal development, and after delivery the relative rate of growth continues to decline. Postnatal growth during infancy and childhood occurs under the direction of circulating hormones, notably growth hormone from the pituitary, adrenal steroid hormones, and thyroid hormones. These hormones affect each tissue and organ in specific ways, depending on the sensitivities of the individual cells. As a result, growth does not occur uniformly, and as Figure 8-7 shows, the body proportions gradually change.

ADOLESCENCE AND MATURITY

Adolescence begins at **puberty**, when three events interact to promote increased hormone production and sexual maturation:

1. The hypothalamus increases its production of *gonadotropin-releasing hormone* (*GnRH*).
2. The anterior pituitary becomes more sensitive to the presence of GnRH, and there is a rapid elevation in the circulating levels of FSH and LH.
3. Ovarian or testicular cells become more sensitive to FSH and LH. These changes initiate the production of male or female gametes and sex hormones that stimulate the appearance of secondary sexual characteristics and behaviors.

In the years that follow, the continual secretion of estrogens or testosterone maintains these sexual characteristics. In addition, the combination of sex hormones and growth hormone, adrenal steroids, and thyroxine leads to a sudden acceleration in the growth rate. The timing of the increase in size varies between the sexes, corresponding to different ages at the onset of puberty. In girls the growth rate is maximum between ages 10 and 13, whereas boys grow most rapidly between ages 12 and 15. Growth continues at a slower pace until ages 18 to 21.

Maturity is often associated with the end of growth in the late teens or early twenties. Although development ends at maturity, functional changes continue. These changes are part of the process of aging, or **senescence**. Aging reduces the efficiency and capabilities of the individual, and even in the absence of other factors will ultimately lead to death.

Concept Questions

✔ How is colostrum different from normal human milk?

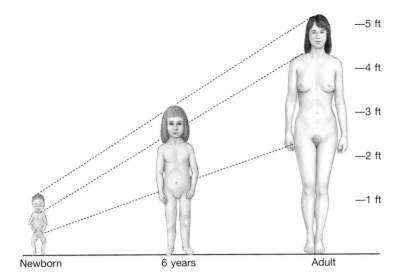

FIGURE 8-7

Growth and Postnatal Changes in Body Form.

Notice the changes in body form and proportions as development proceeds. For example, the head, which contains the brain and sense organs, is relatively large at birth.

—5 ft

—4 ft

—3 ft

—2 ft

—1 ft

Newborn   6 years   Adult

▶ INHERITANCE AND GENES

"People-watching," one of the commonest activities at shopping malls, provides us with abundant examples of the range of human characteristics, or *traits*. Family groups are often obvious because they have similar traits, especially facial features such as eye shape and color. These are examples of inherited traits that are genetically passed on from one generation to the next. The study of *heredity*, or how different traits are inherited, is called **genetics**.

Except for sex cells (sperm and eggs), every cell in the body carries copies of the original 46 chromosomes present in the fertilized egg or zygote. Through development and differentiation, the instructions contained within the genes of the chromosomes are expressed in many different ways. No single living cell or tissue makes use of all its genetic information. For example, in muscle cells the genes important for contractile proteins are active, whereas a different set of genes is operating in neurons.

GENES AND CHROMOSOMES

Chromosomes contain DNA, and genes are segments of DNA. Each gene carries the information needed to direct the synthesis of a specific protein.

The 46 chromosomes of body cells occur in pairs, 23 pairs in all. One member of each pair was contributed by the sperm, and the other by the egg. Twenty-two of those pairs affect only somatic, or general body, characteristics such as hair color or skin pigmentation. The chromosomes of the 23rd pair are called the *sex chromosomes* because they determine whether a person will be male or female.

Except for the sex chromosomes (which are discussed later), both chromosomes in a pair have the same structure and carry genes that affect the same traits. If one member of the chromosome pair contains three genes in a row, with number 1 determining hair color, number 2 eye color, and number 3 skin pigmentation, the other chromosome will carry genes affecting the same traits, and in the same sequence.

Both chromosomes of a pair may carry the same form of a gene for a particular trait. For example, if a zygote receives a gene for curly hair from the sperm and one for curly hair from the egg, the individual will have curly hair. Because the chromosomes that make up a pair have different origins, one paternal and the other maternal, they do not have to carry the same forms of a gene. In that case the trait that is expressed in the individual will be determined by how the two genes interact.

A gene for a particular trait is said to be **dominant** if it is expressed regardless of the instructions carried by the other gene. A **recessive** gene is one that is expressed in the individual only if it is present on both chromosomes of a pair. For example, the albino skin condition is characterized by an inability to synthesize the yellow-brown pigment *melanin*. A single dominant gene determines normal skin coloration; two recessive genes must be present to produce an albino individual.

Not every gene for a trait can be neatly characterized as dominant or recessive. Some that can are included in Table 8-2. If you restrict attention to these genes it is possible to predict the characteristics of individuals based on those of their parents.

Polygenic inheritance involves interactions between two or more different genes. For example, the determination of eye color and skin color involves several genes. Polygenic inheritance is also involved in several important disorders, including hypertension (high blood pressure) and coronary artery disease. In these cases the particular genetic composition of the individual does not by itself determine the onset of the disease. Instead, the genes establish a susceptibility to particular environmental influences. Only if the individual is exposed to these influences will the disease develop. This means that not every individual with the genetic tendency for a disorder will actually get it. This makes it difficult to track polygenic conditions through successive generations and predict which family members might be affected. However, because many inherited polygenic conditions are *likely* but not *guaranteed* to occur, steps can often be taken to prevent the development of disease. For example, hypertension may be prevented or reduced by controlling diet and fluid volume, and coronary artery disease may be prevented by lowering the levels of cholesterol circulating in the blood.

Sex Chromosomes

The **sex chromosomes** determine the genetic sex of the individual. Unlike other chromosomal pairs, the sex chromosomes are not necessarily identical in appearance and in the number of genes they contain.

There are two different sex chromosomes, an **X chromosome** and a **Y chromosome**. The Y chromosome is much smaller than the X chromosome and contains fewer genes. The normal male chromosome pair is *XY*, and the female pair is *XX*. The eggs produced by a woman will always carry

TABLE 8–2   Different Patterns of Inheritance

Dominant Traits

Normal skin coloration
Brachdactyly (short fingers)
Free earlobes
Curly hair
Presence of Rh factor on red blood cell membranes
Presence of A and/or B antigens on red blood cell membranes (in codominance inheritance, both dominant genes may be expressed)

Recessive Traits

Albinism
Blond hair
Red hair
Lack of A, B antigens on red blood cell membranes (Type O blood)
Inability to roll the tongue into a U-shape

Sex-Linked Traits

Color blindness

Polygenic Traits

Eye color
Hair color other than blond or red

chromosome *X*, while a sperm can carry either chromosome *X* or *Y*. As a result, during fertilization, *Y*-carrying sperm will produce a male, and *X*-carrying sperm will produce a female. Figure 8-8 is a photograph of all the chromosomes of a normal male. Note the size difference between the Y and the X chromosomes.

The X chromosome also carries genes that affect body structures. The traits controlled by these genes are usually expressed because in most cases there are no corresponding genes on the Y chromosome. Such traits are known as **sex-linked** traits because the responsible genes are located on the sex chromosomes. The best known sex-linked characteristics are associated with noticeable diseases or disorders.

The inheritance of color blindness is sex-linked. A relatively common form of color blindness is associated with the presence of a dominant or recessive gene

FIGURE 8-8

Chromosomes of a Normal Male.

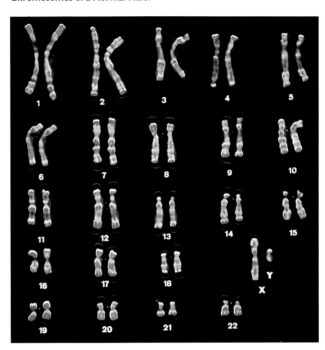

on the X chromosome. Normal color vision is determined by the presence of a dominant gene, *C*, and color blindness results from the presence of the recessive gene *c*. A woman, with her two X chromosomes, can have two dominant genes, *CC*, or one dominant and one recessive, *Cc*, and still have normal color vision. Such an individual (*Cc*) with normal vision and a recessive gene is called a **carrier**. She will be color-blind only if she carries two recessive alleles, *cc*. But a male has only one X chromosome, so whatever that chromosome carries will determine whether he has normal color vision or is color-blind.

A number of other disorders are also X-linked traits, including certain forms of *hemophilia, diabetes insipidus*, and *muscular dystrophy*. In several instances, advances in molecular genetic techniques make it possible to locate specific genes on the X chromosome. This technique provides a relatively direct method of screening for the presence of a particular condition before the symptoms appear and even before birth.

Concept Questions

✔ The ability to roll your tongue is a dominant trait. Would a person with a dominant and recessive gene for that trait be able to roll his tongue? Why, or why not?

✔ Joe has three daughters and complains that it's his wife's fault that he doesn't have any sons. What would you tell him?

☤ Clinical Note

The Human Genome Project

The study of human genetics has long been based on inherited disorders and how they are passed on in families. Because 20 to 25 years can often pass between generations, progress in learning how such disorders are inherited has been generally slow. However, increasing numbers of genes responsible for inherited disorders are now being identified and their locations pinpointed to specific chromosomes. Such accomplishments are due to the activities associated with the **Human Genome Project**. This project, funded by the National Institutes of Health and the Department of Energy, is attempting to identify the complete set of genes, or *genome*, contained in human chromosomes. The project began in October 1990 and was expected to take 10 to 15 years. Progress has been more rapid than expected, and it may actually take considerably less time.

What has been found so far? First, the locations of genes on eight chromosomes have been determined, or mapped, completely, and preliminary maps have been made for all other chromosomes. Over 7400 genes have now been identified. Although a significant number, this is only a small fraction of the estimated 100,000 genes in the human genome. The specific genes responsible for more than 60 inherited disorders have also been identified. Because of these discoveries, *genetic screening*, a technique that can identify specific genes on chromosomes, is now available for many of these conditions.

CHAPTER REVIEW SECTION

KEY WORDS

blastocyst (BLAS-tō-sist):

Early stage in the developing embryo, consisting of an outer cell layer and an inner cell mass.

development:

Growth and expansion from a lower to higher stage of complexity.

embryo (EM-brē-o):

Developmental stage beginning at fertilization and ending at the start of the third developmental month.

fertilization:

Fusion of egg and sperm to form a zygote.

fetus:

Developmental stage lasting from the start of the third developmental month to delivery.

gestation (jes-TĀ-shun):

The period of development within the uterus.

implantation (im-plan-TĀ-shun):

The migration of a blastocyst into the uterine wall.

lactation:

The production of milk by the mammary glands.

parturition (par-tū-RISH-un):

Childbirth, delivery.

placenta:

A complex structure in the uterine wall that permits diffusion between the fetal and maternal circulatory systems; forms the *afterbirth*.

pregnancy:

The condition of having a developing embryo or fetus in the body.

puberty:

Period of rapid growth, sexual maturation, and the appearance of secondary sexual characteristics; usually occurs between the ages of 10 and 15.

STUDY OUTLINE

INTRODUCTION

1. **Development** is the gradual modification of physical characteristics from conception to maturity. **Inheritance** refers to the transfer of parental characteristics to the next generation.

STAGES OF DEVELOPMENT

1. **Prenatal development** occurs before birth and includes development of the **embryo** and **fetus**; **postnatal development** begins at birth and continues to maturity.

FERTILIZATION

1. Fertilization involves the fusion of two gametes, an egg (ovum) and sperm cell.
2. Fertilization normally occurs in the uterine tube within a day after ovulation. *(Figure 8-1a)*
3. The acrosomal caps of the spermatozoa release enzymes that separate follicular cells around the ovum, exposing its membrane. When a single spermatozoon contacts that membrane, fertilization follows.

GESTATION

1. The 9-month (266 days) **gestation period** can be divided into three **trimesters**.

THE FIRST TRIMESTER

1. Major events of this period include (1) cell division and the formation of the embryo, (2) *implantation* of the embryo within the uterine wall, (3) formation of tissues and embryonic membranes, (4) formation of the placenta, and (5) the beginning of organ formation.

EMBRYO FORMATION

2. **Cleavage** subdivides the cytoplasm of the zygote in a series of mitotic divisions; the zygote becomes a **blastocyst**. Its inner cell mass develops into the individual. *(Figure 8-1b)*

IMPLANTATION

3. **Implantation** occurs about 7 days after fertilization as the blastocyst adheres and begins to burrow into the uterine lining. *(Figure 8-1b)*
4. Breakdown of the endometrium is prevented as outer cells of the blastocyst begin secreting a hormone called **human chorionic** (kō-rē-ON-ik) **gonadotropin (hCG)**.

TISSUE AND MEMBRANE FORMATION

5. After implantation, the embryo is composed of three cell layers, an **endoderm**, **ectoderm**, and intervening **mesoderm**. It is from these **germ layers** that the body systems form. *(Table 8-1)*
6. These germ layers help form four **extraembryonic membranes**: the *yolk sac, amnion, allantois,* and *chorion. (Figure 8-2)*
7. The **yolk sac** is an important site of blood cell formation. The **amnion** encloses fluid that surrounds and cushions the developing embryo. The base of the **allantois** later gives rise to the urinary bladder. The **chorion** provides a means of nutrient uptake for the embryo.

THE PLACENTA

8. *Chorionic villi* extend outward into the maternal tissues, forming an intricate, branching network through which maternal blood flows. As development proceeds, the **umbilical cord** connects the fetus to the placenta. *(Figure 8-3)*
9. The placenta also synthesizes hormones such as hCG, estrogens, and progesterones.

THE SECOND AND THIRD TRIMESTERS

1. The organ systems form during the second trimester and become functional during the third trimester. Additionally, the fetus enlarges and becomes more recognizably human. *(Figure 8-4)*

PREGNANCY AND THE MOTHER'S SYSTEMS

2. The developing fetus is totally dependent on maternal organs for nourishment, respiration, and waste removal. Maternal adaptations include increased blood volume, respiratory rate, nutrient intake, and kidney filtration.

CHANGES IN THE UTERUS

3. Progesterone produced by the placenta has an inhibitory effect on uterine muscles; its calming action is opposed by estrogens, oxytocin, and prostaglandins. At some point multiple factors interact to produce **labor contractions** in the uterine wall.

LABOR AND DELIVERY

1. The goal of labor is **parturition** (forcible expulsion of the fetus).

STAGES OF LABOR

2. Labor can be divided into three stages: the **dilation stage**, **expulsion stage**, and **placental stage**. *(Figure 8-5)*

MULTIPLE BIRTHS

3. **Identical** twins are always the same gender. **Fraternal** twins may be the same or different genders.

POSTNATAL DEVELOPMENT

1. Postnatal development involves a series of **life** stages, including the **neonatal period**, **infancy**, **childhood**, **adolescence**, and **maturity**. **Senescence** begins at maturity and ends in the death of the individual.

THE NEONATAL PERIOD, INFANCY, AND CHILDHOOD

2. The **neonatal period** extends from birth to 1 month of age. **Infancy** then continues to 2 years of age, and **childhood** lasts until puberty commences. During these stages major organ systems (other than reproductive) become operational and gradually acquire adult characteristics, and the individual grows rapidly.
3. In the transition from fetus to **neonate** the respiratory, circulatory, digestive, and urinary systems begin functioning independently. The newborn must also begin regulating its body temperature (thermoregulation).
4. Mammary glands produce protein-rich **colostrum** during the infant's first few days and then converts to milk production. These secretions are released as a result of the *milk let-down reflex*. *(Figure 8-6)*
5. Body proportions gradually change during postnatal development. *(Figure 8-7)*

ADOLESCENCE AND MATURITY

6. Adolescence begins at **puberty** when (1) the hypothalamus increases its production of GnRH, (2) circulating levels of FSH and LH rise rapidly, and (3) ovarian or testicular cells become more sensitive to FSH and LH. These changes initiate the production of gametes and sex hormones, and a sudden acceleration in growth rate.

INHERITANCE AND GENES

1. Every body cell, except sex cells, carries copies of the original 46 chromosomes in the zygote. The chromosomes carry the genetic information.

GENES AND CHROMOSOMES

2. Every somatic human cell contains 23 pairs of chromosomes. Of these, 22 pairs affect only somatic, or general body, characteristics. The 23rd pair of chromosomes are the **sex chromosomes** because they determine the genetic sex of the individual.
3. Chromosomes contain DNA, and genes are functional segments of DNA. Both chromosomes of a pair may carry the same or different forms of a particular gene.
4. The different forms of a gene are considered dominant or recessive depending upon how their traits are expressed. *(Table 8-2)*

5. In **simple inheritance** an individual's traits are determined by interactions between a single pair of genes. **Polygenic inheritance** involves interactions among gene pairs on several chromosomes.

6. There are two different sex chromosomes, an **X chromosome** and a **Y chromosome.** The normal male sex chromosome complement is XY; that of females is XX. The X chromosome carries **sex-linked** genes that affect body structures but have no corresponding genes on the Y chromosome. *(Figure 8-8)*

REVIEW QUESTIONS

MATCHING

Match each item in Column A with the most closely related item in Column B. Use letters for answers in the spaces provided.

	Column A	Column B
K	1. gestation	a. blastocyst formation
S	2. cleavage	b. ejection of placenta
M	3. ectoderm	c. forms connective and muscle tissues
C	4. mesoderm	d. indication of pregnancy
A	5. human chorionic gonadotropin	e. embryo-maternal circulatory exchange
D	6. birth	f. XY
A	7. episiotomy	g. time of prenatal development
H	8. afterbirth	h. XX
F	9. senescence	i. perineal musculature incision
C	10. neonate	j. newborn infant
E	11. male sex chromosomes	k. process of aging
M	12. female sex chromosomes	l. parturition
B	13. chorion	m. gives rise to skin and nervous tissue

MULTIPLE CHOICE

14. A zygote forms in the ___A___ .
    (a) vagina
    (b) uterine (fallopian) tube
    (c) ovary
    (e) uterus

15. An embryo becomes a fetus after ___D___ weeks of development.
    (a) 2   (b) 4
    (c) 8   (d) 16

16. The gradual modification of body structures during the period from conception to maturity is ___C___ .
    (a) development   (b) differentiation
    (c) parturition   (d) senescence

17. The membrane that encloses the fluid that surrounds and cushions the developing embryo and fetus is the ___b___ .
    (a) chorion   (b) amnion
    (c) yolk sac   (d) allantois

186. Increased hormone production and sexual maturation during adolescence result from the activity of the ___c___ .
    (a) hypothalamus
    (b) anterior pituitary
    (c) ovaries and testes
    (d) all the above are correct

19. Milk let-down is associated with ___A___ .
    (a) reflex action triggered by suckling
    (b) the release of placental hormones
    (c) implantation
    (d) weaning

20. The normal number of chromosomes in our body cells is ___b___ .
    (a) 23   (b) 24
    (c) 46   (d) 48

TRUE/FALSE

___F___ 21. Implantation refers to the formation of germ layers.

___F___ 22. The first blood cells of the embryo are formed by the yolk sac.

___F___ 23. An individual's gender is determined at birth.

___T___ 24. If both maternal and paternal copies of a gene must be present to express a trait, the genes are recessive.

___T___ 25. Delivery occurs during the third stage of labor.

___F___ 26. The hormone oxytocin stimulates strong contractions of the uterus.

SHORT ESSAY

27. Describe the three life stages that occur between birth and approximately age 10.

28. Identify the three stages of labor, and describe each of their characteristic events.

29. Discuss the changes that occur in the mother's systems during pregnancy.

30. Explain why more men than women are color-blind.

✔ Answers to Concept Check Questions

(p. 220)   **1.** Multiple sperm are required for fertilization because one sperm does not contain enough enzyme to break down the connections between the follicle cells surrounding the egg cell. However, once the egg cell membrane is exposed, only one sperm cell will fertilize the egg. **2.** The inner cell mass of the blastocyst develops into the body. **3.** The amniotic membrane is the extraembryonic membrane that encloses the fluid and developing embryo. **4.** Placental functions include (1) supplying the developing fetus with a route for gas exchange, nutrient transfer, and waste product elimination, and (2) producing hormones that affect the mother's body systems.

(p. 225)   **1.** The glomerular filtration rate increases because of an increase in blood volume. The increased filtration rate speeds up the excretion of the additional metabolic wastes generated by the fetus. **2.** The uterus increases in size as smooth muscle cells enlarge and elongate. **3.** Progesterone decreases uterine contractions. A decrease in progesterone at any time during the pregnancy can lead to uterine contractions and, in late pregnancy, labor.

(p. 226)   **1.** Colostrum contains less fat and more proteins than normal human milk. Many of the proteins are antibodies that help the infant fight off infections prior to the functional development of its own immune system.

(p. 229)   **1.** A person with a dominant and a recessive gene would be able to roll their tongue. As long as a dominant gene is present it will be expressed. **2.** There are two different sex chromosomes, an X chromosome and a Y chromosome. The normal male chromosome pair is XY, and the female pair is XX. The eggs produced by Joe's wife will always carry an X, and the sperm produced during meiosis by Joe may carry X or Y. As a result, the sex of Joe's children depends on which type of sperm cell fertilizes the egg cell.

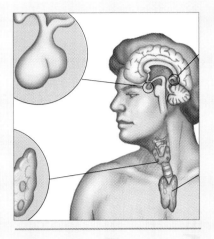

MEDICAL TERMINOLOGY OF THE ENDOCRINE SYSTEM

OBJECTIVES

On completion of this chapter, you should be able to:

- Describe the primary glands of the endocrine system.
- State the primary functions of the endocrine glands.
- Describe the secondary glands of the endocrine system.
- State the vital function of the endocrine system.
- Identify and state the functions of the various hormones secreted by the endocrine glands.
- Analyze, build, spell, and pronounce medical words that relate to surgical procedures and pathology.
- Identify and give the meaning of selected vocabulary words.
- Identify and define selected abbreviations.
- Review Drug Highlights presented in this chapter.
- Provide the description of diagnostic and laboratory tests related to the endocrine system.
- Successfully complete the study and review section.

► ANATOMY AND PHYSIOLOGY OVERVIEW

The endocrine system consists of primary and secondary glands of internal secretion. The primary glands are the *pituitary (hypophysis), pineal, thyroid, parathyroid, pancreas, adrenals (suprarenals), ovaries* and *testes.* The secondary glands of the endocrine system are the thymus, the placenta during pregnancy, and the gastrointestinal mucosa. The endocrine glands are ductless and secrete their hormones directly into the bloodstream. The vital function of the endocrine system involves the production and regulation of chemical substances called *hormones,* which play an essential role in maintaining homeostasis (Fig. 9–1 and Table 9–1).

The word *hormone* is derived from the Greek language and means *to excite* or *to urge on.* A hormone is a chemical transmitter that is released in small amounts and transported via the bloodstream to a target organ or other cells. There are many hormones in the body, and their release is controlled by nerve stimulation. The release of hormones is either stimulated or retarded according to the feedback system regulating supply and demand. Hormones are either proteins, peptides, derivatives of amino acids, or steroids that are synthesized from cholesterol.

The endocrine system and the nervous system closely interact with each other. The *hypothalamus,* located in the brain, plays a vital role in regulating endocrine functions as it synthesizes and secretes releasing hormones such as thyrotropin-releasing hormone (TRH) and gonadotropin-releasing hormone (GnRH) and releasing factors such as corticotropin-releasing factor (CRF), growth hormone-releasing factor (GHRF), prolactin-releasing factor (PRF), and melanocyte-stimulating hormone-releasing factor (MRF). The hypothalamus also synthesizes and secretes release-inhibiting

THE ENDOCRINE SYSTEM

GLAND	PRIMARY FUNCTIONS
Pituitary (Hypophysis)	Master gland; regulatory effects on other endocrine glands
Anterior lobe	Influences growth and sexual development, thyroid function, adrenocortical function; regulates skin pigmentation
Posterior lobe	Stimulates the reabsorption of water and elevates blood pressure; stimulates the release of milk and the uterus to contract during labor, delivery, and parturition
Pineal	Helps regulate the release of gonadotropin and controls body pigmentation
Thyroid	Vital role in metabolism and regulates the body's metabolic processes, influences bone and calcium metabolism, helps maintain plasma calcium homeostasis
Parathyroid	Maintenance of a normal serum calcium level, plays a role in the metabolism of phosphorus
Pancreas (Islets of Langerhans)	Regulates blood glucose levels and plays a vital role in metabolism of carbohydrates, proteins, and fats
Adrenals (Suprarenals)	
Adrenal cortex	Regulates carbohydrate metabolism, anti-inflammatory effect; helps body cope during stress; regulates electrolyte and water balance; promotes development of male characteristics
Adrenal medulla	Synthesizes, secretes, and stores catecholamines (dopamine, epinephrine, norepinephrine)
Ovaries	Promote growth, development, and maintenance of female sex organs
Testes	Promote growth, development, and maintenance of male sex organs

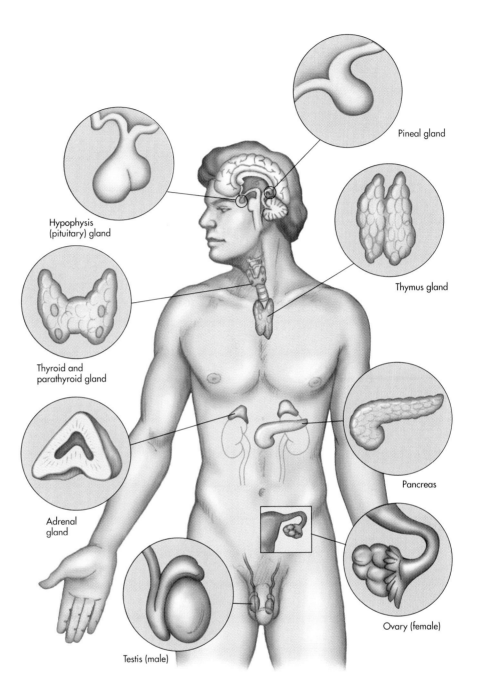

Hypophysis (pituitary) gland

Thyroid and parathyroid gland

Adrenal gland

Testis (male)

Pineal gland

Thymus gland

Pancreas

Ovary (female)

FIGURE 9–1

The primary glands of the endocrine system.

hormones such as growth hormone release-inhibiting hormone. It also produces release-inhibiting factors such as prolactin release-inhibiting factor (PIF) and melanocyte-stimulating hormone release-inhibiting factor (MIF). The hypothalamus also exerts direct nervous control over the anterior pituitary and the adrenal medulla and controls the secretion of the hormones epinephrine and norepinephrine.

TABLE 9–1   Summary of the Endocrine Glands, Hormones, and Hormonal Functions

Endocrine Glands	Hormones	Hormonal Functions
Pituitary Gland		
Anterior lobe	Growth hormone (GH)	Growth and development of bones, muscles, and other organs
	Adrenocorticotropin hormone (ACTH)	Growth and development of the adrenal cortex
	Thyroid-stimulating hormone (TSH)	Growth and development of the thyroid gland
	Follicle-stimulating hormone (FSH)	Stimulates the growth of ovarian follicles in the female and sperm in the male
	Luteinizing hormone (LH)	Stimulates the development of the corpus luteum in the female and the production of testosterone in the male
	Prolactin hormone (PRL)	Stimulates the mammary glands to produce milk after childbirth
	Melanocyte-stimulating hormone (MSH)	Regulates skin pigmentation and promotes the deposit of melanin in the skin after exposure to sunlight
Posterior lobe	Antidiuretic hormone (ADH)	Stimulates the reabsorption of water by the renal tubules and has a pressor effect that elevates the blood pressure
	Oxytocin	Acts on the mammary glands to stimulate the release of milk and stimulates the uterus to contract during labor, delivery, and parturition
Pineal Gland	Melatonin	Helps regulate the release of gonadotropin and influences the body's internal clock
	Serotonin	Neurotransmitter, vasoconstrictor, and smooth muscle stimulant; acts to inhibit gastric secretion
Thyroid Gland	Thyroxine	Maintenance and regulation of the basal metabolic rate (BMR)
	Triiodothyronine	Influences the basal metabolic rate
	Calcitonin	Influences calcium metabolism
Parathyroid Glands	Parathormone hormone (PTH)	Plays a role in maintenance of a normal serum calcium level and in the metabolism of phosphorus
Islets of Langerhans	Glucagon	Facilitates the breakdown of glycogen to glucose
	Insulin	Plays a role in maintenance of normal blood sugar
	Somatostatin	Suppresses the release of glucagon and insulin
Adrenal Glands		
Cortex	Cortisol	Principal steroid hormone. Regulates carbohydrate, protein, and fat metabolism; gluconeogenesis; increases blood sugar level; anti-inflammatory effect; helps body cope during times of stress.
	Corticosterone	Steroid hormone. Essential for normal use of carbohydrates, the absorption of glucose, and gluconeogenesis. Also influences potassium and sodium metabolism.
	Aldosterone	Principal mineralocorticoid. Essential in regulating electrolyte and water balance.
	Testosterone	Development of male secondary sex characteristics
	Androsterone	Development of male secondary sex characteristics

continued

TABLE 9–1   continued

Endocrine Glands	Hormones	Hormonal Functions
Adrenal Glands (cont.)		
Medulla	Dopamine	Dilates systemic arteries, elevates systolic blood pressure, increases cardiac output, increases urinary output
	Epinephrine (adrenaline)	Vasoconstrictor, vasopressor, cardiac stimulant, antispasmodic, and sympathomimetic
	Norepinephrine	Vasoconstrictor, vasopressor, and neurotransmitter
Ovaries	Estrogens (estradiol, estrone, and estriol)	Female sex hormones. Essential for the growth, development, and maintenance of female sex organs and secondary sex characteristics. Promotes the development of the mammary glands, and plays a vital role in a woman's emotional well-being and sexual drive.
	Progesterone	Prepares the uterus for pregnancy
Testes	Testosterone	Essential for normal growth and development of the male accessory sex organs. Plays a vital role in the erection process of the penis and, thus, is necessary for the reproductive act, copulation.
Thymus Gland	Thymosin	Promotes the maturation process of T lymphocytes
	Thymopoietin	Influences the production of lymphocyte precursors and aids in their process of becoming T lymphocytes
Gastrointestinal Mucosa	Gastrin	Stimulates gastric acid secretion
	Secretin	Stimulates pancreatic juice, bile, and intestinal secretion
	Pancreozymin	Stimulates the pancreas to produce pancreatic juice
	Cholecystokinin	Contraction and emptying of the gallbladder
	Enterogastrone	Regulates gastric secretions

▶ THE PITUITARY GLAND (HYPOPHYSIS)

The *pituitary gland* is a small gray gland located at the base of the brain. It lies or rests in a shallow depression of the sphenoid bone known as the *sella turcica*. It is attached by the infundibulum stalk to the hypothalamus. The pituitary is approximately 1 cm in diameter and weighs approximately 0.6 g. It is divided into the anterior lobe or adenohypophysis and the posterior lobe or neurohypophysis. The pituitary is called the *master gland* of the body because of its regulatory effects on the other endocrine glands (see Fig. 9–1).

THE ANTERIOR LOBE

The *adenohypophysis* or anterior lobe secretes several hormones that are essential for the growth and development of bones, muscles, other organs, sex glands, the thyroid gland, and the adrenal cortex. The hormones secreted by the anterior lobe and their functions are described below and shown in Figure 9–2.

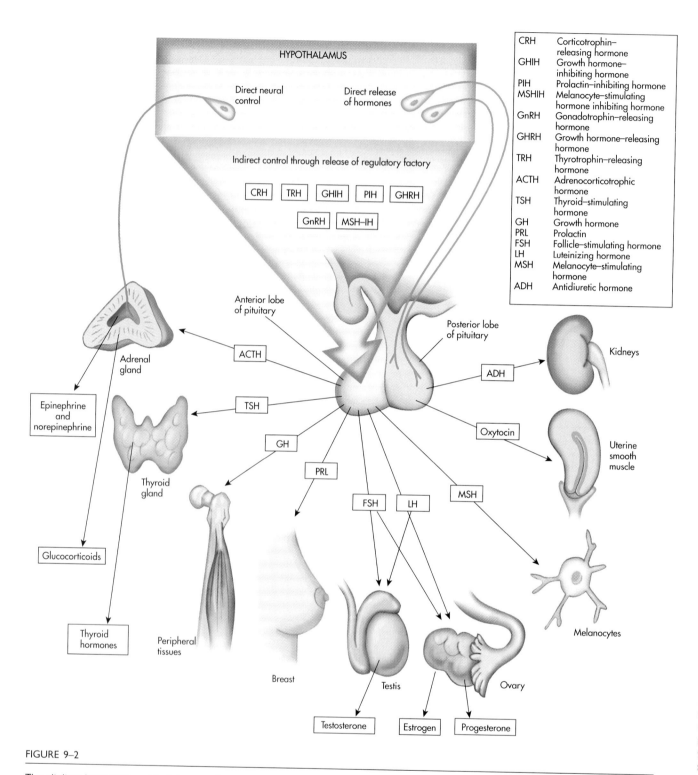

FIGURE 9–2

The pituitary hormones and their target cells, tissues, and/or organs.

GROWTH HORMONE (GH)

Growth hormone, also called somatotropin hormone (STH), is essential for the growth and development of bones, muscles, and other organs. It also enhances protein synthesis, decreases the use of glucose, and promotes fat destruction (lipolysis). Hyposecretion of this hormone may result in *dwarfism* and *Simmonds' disease.* Hypersecretion of the hormone may result in *gigantism* during early life and *acromegaly* in adults.

Adrenocorticotropin (ACTH)

Adrenocorticotropin is essential for growth and development of the middle and inner zones of the adrenal cortex. The adrenal cortex secretes the glucocorticoids cortisol and corticosterone.

Thyroid-Stimulating Hormone (TSH)

Thyroid-stimulating hormone is essential for the growth and development of the thyroid gland. It stimulates the production of thyroxine and triiodothyronine. It also influences the body's metabolic processes and plays an important role in metabolism.

Follicle-Stimulating Hormone (FSH)

Follicle-stimulating hormone is a gonadotropic hormone that is essential in stimulating the growth of ovarian follicles in the female and the production of sperm in the male.

Luteinizing Hormone (LH)

Luteinizing hormone is a gonadotropic hormone that is essential in the maturation process of the ovarian follicles and stimulates the development of the corpus luteum in the female and the production of testosterone in the male.

Prolactin (PRL)

Prolactin is also known as *lactogenic hormone* (LTH). It is a gonadotropic hormone that stimulates the mammary glands to produce milk after childbirth.

Melanocyte-Stimulating Hormone (MSH)

Melanocyte-stimulating hormone regulates skin pigmentation and promotes the deposit of melanin in the skin after exposure to sunlight.

THE POSTERIOR LOBE

The *neurohypophysis* or posterior lobe secretes two known hormones: antidiuretic hormone and oxytocin (see Fig. 9–2). The following is a description of the functions of these hormones.

Antidiuretic Hormone (ADH)

Antidiuretic hormone is also known as *vasopressin* (VP). It stimulates the reabsorption of water by the renal tubules and has a pressor effect that elevates blood pressure. Hyposecretion of this hormone may result in *diabetes insipidus.*

Oxytocin

Oxytocin acts on the mammary glands to stimulate the release of milk and stimulates the uterus to contract during labor, delivery, and parturition.

▶ THE PINEAL GLAND (BODY)

The *pineal gland* is a small, pine cone–shaped gland located near the posterior end of the corpus callosum. It is less than 1 cm in diameter and weighs approximately 0.1 g (see Fig. 9–1). The pineal gland secretes *melatonin* and *serotonin*. Melatonin is a hormone that may be released at night to help regulate the release of gonadotropin. Serotonin is a hormone that is a neurotransmitter, vaso-constrictor, and smooth muscle stimulant and acts to inhibit gastric secretion.

▶ THE THYROID GLAND

The *thyroid gland* is a large, bilobed gland located in the neck. It is anterior to the trachea and just below the thyroid cartilage. The thyroid is approximately 5 cm long and 3 cm wide and weighs approximately 30 g (see Fig. 9–1). It plays a vital role in metabolism and regulates the body's metabolic processes. The hormones described below are stored and secreted by the thyroid gland.

Thyroxine (T$_4$)

Thyroxine is essential for the maintenance and regulation of the *basal metabolic rate* (BMR). It contains four iodine atoms, which are attached to its nucleus. Thyroxine influences growth and development, both physical and mental, and the metabolism of fats, proteins, carbohydrates, water, vitamins, and minerals. It can be synthetically produced or extracted from animal thyroid glands in crystalline form to be used in the treatment of thyroid dysfunction, especially cretinism, myxedema, and Hashimoto's disease.

Triiodothyronine (T$_3$)

Triiodothyronine is an effective thyroid hormone that contains three iodine atoms. It influences the basal metabolic rate and is more biologically active than thyroxine.

Calcitonin

Also known as thyrocalcitonin, *calcitonin* is a thyroid hormone that influences bone and calcium metabolism. It helps maintain plasma calcium homeostasis.

Hyposecretion of the thyroid hormones T$_3$ and T$_4$ results in *cretinism* during infancy, *myxedema* during adulthood, and *Hashimoto's disease*, which is a chronic thyroid disease. Hypersecretion of the thyroid hormones T$_3$ and T$_4$ results in *hyperthyroidism*, which is also called *thyrotoxicosis*, and *Graves' disease, exophthalmic goiter, toxic goiter*, or *Basedow's disease*. Simple or endemic goiter is an enlargement of the thyroid gland caused by a deficiency of iodine in the diet.

▶ THE PARATHYROID GLANDS

The *parathyroid glands* are small, yellowish-brown bodies occurring as two pairs and located on the dorsal surface and lower aspect of the thyroid gland. Each parathyroid gland is approximately 6 mm in diameter and weighs approximately 0.033 g (Fig. 9–1). The hormone secreted by the parathyroids is *parathormone* (PTH). This hormone is essential for the maintenance of a normal serum calcium level. It also plays a role in the metabolism of phosphorus. Hyposecretion of PTH may result in *hypoparathyroidism*, which may result in *tetany*. Hypersecretion of PTH may result in *hyperparathyroidism*, which may result in *osteoporosis, kidney stones*, and *hypercalcemia*.

▶ THE PANCREAS (THE ISLETS OF LANGERHANS)

The *islets of Langerhans* are small clusters of cells located on the surface of the pancreas (see Fig. 9–1). They are composed of three major types of cells: *alpha, beta,* and *delta.* The alpha cells secrete the hormone glucagon, which facilitates the breakdown of glycogen to glucose, thereby elevating blood sugar. The beta cells secrete the hormone insulin, which is essential for the maintenance of normal blood sugar (70–110 mg/100 mL of blood). Insulin is essential to life. It promotes the use of glucose in cells, thereby lowering the blood glucose level, and plays a vital role in carbohydrate, protein, and fat metabolism. Insulin can be synthetically produced in various types and was first discovered and used successfully by Sir F. G. Banting. Hyposecretion or inadequate use of insulin may result in *diabetes mellitus.* Hypersecretion of insulin may result in *hyperinsulinism.* The delta cells secrete a hormone, *somatostatin,* that suppresses the release of glucagon and insulin.

▶ THE ADRENAL GLANDS (SUPRARENALS)

The *adrenal glands* are two small, triangular-shaped glands located on top of each kidney. Each gland weighs about 5 g and consists of an outer portion or *cortex* and an inner portion called the *medulla* (Fig. 9–1).

THE ADRENAL CORTEX

The *cortex* is essential to life as it secretes a group of hormones, the glucocorticoids, the mineralocorticoids, and the androgens. These hormones and their effects on the body are described below.

The Glucocorticoids

The two glucocorticoid hormones are *cortisol* and *corticosterone.*

Cortisol.   *Cortisol* (hydrocortisone) is the principal steroid hormone secreted by the cortex. The following are some of the known influences and functions of this hormone:

- It regulates carbohydrate, protein, and fat metabolism.
- It stimulates output of glucose from the liver (gluconeogenesis).
- It increases the blood sugar level.
- It regulates other physiologic body processes.
- It promotes the transport of amino acids into extracellular tissue, thereby making them available for energy.
- It influences the effectiveness of catecholamines such as dopamine, epinephrine, and norepinephrine.
- It has an anti-inflammatory effect.
- It helps the body cope during times of stress.

Hyposecretion of this hormone may result in *Addison's disease.* Hypersecretion of cortisol may result in *Cushing's disease.*

Corticosterone.   *Corticosterone* is a steroid hormone secreted by the adrenal cortex. It is essential for the normal use of carbohydrates, the absorption of glucose, and the process known as *gluconeogenesis.* It also influences potassium and sodium metabolism.

The Mineralocorticoids

Aldosterone is the principal *mineralocorticoid* secreted by the adrenal cortex. It is essential in regulating electrolyte and water balance by promoting sodium and chloride retention and potassium excretion. Hyposecretion of this hormone may result in a *reduced plasma volume*. Hypersecretion of this hormone may result in a condition known as *primary aldosteronism*.

The Androgens

Androgen refers to a substance or hormone that promotes the development of male characteristics. The two main androgen hormones are *testosterone* and *androsterone*. These hormones are essential for the development of the male secondary sex characteristics.

THE ADRENAL MEDULLA

The *medulla* synthesizes, secretes, and stores catecholamines, specifically, dopamine, epinephrine, and norepinephrine. A discussion of these substances and their effects on the body follows.

Dopamine

Dopamine acts to dilate systemic arteries, elevates systolic blood pressure, increases cardiac output, and increases urinary output. It is used in the treatment of shock and is a neurotransmitter in the nervous system.

Epinephrine

Epinephrine (Adrenalin, adrenaline) acts as a vasoconstrictor, vasopressor, cardiac stimulant, antispasmodic, and sympathomimetic. Its main function is to assist in the regulation of the sympathetic branch of the autonomic nervous system. It can be synthetically produced and may be administered parenterally *(by an injection)*, topically *(on a local area of the skin)*, or by inhalation *(by nose or mouth)*. The following are some of the known influences and functions of this hormone:

- It elevates the systolic blood pressure.
- It increases the heart rate and cardiac output.
- It increases glycogenolysis, thereby hastening the release of glucose from the liver. This action elevates the blood sugar level and provides the body with a spurt of energy; referred to as the "fight-or-flight" syndrome.
- It dilates the bronchial tubes and relaxes air passageways.
- It dilates the pupils so that one can see more clearly.

Norepinephrine

Norepinephrine (noradrenalin) acts as a vasoconstrictor, vasopressor, and neurotransmitter. It elevates systolic and diastolic blood pressure, increases the heart rate and cardiac output, and increases glycogenolysis.

▶ THE OVARIES

The *ovaries* produce *estrogens (estradiol, estrone, and estriol)* and *progesterone*. Estrogen is the female sex hormone secreted by the graafian follicles of the ovaries. Progesterone is a steroid hormone secreted by the corpus luteum. These hormones are essential for promoting the growth, development, and maintenance of secondary female sex organs and characteristics. They also prepare the uterus for pregnancy, promote development of the mammary glands, and play a vital role in a woman's emotional well-being and her sexual drive (see Fig. 9–1).

▶ THE TESTES

The *testes* produce the male sex hormone *testosterone,* which is essential for normal growth and development of the male accessory sex organs. Testosterone plays a vital role in the erection process of the penis and, thus, is necessary for the reproductive act, copulation (see Fig. 9–1).

▶ THE PLACENTA

During pregnancy the *placenta,* a spongy structure joining mother and child, serves as an endocrine gland. It produces chorionic gonadotropin hormone, estrogen, and progesterone.

▶ THE GASTROINTESTINAL MUCOSA

The *mucosa* of the pyloric area of the stomach secretes the hormone *gastrin,* which stimulates gastric acid secretion. Gastrin also affects the gallbladder, pancreas, and small intestine secretory activities.

The mucosa of the duodenum and jejunum secretes the hormone *secretin,* which stimulates pancreatic juice, bile, and intestinal secretion. The mucosa of the duodenum also secretes *pancreozymin-cholecystokinin,* which stimulates the pancreas. *Enterogastrone,* a hormone that regulates gastric secretions, is also secreted by the duodenal mucosa.

▶ THE THYMUS

The *thymus* is a bilobed body located in the mediastinal cavity in front of and above the heart (Fig. 9–3). It is composed of lymphoid tissue and is a part of the lymphoid system. It is a ductless gland-like body and secretes the hormones *thymosin* and *thymopoietin.* Thymosin promotes the maturation process of T lymphocytes (thymus-dependent). Thymopoietin is a hormone that influences the production of lymphocyte precursors and aids in their process of becoming T lymphocytes.

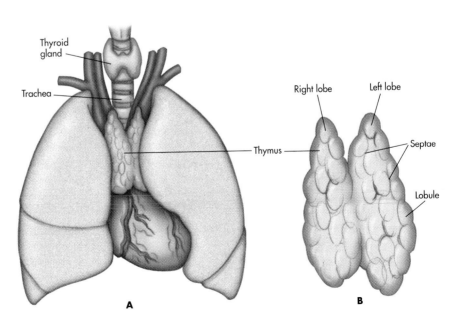

FIGURE 9–3

The thymus gland. **(A)** Appearance and position, **(B)** with anatomic structures.

Life Span Considerations

▶ THE CHILD

Most of the structures and glands of the endocrine system develop during the first 3 months of pregnancy. The endocrine system of the newborn is supplemented by hormones that cross the placental barrier. Both male and female newborns may have swelling of the breast and genitalia from maternal hormones.

Either excessively high or insufficient production of growth hormone (GH) by the anterior lobe of the pituitary gland can cause abnormal growth patterns. Excessive production of GH can cause **gigantism.** Insufficient production of GH can cause **dwarfism.**

Type I—**insulin-dependent diabetes mellitus** (IDDM)—is the most common endocrine system disorder of childhood. The rate of occurrence is highest among 5–7-year-olds and 11–13-year-olds. The classic symptoms of diabetes mellitus—**polyuria, polydipsia,** and **polyphagia**—appear more rapidly in children. Other symptoms seen during childhood are weakness, loss of weight, lethargy, anorexia, irritability, dry skin, vaginal yeast infections in the female child and/or recurrent infections, and abdominal cramps. The management of diabetes mellitus during childhood is very difficult, because diet, exercise, and medication have to be adjusted and regulated according to the various stages of growth and development of the child.

▶ THE OLDER ADULT

With aging, **hormonal changes** vary with each individual. Generally the number of tissue receptors decreases, thus diminishing the body's response to hormones. This is especially the case with older adults who develop Type II—**non-insulin-dependent diabetes mellitus** (NIDDM). In this condition sufficient insulin is produced, but because the number of cell receptors is reduced, glucose does not enter the cells.

An older adult may not be diagnosed with diabetes until he or she goes in for a regular eye exam and the ophthalmologist discovers a problem and/or one goes in for a physical examination and the blood test indicates an elevated blood glucose level. There are multiple risk factors associated with the older adult and the development of diabetes; these are:

- Age-related decreased insulin production
- Age-related insulin resistance
- Heredity
- Decreased physical activity
- Multiple diseases
- Polypharmacy
- Obesity
- New stressors in life

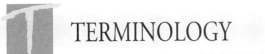

TERMINOLOGY

WITH SURGICAL PROCEDURES & PATHOLOGY

TERM	WORD PARTS			DEFINITION
acidosis (ăs″ ĭ-dō′ sĭs)	acid osis	R S	acid condition of	A condition of excessive acidity of body fluids
acromegaly (ăk″ rō-měg′ ă-lē)	acro megaly	CF S	extremity enlargement, large	Enlargement of the extremities caused by excessive growth hormone
adenalgia (ăd″ ēn -ăl′ jĭ-ă)	aden algia	R S	gland pain	Pain in a gland
adenectomy (ăd″ ĕn-ĕk′ tō-mē)	aden ectomy	R S	gland excision	Surgical excision of a gland
adenoma (ăd″ ĕ-nō′ mă)	aden oma	R S	gland tumor	A tumor of a gland
adenomalacia (ăd″ ĕ-nō-mă-lā′ shĭ-ă)	adeno malacia	CF S	gland softening	A softening of a gland
adenosclerosis (ăd″ ĕ-nō-sklĕ-rō′ sĭs)	adeno scler osis	CF R S	gland hardening condition of	A condition of hardening of a gland
adenosis (ăd″ ĕ-nō′ sĭs)	aden osis	R S	gland condition of	Any disease condition of a gland
adrenal (ăd-rē′ năl)	ad ren al	P R S	toward kidney pertaining to	Pertaining to toward the kidney
adrenalectomy (ăd-rē″ năl-ĕk′ tō-mē)	ad ren al ectomy	P R S S	toward kidney pertaining to excision	Surgical excision of the adrenal gland
adrenopathy (ăd″ rĕn-ŏp′ ă-thē)	ad reno pathy	P CF S	toward kidney disease	Any disease of the adrenal gland
adrenotropic (ăd-rē″ nō-trōp′ ĭk)	ad reno trop ic	P CF R S	toward kidney nourishment pertaining to	Pertaining to the nourishment of the adrenal glands

continued

Terminology - continued

TERM	WORD PARTS			DEFINITION
cretinism (krē′ tĭn-ĭzm)	cretin ism	R S	cretin condition of	A congenital deficiency in secretion of the thyroid hormones T$_3$ and T$_4$
diabetes (dī″ ă-bē′ tēz)	dia betes	P S	through to go	Chronic disease of insulin deficiency or resistance

TERMINOLOGY SPOTLIGHT

Diabetes mellitus is a complex disorder of metabolism. It affects 14 million Americans, with care and treatment costing $20 billion annually.

The National Diabetes Data Group of the National Institutes of Health has categorized the various forms of diabetes mellitus: Type I—insulin-dependent diabetes mellitus (IDDM); Type II—non-insulin-dependent diabetes mellitus (NIDDM); Type III—women who have developed glucose intolerance in association with pregnancy; and Type IV—diabetes associated with pancreatic disease, hormonal changes, the adverse effects of drugs, and other anomalies. One in 10 people who have diabetes are Type I diabetics and must take insulin on a regular basis.

The American Diabetes Association estimates that 7 million American have diabetes and do not know it. Are you at risk for diabetes? Do you have any, some, or many of the signs and symptoms of diabetes? See Table 9–2 for the warning signs and symptoms of diabetes mellitus.

TABLE 9–2   Warning Signs and Symptoms of Diabetes Mellitus

Type I IDDM	Type II NIDDM
Frequent urination (polyuria) Excessive thirst (polydipsia) Extreme hunger (polyphagia) Unexplained weight loss Extreme fatigue Blurred vision	Any Type I symptom Tingling or numbing in the feet Frequent vaginal or skin infection

TERM	WORD PARTS			DEFINITION
dwarfism (dwar′ fizm)	dwarf ism	R S	small condition of	A condition of being abnormally small
endocrine (ĕn′ dō-krĭn)	endo crine	P R	within to secrete	A ductless gland that produces an internal secretion
endocrinologist (ĕn″ dō-krĭn-ŏl′ ō-gĭst)	endo crino log ist	P CF R S	within to secrete study of one who specializes	One who specializes in the study of the endocrine glands
endocrinology (ĕn″ dō-krĭn-ŏl′ ō-jē)	endo crino logy	P CF S	within to secrete study of	The study of the endocrine glands

Terminology - continued

TERM	WORD PARTS			DEFINITION
endocrinopathy (ĕn″ dō-krĭn-ŏp′ ă-thē)	endo crino pathy	P CF S	within to secrete disease	A disease of an endocrine gland or glands
endocrino- therapy (ĕn″ dō-krĭn″ ō-thĕr′ ă-pē)	endo crino therapy	P CF S	within to secrete treatment	Treatment with endocrine preparations
euthyroid (ū-thī′ royd)	eu thyr oid	P R S	good, normal thyroid, shield resemble	Normal activity of the thyroid gland
exocrine (ĕks′ ō-krĭn)	exo crine	P R	out, away from to secrete	External secretion of a gland
exophthalmic (ĕks″ŏf-thăl′ mĭk)	ex ophthalm ic	P R S	out, away from eye pertaining to	Pertaining to an abnormal protrusion of the eye
galactorrhea (gă-lăk″ tō-rĭ′ ă)	galacto rrhea	CF S	milk flow, discharge	Excessive secretion of milk after cessation of nursing
gigantism (jī′ găn-tĭzm)	gigant ism	R S	giant condition of	A condition of being abnormally large
glandular (glăn′ dū-lăr)	glandul ar	R S	little acorn pertaining to	Pertaining to a gland
glucocorticoid (glū″ kō-kŏrt′ ĭ-koyd)	gluco cortic oid	CF R S	sweet, sugar cortex resemble	A general classification of the adrenal cortical hormones
hirsutism (hŭr′ sūt-ĭzm)	hirsut ism	R S	hairy condition of	An abnormal condition characterized by excessive growth of hair, especially in women. See Figure 11–4.
hypergonadism (hī″ pĕr-gō′ năd-ĭzm)	hyper gonad ism	P R S	excessive seed condition of	A condition of excessive secretion of the sex glands
hyperinsulinism (hī″ pĕr-ĭn′ sū-lĭn-ĭzm)	hyper insulin ism	P R S	excessive insulin condition of	A condition of excessive amounts of insulin in the blood
hyperkalemia (hī″ pĕr-kă-lē′ mĭ-ă)	hyper kal emia	P R S	excessive potassium (K) blood condition	A condition of excessive amounts of potassium in the blood

continued

Terminology - continued

TERM	WORD PARTS			DEFINITION
hyperthyroidism (hī″ pĕr-thī′ royd-ĭzm)	hyper thyr oid ism	P R S S	excessive thyroid, shield resemble condition of	A condition caused by excessive secretion of the thyroid gland
hypocrinism (hī″ pō-krī′ nĭzm)	hypo crin ism	P R S	deficient to secrete condition of	A condition caused by deficient secretion of any gland
hypogonadism (hī″ pō-gō′ năd-ĭzm)	hypo gonad ism	P R S	deficient seed condition of	A condition caused by deficient internal secretion of the gonads
hypoparathyroid-ism (hī″ pō-păr″ă-thī′ royd-ĭzm)	hypo para thyr oid ism	P P R S S	deficient beside thyroid, shield resemble condition of	Deficient internal secretion of the parathyroid glands
hypophysis (hī-pŏf′ ĭ-sĭs)	hypo physis	P S	deficient, under growth	Any undergrowth; the pituitary body
hypothyroidism (hī″ pō-thī′ royd-ĭzm)	hypo thyr oid ism	P R S S	deficient thyroid, shield resemble condition of	Deficient secretion of the thyroid gland
insulinogenic (ĭn″ sū-lĭn″ ō-jĕn′ ĭk)	insulino genic	CF S	insulin formation produce	The formation or production of insulin
insulinoid (ĭn′ sū-lĭn-oyd″)	insulin oid	R S	insulin resemble	Resembling insulin
insuloma (ĭn′ sū-lō″ mă)	insul oma	R S	insulin tumor	A tumor of the islets of Langerhans
lethargic (lĕ-thar′ jĭk)	letharg ic	R S	drowsiness pertaining to	Pertaining to drowsiness, sluggish
myxedema (mĭks″ ĕ-dē′ mă)	myx edema	R S	mucus swelling	A condition of mucus swelling resulting from hypofunction of the thyroid gland. See Figure 9–5.
pancreatic (păn″ krē-ăt′ ĭk)	pan creat ic	P R S	all flesh pertaining to	Pertaining to the pancreas

Terminology - continued

TERM	WORD PARTS			DEFINITION
parathyroid (păr″ă-thī′ royd)	para thyr oid	P R S	beside thyroid, shield resemble	An endocrine gland located beside the thyroid gland
pineal (pĭn′ ē-ăl)	pine al	R S	pine cone pertaining to	An endocrine gland that is shaped like a small pine cone
pinealectomy (pĭn″ ē-ăl-ĕk′ tō-mē)	pineal ectomy	R S	pineal body excision	Surgical excision of the pineal body
pinealoma (pĭn″ ē-ă-lō′ mă)	pineal oma	R S	pineal body tumor	A tumor of the pineal body
pituitarism (pĭt-ū′ ĭ-tă-rĭzm)	pituitar ism	R S	phlegm condition	Any condition of the pituitary gland
pituitary (pĭ-tū′ ĭ-tăr″ ē)	pituitar y	R S	phlegm pertaining to	Pertaining to phlegm; the pituitary body or gland, the hypophysis
progeria (prō-jē′ rĭ-ă)	pro ger ia	P R S	before old age condition	A condition of premature old age occurring in childhood
thymectomy (thī-mĕk′ tō-mē)	thym ectomy	R S	thymus excision	Surgical excision of the thymus gland
thymitis (thī-mī′ tĭs)	thym itis	R S	thymus inflammation	Inflammation of the thymus gland
thymopexy (thī′ mō-pĕks″ ē)	thymo pexy	CF S	thymus fixation	Surgical fixation of an enlarged thymus in a new position
thyroid (thī′ royd)	thyr oid	R S	thyroid, shield resemble	Resembling a shield; one of the endocrine glands
thyroidectomy (thī″ royd-ĕk′ tō-mē)	thyr oid ectomy	R S S	thyroid, shield resemble excision	Surgical excision of the thyroid gland
thyroiditis (thī″ royd′ī′ tĭs)	thyr oid itis	R S S	thyroid, shield resemble inflammation	Inflammation of the thyroid gland
thyroptosis (thī″ rŏp-tō′ sĭs)	thyro ptosis	CF S	thyroid, shield drooping	Downward drooping of the thyroid into the thorax
thyrosis (thī-rō′ sĭs)	thyr osis	R S	thyroid, shield condition of	Any condition of abnormal functioning of the thyroid

continued

Terminology - continued

TERM	WORD PARTS			DEFINITION
thyrotherapy (thī″ rō-thĕr′ ă-pē)	thyro therapy	CF S	thyroid, shield treatment	Pertaining to the treatment using thyroid gland extracts
thyrotome (thī″ rō-tōm)	thyro tome	CF S	thyroid, shield instrument to cut	An instrument used to cut the thyroid cartilage
thyrotoxicosis (thī″ rō-tŏks″ ĭ-kō′ sĭs)	thyro toxic osis	CF R S	thyroid, shield poison condition of	A poisonous condition of the thyroid gland caused by hyperactivity
virilism (vĭr′ ĭl-ĭzm)	viril ism	R S	masculine condition of	The condition of masculinity developed in a woman

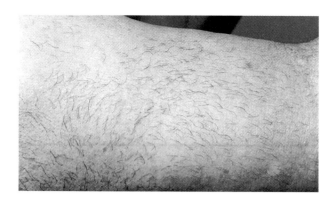

FIGURE 9–4

Hirsutism. *(Courtesy of Jason L. Smith, MD.)*

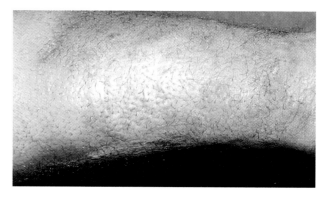

FIGURE 9–5

Pretibial myxedema. *(Courtesy of Jason L. Smith, MD.)*

VOCABULARY WORDS

Vocabulary words are terms that have not been divided into component parts. They are common words or specialized terms associated with the subject of this chapter. These words are provided to enhance your medical vocabulary.

WORD	DEFINITION
aldosterone (ăl-dŏs′ tĕr-ōn)	A mineralocorticoid hormone secreted by the adrenal cortex that helps regulate metabolism of sodium, chloride, and potassium

Vocabulary - continued

WORD	DEFINITION
androgen (ăn′ drō-jĕn)	Hormones that produce or stimulate the development of male characteristics. The two major androgens are testosterone and androsterone.
catecholamines (kăt″ ĕ-kōl′ ăm-ēns)	Biochemical substances, epinephrine, norepinephrine, and dopamine
cortisone (kŏr′ tĭ-sōn)	A glucocorticoid hormone that is isolated from the adrenal cortex; *used as an anti-inflammatory agent*
dopamine (dō′ pă-mēn)	An intermediate substance in the synthesis of norepinephrine; used in the treatment of shock as it acts to elevate blood pressure and increase urinary output
epinephrine (ĕp″ ĭ-nĕf′ rĭn)	A hormone produced by the adrenal medulla; used as a vasoconstrictor, as a cardiac stimulant, to relax bronchospasm, and to relieve allergic symptoms; *also called adrenaline, Adrenalin*
estrogen (ĕs′ trō-jĕn)	Hormones produced by the ovaries, including estradiol, estrone, and estriol; female sex hormones important in the development of secondary sex characteristics and regulation of the menstrual cycle
hormone (hor′ mōn)	A chemical substance produced by the endocrine glands
hydrocortisone (hī‴ drō-kŏr′ tĭ-sōn)	A glucocorticoid hormone produced by the adrenal cortex; *used as an anti-inflammatory agent*
insulin (in′ sū-lĭn)	A hormone produced by the beta cells of the islets of Langerhans of the pancreas; essential for the metabolism of carbohydrates and fats; *used in the management of diabetes mellitus*
iodine (ī′ ō-dīn)	A trace mineral that aids in the development and functioning of the thyroid gland
necrobiosis lipoidica diabeticorum (nĕk-rō-bī-ō′sĭs lĭp-oyd′īcă dī-ă-bĕt′ĭk′-ō″rŭm)	A skin disease commonly found in diabetics; it is marked by gradual degeneration and swelling of connective and elastic tissue; the lesions have a central yellowish area surrounded by a brownish border and are usually present on the anterior surface of the legs. See Figures 9–6 and 9–7.
norepinephrine (nŏr-ĕp″ ĭ-nĕf′ rĭn)	A hormone produced by the adrenal medulla; used as a vasoconstrictor of peripheral blood vessels in acute hypotensive states
oxytocin (ŏk″ sĭ-tō′ sĭn)	A hormone produced by the pituitary gland that stimulates uterine contraction during childbirth and stimulates the release of milk during nursing

continued

Vocabulary - continued

WORD	DEFINITION
progesterone (prō-jĕs′ tĕr-ōn)	A hormone produced by the corpus luteum of the ovary, the adrenal cortex, or the placenta; released during the second half of the menstrual cycle
somatotropin (sō-măt′ ō-trō″ pĭn)	Growth-stimulating hormone produced by the anterior lobe of the pituitary gland
steroids (stĕr′ oydz)	A group of chemical substances that includes hormones, vitamins, sterols, cardiac glycosides, and certain drugs
testosterone (tĕs-tŏs′ tĕr-ōn)	A hormone produced by the testes; male sex hormone important in the development of secondary sex characteristics and masculinization
thyroxine (thī-rŏks′ ēn)	A hormone produced by the thyroid gland; important in growth and development and regulation of the body's metabolic rate and metabolism of carbohydrates, fats, and proteins
vasopressin (văs″ ō-prĕs′ ĭn)	A hormone produced by the hypothalamus and stored in the posterior lobe of the pituitary gland; also called antidiuretic hormone, ADH

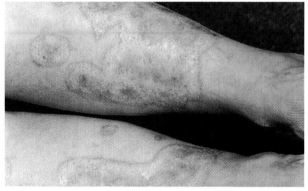

FIGURE 9–6

Necrobiosis lipoidica diabeticorum. *(Courtesy of Jason L. Smith, MD.)*

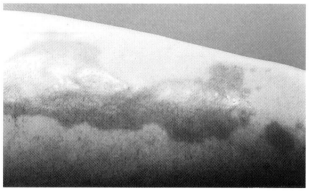

FIGURE 9–7

Necrobiosis lipoidica diabeticorum. *(Courtesy of Jason L. Smith, MD.)*

 # ABBREVIATIONS

ACTH	adrenocorticotropic hormone	**CRF**	corticotropin-releasing factor
ADA	American Diabetes Association	**DI**	diabetes insipidus
ADH	antidiuretic hormone	**DM**	diabetes mellitus
BG, bG	blood glucose	**FBS**	fasting blood sugar
BMR	basal metabolic rate	**FSH**	follicle-stimulating hormone

GH	growth hormone	**PBI**	protein-bound iodine
GHb	glycosylated hemoglobin	**PIF**	prolactin release-inhibiting factor
GHRF	glycosylated hemoglobin-releasing factor	**PRF**	prolactin-releasing factor
		PTH	parathormone
GnRF	gonadotropin-releasing factor	**RAIU**	radioactive iodine uptake
GTT	glucose tolerance test	**RIA**	radioimmunoassay
IDDM	insulin-dependent diabetes mellitus	**SMBG**	self-monitoring of blood glucose
		STH	somatotropin hormone
K	potassium	**T₃**	triiodothyronine
LH	luteinizing hormone	**T₃RU**	triiodothyronine resin uptake
LTH	lactogenic hormone	**T₄**	thyroxine
MIF	melanocyte-stimulating hormone release-inhibiting factor	**TFS**	thyroid function studies
		TSH	thyroid-stimulating hormone
MSH	melanocyte-stimulating hormone	**VMA**	vanillylmandelic acid
NIDDM	non-insulin-dependent diabetes mellitus	**VP**	vasopressin

DRUG HIGHLIGHTS

Drugs that are generally used for endocrine system diseases and disorders include thyroid hormones, antithyroid hormones, insulin, and oral hypoglycemic agents.

Thyroid Hormones Increase metabolic rate, cardiac output, oxygen consumption, body temperature, respiratory rate, blood volume, and carbohydrate, fat, and protein metabolism, and influence growth and development at cellular level. Thyroid hormones are used as supplements or replacement therapy in hypothyroidism, myxedema, and cretinism.
Examples: Levothroid and Synthroid (levothyroxine sodium), Cytomel (liothyronine sodium), Euthroid and Thyrolar (liotrix), and thyroid, USP.

Antithyroid Hormones Inhibit the synthesis of thyroid hormones by decreasing iodine use in manufacture of thyroglobin and iodothyronine. They do not inactivate or inhibit thyroxine or triiodothyronine. They are used in the treatment of hyperthyroidism.
Example: Tapazole (methimazole), potassium iodide solution, Lugol's solution (strong iodine solution), and Iodotope I-131 (sodium iodide).

Insulin Stimulates carbohydrate metabolism by increasing the movement of glucose and other monosaccharides into cells. It also influences fat and carbohydrate metabolism in the liver and adipose cells. It decreases blood sugar, phosphate, and potassium, and increases blood pyruvate and lactate. *Insulin* is used in the treatment of insulin-dependent diabetes mellitus (Type I—IDDM), non-insulin-dependent diabetes mellitus (Type II—NIDDM) when other regimens are not effective, and to treat ketoacidosis.

Insulin Preparations Insulin is given by subcutaneous injection and is available in rapid-acting, intermediate-acting, and long-acting preparations.

  Rapid-acting *Examples: Regular Novolin R, Humulin R, and Velosulin BR*
Onset of Action ½ hour   Appearance—clear

Intermediate-acting	*Examples: NPH, Novolin N, Humulin L, Iletin II, Lente Insulin, and Novolin L.*
	Onset of Action 1–1½ hours Appearance—cloudy
Long-acting	*Examples: Ultralente and Humulin U*
	Onset of Action 4–8 hours Appearance—cloudy

Oral Hypoglycemic Agents
Are agents of the sulfonylurea class and are used to stimulate insulin secretion from pancreatic cells in non-insulin-dependent diabetics with some pancreatic function.
Examples: Dymelor (acetohexamide), Diabinese (chlorpropamide), Glucotrol (glipizide), DiaBeta and Micronase (glyburide), Tolinase (tolazamide), and Orinase (tolbutamide).

DIAGNOSTIC AND LABORATORY TESTS

Test	Description
catecholamines (kăt″ ĕ-kōl′ ă-mēns)	A test performed on urine to determine the amount of epinephrine and norepinephrine present. These adrenal hormones increase in times of stress.
corticotropin, corticotropin-releasing factor (CRF) (kor″ tĭ-kō-trō′ pin)	A test performed on blood plasma to determine the amount of corticotropin present. Increased levels may indicate stress, adrenal cortical hypofunction, and/or pituitary tumors. Decreased levels may indicate adrenal neoplasms and/or Cushing's syndrome.
fasting blood sugar (FBS) (făs-tĭng blod shoog′ ar)	A test performed on blood to determine the level of sugar in the bloodstream. Increased levels may indicate diabetes mellitus, diabetic acidosis, and many other conditions. Decreased levels may indicate hypoglycemia, hyperinsulinism, and many other conditions.
glucose tolerance test (GTT) (gloo′ kōs tŏl′ ĕr-ăns test)	A blood sugar test performed at specified intervals after the patient has been given a certain amount of glucose. Blood samples are drawn, and the blood glucose level of each sample is determined. It is more accurate than other blood sugar tests, and it is used to diagnose diabetes mellitus.
hemoglobin (A₁C) (hē″mō-glō bĭn)	A test that measures the amount of glycosylated hemoglobin found and stored in red blood cells. This test determines how well blood glucose levels have been controlled for up to a prior of four months. An elevated level indicates uncontrolled diabetes.
17-hydroxycorticosteroids (17-OHCS) (hī-drŏk″ sē-kor″ tĭ-kō-stĕr′ oyd)	A test performed on urine to identify adrenocorticosteroid hormones. It is used to determine adrenal cortical function.

17-ketosteroids (17-KS)
(kē″ tō-stĕr′ oyd)

A test performed on urine to determine the amount of 17-KS present. 17-KS is the end product of androgens and is secreted from the adrenal glands and testes. It is used in the diagnosing of adrenal tumors.

Test	Description

protein-bound iodine (PBI)
(prō′ tēn bound ī′ ō-dīn)

A test performed on serum to indicate the amount of iodine that is attached to serum protein. It may be used to indicate thyroid function.

radioactive iodine uptake (RAIU)
(rā″ dē-ō-ăk′ tīv ī′ ō-dīn ŭp′ tāk)

A test to measure the ability of the thyroid gland to concentrate ingested iodine. Increased level may indicate hyperthyroidism, cirrhosis, and/or thyroiditis. Decreased level may indicate hypothyroidism.

radioimmunoassay
(rā″ dē-ō-ĭm″ū-nō-ăs′ā)

A standard assay method that is used for the measurement of minute quantities of specific antibodies and/or antigens. It may be used for clinical laboratory measurements of hormones, therapeutic drug monitoring, and substance abuse screening.

thyroid scan
(thī′ royd skăn)

A test to detect tumors of the thyroid gland. The patient is given radioactive iodine 131, which localizes in the thyroid gland, and the gland is then visualized with a scanner device.

thyroxine (T$_4$)
(thī-rōks′ ĭn)

A test performed on blood serum to determine the amount of thyroxine present. Increased levels may indicate hyperthyroidism. Decreased levels may indicate hypothyroidism.

triiodothyronine uptake (T$_3$)
(trī″ ī-ō″ dō-thī′ rō-nĭn ŭp′ tāk)

A test performed on blood serum to determine the amount of triiodothyronine present. Increased levels may indicate thyrotoxicosis, toxic adenoma, and/or Hashimoto's struma. Decreased levels may indicate starvation, severe infection, and severe trauma.

total calcium
(tōt′ l kăl′ sē-ŭm)

A test performed on blood serum to determine the amount of calcium present. Increased levels may indicate hyperparathyroidism. Decreased levels may indicate hypoparathyroidism.

ultrasonography
(ŭl-tră-sŏn-ŏg′ ră-fē)

The use of high-frequency sound waves to visualize the structure being studied. May be used to visualize the pancreas, thyroid, and any other gland. It is used as a screening test or as a diagnostic tool.

COMMUNICATION ENRICHMENT

This segment is provided for those who wish to enhance their ability to communicate in either English or Spanish.

▶ **Related Terms**

English	Spanish	English	Spanish
adrenal	adrenal (ă-*drĕ*-năl)	harden	endurecer (ĕn-*dŭ*-rĕ-sĕr)
diabetes	diabetes (dĭ-ă-*bĕ*-tĕs)	small	pequeño (pĕ-*kĕ*-ñō)
endocrine system	sistema endocrino (sĭs-*tĕ*-mă ĕn-dō-crĭ-nō)	large	grande (*grănd*-ĕ)
gland	glándula (glăn-*dŭ*-lă)	giant	gigante (hĭ-*găn*-tĕ)
goiter	bocio (*bŏ*-sĭ-ō)	thyroidectomy	tiroidectomía (tĭ-rō-ĭ-dĕc-tō-mĭ-ă)
insulin	insulina (ĭn-sŭ-*lĭ*-nă)	thyroxine	tiroxina (tĭ-rōx-*sĭ*-nă)
pancreas	pancreas (păn-*krĕ*-ăs)	hairy	peludo (pĕ-*lŭ*-dō)
parathyroids	paratiroides (pă-*ră*-tĭ-rō-ĭ-dĕs)	sweet	dulce (*dŭl*-sĕ)
pituitary	pituitario (pĭ-tŭ-ĭ-*tă*-rĭ-ō)	excessive	excesivo (ĕx-sĕ-*sĭ*-vō)
thyroid	tiroides (tĭ-rō-ĭ-*dĕs*)	seed	semilla (sĕ-mĭ-jă)
adrenalin	adrenalina (ă-*drĕ*-nă-lĭ-nă)	potassium	potasio (pō-*tă*-sĭ-ō)
hormone	hormona (ōr-mō-nă)	deficient	deficiente (dĕ-fĭ-sĭ-*ĕn*-tĕ)
iodine	iodo (ĭ-ō-dō)	phlegm	flema (*flĕ*-mă)
acidosis	acidismo (ă-sĭ-dĭs-mō)	masculine	masculino (*măs*-kŭ-lĭ-nō)
extremity	extremidad (ĕx-trĕ-*mĭ*-dăd)	within	dentro (*dĕn*-trō)
soften	ablandar (ă-blăn-dăr)		

CHAPTER REVIEW SECTION

LEARNING EXERCISES

▶ **Anatomy and Physiology**

Write your answers to the following questions. Do not refer back to the text.

1. Name the primary glands of the endocrine system.

   a. _____   b. _____

   c. _____   d. _____

   e. _____   f. _____

   g. _____   h. _____

2. Name the secondary glands of the endocrine system.

   a. _____   b. _____

   c. _____

3. State the vital function of the endocrine system. _____

   _____

4. Define hormone. _____

5. State the vital role of the hypothalamus in regulating endocrine functions.

   _____

   _____

   _____

6. Why is the pituitary gland known as the master gland of the body? _____

   _____

7. Name the hormones secreted by the adenohypophysis.

   a. _____   b. _____

   c. _____   d. _____

   e. _____   f. _____

   g. _____

8. Name the hormones secreted by the neurohypophysis.

   a. _____   b. _____

9. The pineal gland secretes the hormones _____

   and _____.

10. State the vital role of the thyroid gland. _____

    _____

11. Name the hormones stored and secreted by the thyroid gland.

    a. _____   b. _____

    c. _____

12. Parathormone is essential for the maintenance of a normal level of _____

    _____ and also plays a role in the metabolism of _____.

13. Insulin is essential for the maintenance of a normal level of _____.

14. The adrenal cortex secretes a group of hormones known as the _____,

    the _____, and the _____.

15. Name four functions of cortisol.

    a. _____   b. _____

    c. _____   d. _____

16. Name four functions of corticosterone.

    a. _____   b. _____

    c. _____   d. _____

17. _____ is the principal mineralocorticoid secreted by the adrenal cortex.

18. Define androgen. _____

    _____

19. Name the three main catecholamines synthesized, secreted, and stored by the adrenal medulla.

    a. _____   b. _____

    c. _____

20. Name three functions of the hormone epinephrine.

    a. _____

    b. _____

    c. _____

21. The ovaries produce the hormones _____ and _____.

22. The testes produce the hormone _____.

23. Name the two hormones secreted by the thymus.

   a. _____   b. _____

24. Name the four hormones secreted by the gastrointestinal mucosa.

   a. _____   b. _____

   c. _____   d. _____

▶   Word Parts
_____

1. In the spaces provided, write the definitions of these prefixes, roots, combining forms, and suffixes. Do not refer to the listings of terminology words. Leave blank those terms you cannot define.

2. After completing as many as you can, refer back to the terminology word listings to check your work. For each word missed or left blank, write the term and its definition several times on the margins of these pages or on a separate sheet of paper.

3. To maximize the learning process, it is to your advantage to do the following exercises as directed. To refer to the terminology listings before completing these exercises invalidates the learning process.

Prefixes
Give the definitions of the following prefixes:

1. ad- _____   2. dia- _____

3. endo- _____   4. eu- _____

5. ex- _____   6. exo- _____

7. hyper- _____   8. hypo- _____

9. pan- _____   10. para- _____

11. pro- _____

Roots and Combining Forms
Give the definitions of the following roots and combining forms:

1. acid _____   2. acro _____

3. aden _____   4. adeno _____

5. cortic _____   6. creat _____

7. cretin _____   8. crin _____

9. crine _____

10. crino _____

11. dwarf _____

12. galacto _____

13. ger _____

14. gigant _____

15. glandul _____

16. gluco _____

17. gonad _____

18. hirsut _____

19. insul _____

20. insulin _____

21. insulino _____

22. kal _____

23. letharg _____

24. log _____

25. myx _____

26. ophthalm _____

27. pine _____

28. pineal _____

29. pituitar _____

30. ren _____

31. reno _____

32. scler _____

33. thym _____

34. thymo _____

35. thyr _____

36. thyro _____

37. toxic _____

38. trop _____

39. viril _____

Suffixes

Give the definitions of the following suffixes:

1. -al _____

2. -algia _____

3. -ar _____

4. -betes _____

5. -ectomy _____

6. -edema _____

7. -emia _____

8. -genic _____

9. -ia _____

10. -ic _____

11. -ism _____

12. -ist _____

13. -itis _____

14. -logy _____

15. -malacia _____

16. -megaly _____

17. -oid _____

18. -oma _____

19. -osis _____

20. -pathy _____

21. -pexy _____

22. -physis _____

23. -ptosis _____   24. -rrhea _____

25. -therapy _____   26. -tome _____

27. -y _____

▶ **Identifying Medical Terms**

In the spaces provided, write the medical terms for the following meanings:

1. _____   Any disease condition of a gland

2. _____   A congenital deficiency in secretion of the thyroid hormone

3. _____   A disease characterized by excessive discharge of urine

4. _____   The study of the endocrine system

5. _____   Normal activity of the thyroid gland

6. _____   External secretion of a gland

7. _____   A condition of being abnormally large

8. _____   A general classification of the adrenal cortex hormones

9. _____   An excessive amount of potassium in the blood

10. _____   Deficient secretion of any gland

11. _____   Deficient internal secretion of the gonads

12. _____   Pertaining to drowsiness; sluggishness

13. _____   A tumor of the pineal body

14. _____   Inflammation of the thymus

▶ **Spelling**

In the spaces provided, write the correct spelling of these misspelled terms:

1. adensclrosis _____   2. crtinism _____

3. exopthalmic _____   4. hypthyoidism _____

5. myexdema _____   6. pinael _____

7. pitutary _____   8. thyoid _____

9. thyrtome _____   10. virlism _____

WORD PARTS STUDY SHEET

Word Parts	Give the Meaning
endo-	
eu-	
ex-, exo-	
hyper-	
hypo-	
pan-	
pro-	
acro-	
aden-, adeno-	
creat-	
crin-, crine-, crino-	
dwarf-	
ger-	
gigant-	
insul-, insulin-, insulino-	
letharg-	
myx-	
pine-	
pituitar-	
ren-	
scler-	
thym-, thymo-	
thyr-, thyro-	
trop-	
viril-	
-betes	
-edema	

-emia   _____

-genic   _____

-ia, -ism, -osis   _____

-malacia   _____

-megaly   _____

-oid   _____

-oma   _____

-pathy   _____

-pexy   _____

-physis   _____

-ptosis   _____

-rrhea   _____

-therapy   _____

REVIEW QUESTIONS

▶ Matching

Select the appropriate lettered meaning for each numbered line.

_____ 1. aldosterone

_____ 2. androgen

_____ 3. catecholamines

_____ 4. cortisone

_____ 5. dopamine

_____ 6. epinephrine

_____ 7. insulin

_____ 8. iodine

_____ 9. thyroxine

_____ 10. vasopressin

a. Also called antidiuretic hormone, ADH
b. Biochemical substances, epinephrine, norepinephrine, and dopamine
c. A hormone essential for the metabolism of carbohydrates and fats
d. A hormone produced by the thyroid gland
e. The principal mineralocorticoid secreted by the adrenal cortex
f. Hormones that produce or stimulate the development of male characteristics
g. A glucocorticoid hormone used as an anti-inflammatory agent
h. An intermediate substance in the synthesis of norepinephrine
i. Also called adrenaline, Adrenalin
j. A trace mineral that aids in the development and functioning of the thyroid gland
k. A hormone produced by the testes

▶ **Abbreviations**

Place the correct word, phrase, or abbreviation in the space provided.

1. basal metabolic rate ___BMR___

2. diabetes mellitus ___IDDM___

3. FBS ___Fasting Blood Sugar___

4. GTT ___glucose tolerance test___

5. protein-bound iodine ___PBI___

6. PTH ___Parathorme___

7. RIA ___radioimmunoassy___

8. somatotropin hormone ___STH___

9. TFS ___Thyroid Function studies___

10. VP ___Vasopressin___

▶ **Diagnostic and Laboratory Tests**

Select the best answer to each multiple choice question. Circle the letter of your choice.

1. A test performed on urine to determine the amount of epinephrine and norepinephrine present.
   a. catecholamines
   b. corticotropin
   c. protein-bound iodine
   d. total calcium

2. Increased levels may indicate diabetes mellitus, diabetes acidosis, and many other conditions.
   a. protein-bound iodine
   b. total calcium
   c. fasting blood sugar
   d. thyroid scan

3. A test used to detect tumors of the thyroid gland.
   a. thyroxine
   b. total calcium
   c. thyroid scan
   d. protein-bound iodine

4. A blood sugar test performed at specific intervals after the patient has been given a certain amount of glucose.
   a. fasting blood sugar
   b. glucose tolerance test
   c. protein-bound iodine
   d. corticotropin

5. A test used in the diagnosing of adrenal tumors.
    a. 17-HCS
    b. 17-OHCS
    c. 17-KS
     17-HDL

CRITICAL THINKING ACTIVITY

▶ **Case Study**

Diabetes Mellitus Type I—IDDM

Please read the following case study and then answer the questions that follow.

A 20-year-old female was seen by a physician and the following is a synopsis of the visit.

Present History: The patient states that she has been very thirsty and hungry and urinating a lot. She says that diabetes runs in her family, and she is concerned that she may be developing the disease.

Signs and Symptoms: Chief complaints: polydipsia, polyphagia, polyuria.

Diagnosis: Diabetes mellitus Type I—IDDM. The diagnosis was determined by the characteristic symptoms, family history, a blood glucose test, and a glucose tolerance test.

Treatment: The management of diabetes mellitus Type I is based on trying to normalize insulin activity and blood glucose levels to reduce the development of complications of the disease. The patient was instructed in insulin therapy, diet therapy, an exercise program, and lifestyle modifications. The patient was taught how to properly administer insulin, with dosage based on her blood glucose test performed before breakfast, lunch, and dinner. A follow-up visit was scheduled for 2 weeks with instructions to call if there were any questions or problems.

Critical Thinking Questions

1. Signs and symptoms of diabetes mellitus Type I include _____, polyphagia, and polyuria.

2. The diagnosis was determined by the characteristic symptoms, family history, a blood glucose test, and a _____ tolerance test.

3. Treatment for diabetes mellitus Type I includes insulin therapy, _____ therapy, an exercise program, and lifestyle changes.

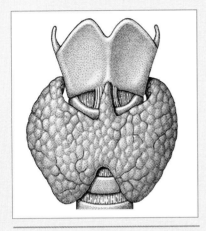

ANATOMY AND PHYSIOLOGY OF THE ENDOCRINE SYSTEM

OBJECTIVES

- Contrast the response times to changing conditions by the nervous and endocrine systems.

- List the types of molecules that form the two main groups of hormones.

- Explain the general actions of hormones.

- Describe how endocrine organs are controlled by negative feedback.

- Discuss the location, hormones, and functions of the following endocrine glands and tissues: pituitary, thyroid, parathyroids, thymus, adrenals, pancreas, testes, ovaries, and pineal gland.

- Briefly describe the functions of the hormones secreted by the kidneys, heart, digestive system, and adipose tissue.

- Explain how the endocrine system responds to stress.

The body adapts to changing conditions through a combination of rapid, short-term and slower, long-term responses. As we learned in the last two chapters, the nervous system allows us to respond quickly to changing internal and external stimuli. In contrast, the responses of the **endocrine system** are slower and longer lasting. Some of the endocrine responses aid in maintaining homeostasis, such as the control of blood sugar (glucose) and calcium ion levels, while others promote permanent structural changes, such as those associated with growth and development.

This chapter introduces the wide range of structures and functions of the endocrine system. It will also show the close working relationship between the nervous and endocrine systems.

▶ SYSTEM BRIEF

The endocrine system includes all the endocrine cells and tissues of the body. As noted in Chapter 4, *endocrine cells* are secretory cells that release their secretions into the bloodstream, where they can reach all parts of the body. In contrast, the secretions of *exocrine cells* travel through ducts to specific locations. *Endocrine glands* are ductless glands made up of groups of endocrine cells and other tissues. They form the organs of the endocrine system.

The cells of endocrine glands secrete chemicals called **hormones**, a word that means "to set in motion." Hormones are chemical compounds that travel in the circulatory system and affect the activities of other cells.

The major glands of the endocrine system are shown in Figure 10-1. Some of these organs, such as the pituitary gland, only secrete hormones; others, such as the pancreas, have many other functions in addition to hormone secretion.

Table 10-1 lists the major glands of the endocrine system and the hormones they secrete, and contains brief remarks about their general effects on body functions.

▶ HORMONES

CHEMICAL MAKEUP

Most hormones are composed of amino acids, the building blocks of proteins. These **amino acid–based hormones** range in size from hormones derived from single amino acids to large protein hormones. This is by far the largest category of hormones, and it includes the hormones of most endocrine organs other than the reproductive organs (ovaries, testes, and placenta) and the outer portion of the adrenal gland (the adrenal cortex).

Lipid-based hormones include *steroid hormones* and *prostaglandins*. **Steroid hormones** are built from molecules of cholesterol. Steroid hormones are released by the reproductive organs and the adrenal cortex. **Prostaglandins** are produced from fatty acids

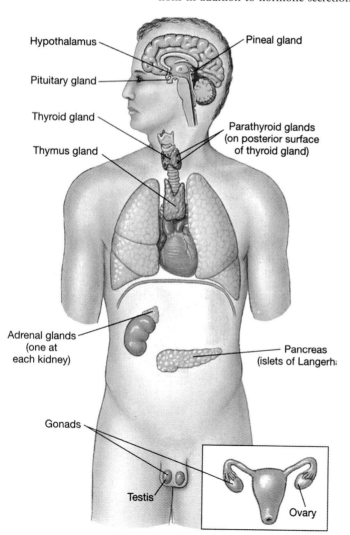

Hypothalamus
Pituitary gland
Thyroid gland
Thymus gland
Pineal gland
Parathyroid glands (on posterior surface of thyroid gland)
Adrenal glands (one at each kidney)
Pancreas (islets of Langerh
Gonads
Testis
Ovary

FIGURE 10-1

The Endocrine System.

Table 10-1	Endocrine Hormones: Their Sources and Effects
Gland/Hormone	**Effects**
Hypothalamus	
Releasing hormones	Stimulate hormone production in anterior pituitary
Inhibiting hormones	Prevent hormone production in anterior pituitary
Anterior Pituitary	
Thyroid-stimulating hormone (TSH)	Triggers release of thyroid hormones
Adrenocorticotropic hormone (ACTH)	Stimulates adrenal cortex cells to secrete glucocorticoids
Follicle-stimulating hormone (FSH)	*Female*: promotes egg development; stimulates estrogen production *Male*: promotes sperm production
Luteinizing hormone (LH)	*Female*: produces ovulation (egg release); stimulates ovaries to produce estrogen and progesterone *Male*: stimulates testes to produce androgens (e.g., testosterone)
Prolactin (PRL)	Stimulates mammary gland development and production of milk
Growth hormone (GH)	Stimulates cell growth and division
Posterior Pituitary	
Antidiuretic hormone (ADH)	Reduces water loss at kidneys
Oxytocin	Stimulates contraction of smooth muscles of uterus and release of milk in females; stimulates prostate gland contraction in males
Thyroid	
Thyroxine	Stimulates general rate of body metabolism
Calcitonin	Reduces calcium ion levels in blood
Parathyroid	
Parathyroid hormone (PTH)	Increases calcium ion levels in the blood
Thymus	
Thymosins	Stimulate development of white blood cells (lymphocytes) in early life
Adrenal Cortex	
Glucocorticoids	Stimulate glucose synthesis and storage (as glycogen) by liver
Mineralocorticoids	Cause the kidneys to retain sodium ions and water and excrete potassium ions
Androgens	Produced in both sexes, but functions uncertain
Adrenal Medullae	
Epinephrine (E)	Also known as *adrenaline*; stimulates use of glucose and glycogen and release of lipids by adipose tissue; increases heart rate and blood pressure
Norepinephrine (NE)	Also known as *noradrenaline*; effects similar to epinephrine
Pancreas	
Insulin	Decreases glucose levels in blood
Glucagon	Increases glucose levels in blood
Testes	
Testosterone	Promotes production of sperm and development of male sex characteristics
Ovaries	
Estrogens	Support egg development, growth of uterine lining, and development of female sex characteristics
Progesterones	Prepare uterus for arrival of developing embryo and support of further embryonic development
Pineal Gland	
Melatonin	Delays sexual maturation; establishes day/night cycle
Adipose Tissue	
Leptin	Promotes weight loss; stimulates metabolism

by most tissues of the body. Locally, prostaglandins coordinate cellular activities within the tissue. For this reason, they are sometimes called "local hormones." However, some prostaglandins enter the circulation and have more widespread effects on body processes.

ACTIONS ON CELLS

Each hormone has specific **target cells** that respond to its presence. As Figure 10-2 shows, such cells have the appropriate receptor molecules in their cell membranes. Because the target cells may be anywhere in the body, a single hormone can affect the activities of multiple tissues and organs simultaneously.

All the structures and functions of cells depend on proteins. Structural proteins determine the general shape and internal structure of a cell, and enzymes (which are proteins as well) control its metabolic activities. Hormones alter the workings of a target cell by changing the dominant *types, activities,* or *quantities* of important enzymes and structural proteins. For example, the hormone *testosterone,* the dominant sex hormone in males, stimulates the production of enzymes and proteins in skeletal muscle fibers, increasing muscle size and strength.

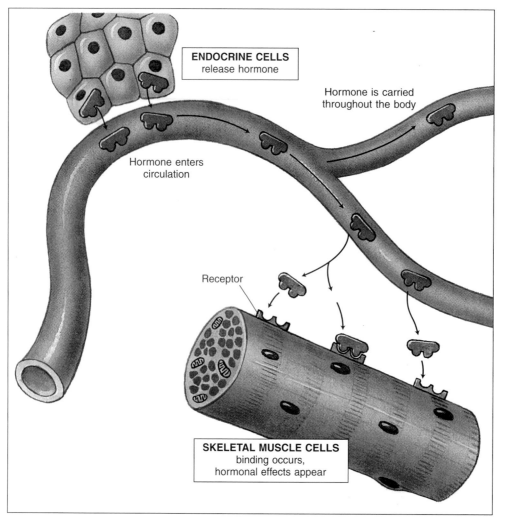

ENDOCRINE CELLS
release hormone

Hormone is carried
throughout the body

Hormone enters
circulation

Receptor

SKELETAL MUSCLE CELLS
binding occurs,
hormonal effects appear

FIGURE 10-2

Hormones and Target Cells.

For a hormone to affect a target cell, that cell must have receptors that can bind the hormone and initiate a change in cellular activity. This hormone affects skeletal muscle cells because the muscle cells have the appropriate receptors.

CONTROL OF HORMONE SECRETION

The rate of hormone secretion varies from hour to hour and day to day. The control of hormone secretion is based on negative feedback. Recall that in negative feedback processes, actions are taken that reduce or eliminate the effects of a stimulus. Hormone secretions occur in response to changes in the composition of blood or surrounding tissue fluid. Once in circulation, the hormone stimulates a target cell to restore normal conditions (homeostasis).

Some endocrine glands respond directly to changes in the composition of body fluids. For example, the parathyroid and thyroid glands control calcium ion levels in this manner. When circulating calcium levels decline, the parathyroid glands release *parathyroid hormone*, and target cells respond by elevating blood calcium ion levels. When calcium levels rise, the thyroid gland releases *calcitonin*, and target cells respond by lowering blood calcium ion levels.

Other endocrine glands respond indirectly to changes in the composition of body fluids. The activities of these endocrine glands are regulated by the hypothalamus. The hypothalamus provides the link between the nervous and endocrine systems.

The Hypothalamus and Hormone Secretion

Neurons in the hypothalamus regulate the activities of the nervous and endocrine systems in three ways (see Figure 10-3).

1. The hypothalamus contains autonomic nervous system centers that control the endocrine cells of the adrenal medullae through sympathetic innervation. When the sympathetic division of the ANS is activated, the adrenal medullae release hormones into the bloodstream. These hormones, epinephrine and norepinephrine, increase heart rate, and blood pressure, and free up energy reserves for immediate use.
2. The hypothalamus itself acts as an endocrine organ, releasing the hormones *ADH* and *oxytocin*. ADH reduces water losses at the kidneys; oxytocin stimulates smooth muscle contractions in the uterus and mammary glands (women) and the prostate gland (men).
3. The hypothalamus also secretes **regulatory hormones**, special hormones that regulate the secretions of endocrine cells in the anterior pituitary gland. There are two classes of regulatory hormones: *Releasing hormones (RH)* stimulate the production of pituitary hormones, and *inhibiting hormones (IH)* prevent the synthesis and secretion of pituitary hormones.

Concept Questions

✔ How does a hormone affect a target cell?

✔ What do the regulatory hormones of the hypothalamus regulate?

▶ MAJOR ENDOCRINE GLANDS

THE PITUITARY GLAND

hypo, below + *physis*, growth
hypophysis: the pituitary gland, which lies beneath the diencephalon and is connected to the hypothalamus

The pituitary gland, or **hypophysis** (hī-POF-i-sis), secretes eight different hormones. Many of the pituitary's hormones "turn on" other endocrine glands, and are called *-tropins*. This name comes from the Greek word *tropos*, which means "to turn" or "change." As a result, the pituitary is often called the "master gland" of the body. Figure 10-3 shows the hormones released by the pituitary gland and their target organs.

The pituitary is a small, oval gland that lies under the brain, where it is nestled within a depression in the sphenoid bone of the skull. It is connected to the overlying hypothalamus by a slender stalk called the **infundibulum** (in-fun-DIB-ū-lum). The pituitary gland is divided into distinct anterior and posterior regions.

infundibulum: a funnel-shaped structure, in this case the stalk attaching the pituitary gland to the hypothalamus

Anterior Pituitary

The endocrine cells of the **anterior pituitary** are surrounded by a network of capillaries. Those capillaries are also connected to another capillary network within the hypothalamus. These two networks, along with the connecting blood vessels, make up the *hypophyseal portal system*. The two groups of capillaries provide a direct route that carries hormones from the hypothalamus to the anterior pituitary gland, and from there into the general circulation.

FIGURE 10-3

Hormones of the Hypothalamus and
Pituitary Gland, and Their Targets.

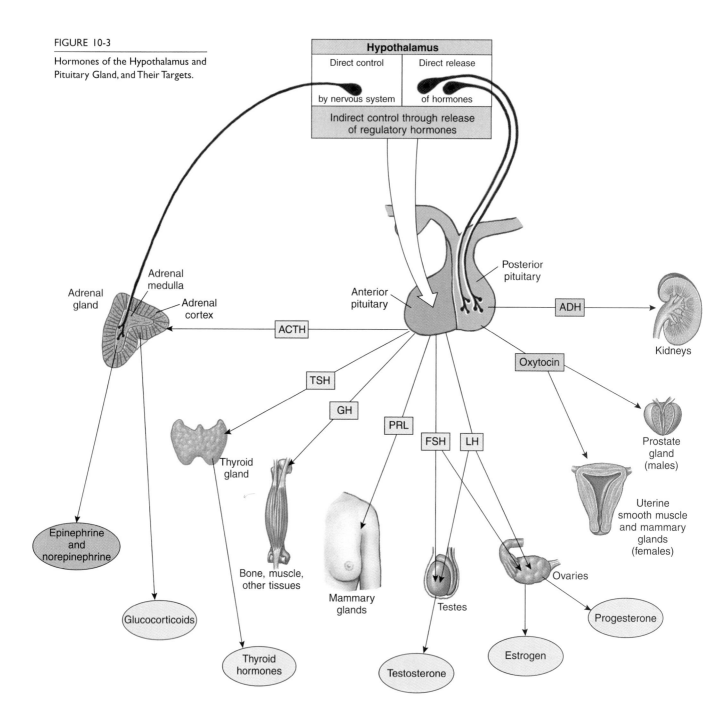

The regulatory hormones produced by the hypothalamus control the secretions of the anterior pituitary gland. An endocrine cell in the anterior pituitary may be controlled by releasing hormones, inhibiting hormones, or some combination of the two. These regulatory hormones are released by neurons in the hypothalamus and carried directly to the anterior pituitary gland by the hypophyseal portal system.

Six hormones are produced by the anterior pituitary. Of these, four regulate the production of hormones by other endocrine glands.

1. Thyroid-stimulating hormone (**TSH**) targets the thyroid gland and triggers the release of thyroid hormones.

2. **Adrenocorticotropic hormone** (**ACTH**) stimulates the release of steroid hormones by the adrenal cortex. In particular, it stimulates the cells producing hormones called **glucocorticoids** (gloo-kō-KŌR-ti-koyds).

3. **Follicle-stimulating hormone** (**FSH**) promotes oocyte development in women and stimulates the secretion of **estrogens**, steroid hormones produced by cells of the ovary. In men, FSH production supports sperm production in the testes.

4. **Luteinizing** (LOO-tē-in-ī-zing) **hormone** (**LH**) induces ovulation (egg release) in women and promotes the ovarian secretion of estrogens and the **progestins** (such as *progesterone*) that prepare the body for possible pregnancy. In men the same hormone stimulates the production of male sex hormones by the *interstitial cells* of the testes. FSH and LH are called **gonadotropins** (gō-nad-ō-TRŌ-pinz) because they regulate the activities of the male and female sex organs (gonads).

5. **Prolactin** (prō-LAK-tin), or **PRL**, which means "before milk," stimulates the development of the mammary glands and their production of milk in the female. It has other stimulatory effects on cell growth and development in both sexes.

6. **Growth hormone** (**GH**), also called *human growth hormone* (hGH) or *somatotropin*, stimulates overall body growth through cell growth and cell division by increasing the rate of protein synthesis. Its greatest effects are on muscular and skeletal development, especially in children.

Posterior Pituitary

The **posterior pituitary** stores hormones produced by two different groups of neurons within the hypothalamus. One group manufactures antidiuretic hormone *(ADH)* and the other, *oxytocin*. Their secretions are transported within axons that extend through the infundibulum to the posterior pituitary.

anti, against + *dia*, through + *ouresis*, urination
antidiuretic hormone: a hormone that reduces the water content of urine

Antidiuretic hormone (**ADH**) is released when there is a rise in the concentration of electrolytes (ions) in the blood or a fall in blood volume or pressure. ADH acts to decrease the amount of water lost at the kidneys. With losses minimized, any water absorbed from the digestive tract will be retained, reducing the concentration of electrolytes. ADH also causes the constriction of blood vessels, which helps increase blood pressure. Alcohol interferes with the production of ADH, which explains why the excretion of urine increases after the consumption of alcoholic beverages.

In women, **oxytocin**, which means "quick childbirth," stimulates smooth muscle cells in the uterus and special cells surrounding the secretory cells of the mammary glands. The stimulation of uterine muscles by oxytocin helps maintain and complete normal labor and childbirth. After delivery, oxytocin triggers the release of milk from the breasts.

In the male, oxytocin stimulates the smooth muscle contraction in the walls of the *prostate gland*. This action may be important prior to ejaculation.

Figure 10-3 and Table 10-1 summarize important information about the hormones of the pituitary gland.

Concept Questions

✔ Why is the pituitary gland referred to as the "master gland" of the body?

✔ How would dehydration affect the level of ADH released by the posterior pituitary?

THE THYROID GLAND

The thyroid gland is located just below the **thyroid** ("shield-shaped") **cartilage**, or "Adam's apple" in the neck (Figure 10-4). Its left and right lobes wrap around the *larynx*, or "voice box." The thyroid gland has a deep red color because of its large number of blood vessels.

The thyroid gland contains large numbers of spherical **thyroid follicles**. Thyroid follicles release two main types of hormones into the circulation. The most important of these is **thyroxine** (T_4) (thī-ROKS-in). Thyroxine production depends on a regular supply of iodine. In many parts of the world, inadequate dietary iodine leads to an inability to synthesize thyroid hormones. Under these conditions, the thyroid follicles swell up, resulting in an enlarged thyroid gland, or *goiter*. This is seldom a problem in the United States because the typical American diet provides roughly three times the minimum daily requirement of iodine, thanks to the addition of iodine to table salt ("iodized salt").

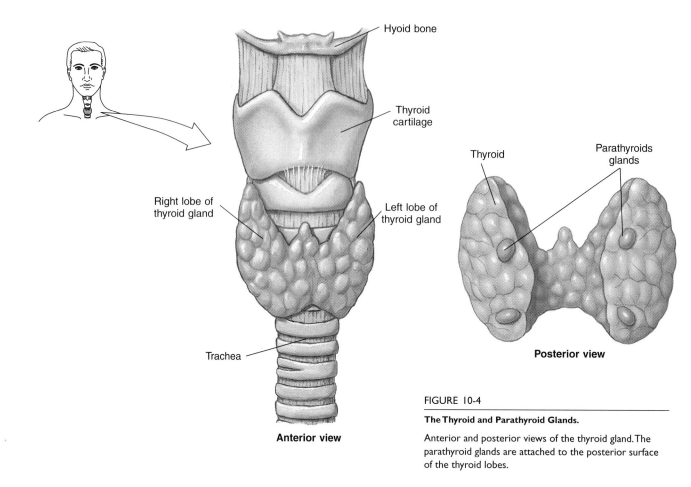

Hyoid bone

Thyroid cartilage

Thyroid

Parathyroids glands

Right lobe of thyroid gland

Left lobe of thyroid gland

Trachea

Posterior view

FIGURE 10-4

The Thyroid and Parathyroid Glands.

Anterior and posterior views of the thyroid gland. The parathyroid glands are attached to the posterior surface of the thyroid lobes.

Anterior view

Thyroxine affects almost every cell in the body. It stimulates energy production in cells, resulting in an increase in cellular metabolism and oxygen consumption. In growing children, thyroid hormones are essential to normal development of the skeletal, muscular, and nervous systems. They also help them adapt to cold temperatures. When the metabolic rate increases, cells consume more energy and more heat is generated, replacing the heat lost to a chilly environment.

The thyroid gland also produces the hormone **calcitonin** (kal-si-TŌ-nin) (**CT**). Calcitonin helps regulate calcium ion concentrations in body fluids. This hormone is released when the calcium ion concentration of the blood rises above normal. The target organs are the bones, the digestive tract, and the kidneys. Calcitonin reduces calcium levels by stimulating bone-building cells (osteoblasts), reducing calcium absorption by the intestine, and stimulating calcium excretion at the kidneys. The resulting reduction in the calcium ion concentrations eliminates the stimulus and "turns off" calcitonin secretion.

THE PARATHYROID GLANDS

Two tiny pairs of parathyroid glands are embedded in the posterior surfaces of the thyroid gland (Figure 10-4). The parathyroid glands produce **parathyroid hormone** (**PTH**) when the calcium concentration falls below normal. Although parathyroid hormone acts on the same target organs as does calcitonin, it produces the opposite effects. PTH stimulates bone-dissolving cells (osteoclasts), promotes intestinal absorption of calcium, and reduces urinary excretion of calcium ions until blood concentrations return to normal.

Concept Questions

✔ What element needs to be supplied in the diet for the thyroid to manufacture thyroxine hormone?

✔ Which glands regulate the concentration of calcium in the body?

THE THYMUS

The thymus is embedded in a mass of connective tissue inside the thoracic cavity, just posterior to the sternum. In a newborn infant the thymus is relatively enormous, often extending from the base of the neck to the upper border of the heart. As the child grows, the thymus continues to enlarge slowly, reaching its maximum size just before puberty. After puberty it gradually atrophies.

The thymus produces several hormones, collectively known as **thymosins** (thī-MŌ-sins). The thymosins promote the development and maturation of white blood cells called *lymphocytes*. These cells play a key role in the body's immune defenses.

THE ADRENAL GLAND

Each kidney is topped by an **adrenal gland**. Each adrenal gland can be divided into two parts, an outer **adrenal cortex** and an inner **adrenal medulla**.

Adrenal Cortex

The adrenal cortex has a grayish yellow coloration because of the presence of stored lipids, especially cholesterol and various fatty acids. The adrenal cortex produces three different classes of steroid hormones, collectively called *corticosteroids*.

1. **Glucocorticoids:** The **glucocorticoids** (glū-kō-KŌR-ti-koyds) (**GC**) are steroid hormones that affect glucose metabolism through a *glucose-sparing effect*. These hormones speed up the rates of glucose synthesis and glycogen formation, especially in the liver. In addition, fatty tissue responds by releasing fatty acids into the blood, and other tissues begin to break down fatty acids and proteins for energy instead of glucose. The net result of all this activity is that more glucose is available to the brain. This is important because glucose is the sole source of energy for neurons.

   Glucocorticoids also have *anti-inflammatory activity*; they suppress the activities of white blood cells and other components of the immune system. Glucocorticoid creams are often used to control irritating allergic rashes, such as those produced by poison ivy, and injections of glucocorticoids may be used to control more severe allergic reactions. *Cortisol* (KŌR-ti-sol), also called *hydrocortisone*, is one of the most important glucocorticoids.

2. **Mineralocorticoids:** Corticosteroids known as mineralocorticoids (min-er-al-ō-KŌR-ti-koyds) (**MC**) affect the concentrations of sodium and potassium ions in body fluids. **Aldosterone** (al-DOS-ter-ōn), the main mineralocorticoid, targets kidney cells that regulate the composition of urine. It causes the retention of sodium ions and water, reducing fluid loss in the urine. Aldosterone also reduces sodium and water loss at the sweat glands, salivary glands, and along the digestive tract. The sodium ions recovered are exchanged for potassium ions, so aldosterone also lowers potassium ion concentrations in body fluids.

3. **Androgens:** The adrenal cortex in both sexes produces small quantities of sex hormones called androgens. Androgens are produced in large quantities by the testes of males, and the importance of the small adrenal production in both sexes remains uncertain.

Adrenal Medulla

Each adrenal medulla has a reddish brown coloration partly because of the many blood vessels in this area. Its cells are targets of sympathetic nerve fibers that extend from the spinal cord.

The adrenal medullae contain secretory cells that produce **epinephrine** *(adrenaline)* and **norepinephrine** *(noradrenaline)*. These hormones are normally released at a low rate, but nerve impulses from the sympathetic nervous system speed up their rate of secretion dramatically. The sudden release of these hormones rapidly prepares the body for emergency "fight-or-flight" situations.

Epinephrine and norepinephrine speed up the use of cellular energy and free up energy reserves. They accomplish this by targeting receptors on skeletal muscle, fat, and liver cells. Skeletal muscles release glucose from their glycogen reserves and, in turn, produce energy from the glucose. This increases muscular power and endurance. In fatty tissue, stored fats are broken down, releasing fatty acids, and in the liver, glycogen molecules are converted to glucose. The fatty acids and glucose are then released into the bloodstream for use by other body tissues. The heart responds to epinephrine and norepinephrine with an increase in the rate and strength of cardiac contractions. This elevates blood pressure.

THE PANCREAS

The **pancreas** lies between the stomach and small intestine (Figure 10-5a). It is a slender, usually pink organ with a lumpy consistency that contains both exocrine and endocrine cells. The **exocrine pancreas** produces large quantities of *pancreatic juice* that is secreted into the digestive tract.

Cells of the **endocrine pancreas** form clusters known as **pancreatic islets**, or the *islets of Langerhans* (LAN-ger-hanz) (Figure 10-5b). Like small islands, the islets are scattered among the exocrine cells that make up most of the pancreas. Each islet contains different cell types that produce different hormones. The two most important hormones are **glucagon** (GLOO-ka-gon) and **insulin** (IN-su-lin). Glucagon and insulin regulate blood glucose concentrations in the same way that parathyroid hormone and calcitonin control blood calcium levels.

Regulation of Blood Glucose

When glucose levels in the blood rise, certain islet cells release insulin, which stimulates the transport of glucose across cell membranes into most body cells. As cells absorb glucose from the bloodstream, circulating glucose concentrations decline.

In summary, insulin lowers blood glucose by shifting the glucose into cells. While glucose levels remain high most cells use it as an energy source instead of breaking down fatty acids or amino acids. The energy generated by the breakdown of glucose molecules is then used to build proteins and enhance energy reserves in the form of fats or glycogen. Thus insulin stimulates cell growth throughout the body. In adipose tissues, fat cells enlarge as they synthesize additional triglycerides; in the liver and in skeletal muscles, glycogen formation accelerates.

When blood glucose concentrations fall below normal, other islet cells release glucagon, and energy reserves are used. Skeletal muscles and liver cells break down glycogen to release glucose, fatty

FIGURE 10-5

The Pancreas and Its Endocrine Cells.

(a) Orientation of the pancreas. **(b)** A pancreatic islet surrounded by exocrine-secreting cells.

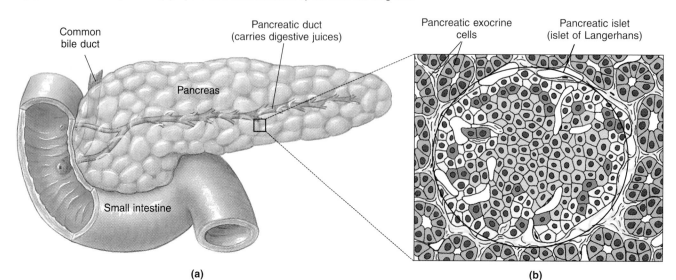

(a)

(b)

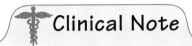

Clinical Note

Diabetes Mellitus

Diabetes mellitus (dī-a-BĒ-tēs me-LĪ-tus) is characterized by high glucose concentrations in the blood and urine. The high levels of glucose in the kidney limits its ability to conserve water, and as a result excessive amounts of urine are produced. Diabetes mellitus occurs when islet cells produce inadequate amounts of insulin or when cells have too few insulin receptors (or abnormal receptors). Insulin stimulates cells to absorb glucose from their surroundings. When insulin levels are low, or cells are unable to detect it, the cells start breaking down fatty acids and even proteins to obtain energy. Because most tissues can no long absorb glucose, circulating glucose levels climb after every meal, and then remain elevated between meals. Over time, the combination of metabolic changes and water losses cause a variety of problems in virtually all body systems. Some examples of these problems include disturbances of vision; kidney failure; nervous system disorders; and an increased risk of heart attacks.

tissues release fatty acids, and proteins are broken down into their component amino acids. The fatty acids are absorbed by many cells, and used for energy production instead of glucose. The liver absorbs the amino acids and converts them to glucose, which can be released into the circulation. As a result, blood glucose concentrations rise toward normal levels.

Some cells, such as brain and kidney cells, do not have insulin receptors. These cells can absorb and use glucose without the presence of insulin. When blood glucose levels fall below normal, and insulin secretion is minimal, other tissues stop using glucose. The glucose that remains in circulation then remains available for brain and kidney cells.

Under normal conditions, glucose is conserved at the kidneys, and glucose is not lost in the urine. A lack of insulin or an inability to respond normally to insulin will prevent most cells from absorbing glucose, even after a meal rich in sugars. As a result, the glucose concentration in the blood can rise to very high levels (several times normal levels). When this happens, the kidneys can no longer prevent the loss of glucose in the urine. This is a characteristic symptom of the condition called *diabetes mellitus*.

THE REPRODUCTIVE ORGANS

The male and female reproductive organs, the testes and ovaries, produce sex cells and hormones.

The Testes

In the male, the *interstitial cells* of the testes produce the steroid hormones known as **androgens** (from the word *andros,* meaning male). **Testosterone** (tes-TOS-ter-ōn) is the most important androgen. During embryonic development, the production of testosterone causes the development of male reproductive ducts and external genital organs, such as the penis and scrotum. Later in life testosterone stimulates the production of sperm cells, maintains the secretory glands of the male reproductive tract, and determines other male traits, called *secondary sexual characteristics*, such as muscle mass, sexual drive, and the distribution of facial hair and body fat.

The Ovaries

In the ovaries, eggs develop in specialized structures called *follicles*, under stimulation by FSH. Follicle cells surrounding the developing eggs produce **estrogens** (ES-trō-jenz). These steroid hormones support the development of the eggs and stimulate the growth of the uterine lining during the uterine cycle. They are also responsible for determining female *secondary sexual characteristics* such as breast development and body fat distribution. After ovulation has occurred, the cells making up the follicle also begin to secrete **progesterone** (prō-JES-ter-ōn). Progesterone prepares the uterus for the arrival of a developing embryo. Along with other hormones, it also causes an enlargement of the mammary glands.

Concept Questions

✔ What effect would elevated cortisol levels have on the level of glucose in the blood?

✔ How do insulin and glucagon control the levels of glucose in blood?

✔ What hormones are secreted by the testes and ovaries?

✔ Increased amounts of light would reduce the production of which hormone?

During pregnancy the placenta itself functions as an endocrine organ, working together with the ovaries and the pituitary gland to promote normal fetal development and delivery. The placenta secretes estrogen, progesterone, and other hormones. The presence of a placental hormone in the urine is the basis of home pregnancy tests.

THE PINEAL GLAND

The pineal gland lies in the roof of the diencephalon superior to the third ventricle. This gland synthesizes the hormone **melatonin** (mel-a-TŌ-nin). Visual information is relayed to the pineal gland, and light/dark cycles affect the rate of melatonin production. Melatonin production is lowest during daylight hours and highest in the dark of night.

Melatonin has several functions. It plays a role in the timing of puberty and human sexual maturation. In addition, because its rate of secretion varies with the day/night cycle, the pineal gland helps set a basic 24-hour rhythm to bodily processes.

▶ OTHER HORMONE SOURCES

THE KIDNEYS

The kidneys release three hormones. One is important in balancing the levels of calcium, and the other two help regulate blood pressure and blood volume.

Calcitriol (kal-si-TRĪ-ol) is a hormone secreted by the kidney in response to the presence of parathyroid hormone (PTH). Calcitriol stimulates the absorption of calcium ions along the digestive tract.

Erythropoietin (e-rith-rō-POY-e-tin), or **EPO**, is released by the kidney in response to low oxygen levels in kidney tissues. Its name, derived from terms that mean "red making," refers to its function: EPO stimulates the production of red blood cells by the bone marrow. The increase in the number of erythrocytes increases the amount of oxygen carried to body tissues.

Renin is released by kidney cells in response to a drop in blood volume and/or blood pressure. Once in the bloodstream, renin acts as an enzyme, and it starts a chemical chain reaction that leads to the formation of the hormone *angiotensin II*. **Angiotensin** (an-jē-ō-TEN-sin) **II** has several functions, including the stimulation of aldosterone production by the adrenal cortex.

THE HEART

The endocrine cells in the heart are cardiac muscle cells in the walls of the *atria*, chambers that receive venous blood. If the blood volume becomes too great, these cardiac muscle cells are excessively stretched. Under these conditions, they release **atrial natriuretic** (nā-trē-ū-RET-ik) **peptide (ANP)**. This hormone lowers blood volume by increasing the loss of sodium and water at the kidneys and suppressing thirst.

THE DIGESTIVE SYSTEM

In addition to the pancreatic islets, the lining of the digestive tract produces a variety of endocrine secretions that are essential to the normal breakdown and absorption of food. Although the pace of digestive activities can be affected by the autonomic nervous system, most digestive processes are controlled locally. The various components of the digestive tract communicate with one another by means of hormones.

Concept Questions

✔ Low oxygen concentrations at the kidneys stimulate the release of EPO. What is the function of this kidney hormone?

✔ How would an increase in the amount of atrial natriuretic peptide affect the volume of urine?

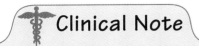

Clinical Note

Anabolic Steroids and Athletes

In order to enhance their performances (and future earnings potential), significant numbers of athletes around the world have turned to the use of **anabolic steroids**. These are synthetic molecules of the male hormone testosterone. Normally, testosterone stimulates muscle building and secondary sex effects during puberty.

Although the use of anabolic steroids is banned by many national and international athletic organizations, it is estimated that 10 to 20 percent of male high school athletes, up to 30 percent of college and professional athletes, and up to 80 percent of bodybuilders use anabolic steroids to "bulk up." Known health risks associated with such use include premature stoppage of bone growth, liver problems (including jaundice and tumors), enlargement of the prostate gland, shrink-age of the testes, and sterility. A link to heart attacks and strokes has also been suggested.

In males, high doses of anabolic steroids can also depress the normal production of testosterone. This effect, which can be permanent, can occur by interference with the production of the hypothalamic releasing hormone that stimulates LH secretion.

Anabolic steroids also add muscle mass to female bodies. However, women taking these hormones can develop irregular menstrual periods, reduced breasts, changes in body hair distribution (including baldness), and a lowered voice. In both genders, androgen abuse may cause a depression of the immune system.

THE ADIPOSE TISSUE

Leptin is a recently discovered weight-control hormone produced by adipose tissue. Its name means "slender." Released into the blood by fat cells, leptin binds to the appetite control centers of the hypothalamus. It acts to control weight gain by (1) suppressing appetite and (2) stimulating metabolic processes that burn energy.

HORMONES AND STRESS

Any condition within the body that threatens its steady state, or homeostasis, is a form of **stress**. Causes of stress may be (1) physical, such as illness or injury; (2) emotional, such as depression or anxiety; (3) environmental, such as extreme heat or cold; or (4) metabolic, such as starvation. The stresses produced may be opposed by specific homeostatic adjustments. For example, a decline in body temperature will result in responses, such as changes in the pattern of circulation or shivering, that attempt to restore normal body temperature.

In addition, the body has a general, or standard, response to different types of stress that involves both the endocrine and nervous systems.

The first, or immediate, response to the stress involves the sympathetic division of the autonomic nervous system. During this phase, energy reserves are mobilized, mainly in the form of glucose, and the body prepares for any physical activities needed to eliminate or escape from the source of the stress with increases in heart and breathing rates. Epinephrine is the dominant hormone of the alarm phase, and its secretion by the adrenal medullae accompanies the sympathetic activation that produces the "fight or flight" response.

If a stress lasts longer than a few hours, other hormones become involved in maintaining the higher energy demands placed on the body. Although epinephrine, growth hormone, and thyroid hormones are released, the dominant hormones of this period are the glucocorticoids. As discussed earlier, glucocorticoids are important in maintaining adequate levels of glucose in the blood, primarily for use by the nervous tissue of the brain and spinal cord. At the same time, however, these secretions have side effects that decrease the immune response and increase the chances of infection.

After extended periods of time under continual stress, organ systems begin to fail due to a lack of lipids, a lack of glucocorticoids, high blood pressure, a failure to balance electrolytes, and mounting damage to vital organs. Although a single cause, such as heart failure, may be listed as the official cause of death, the underlying problem is the inability to support the endocrine and metabolic responses to stress.

Concept Question

✔ What is a negative side effect of continuing glucocorticoid release during periods of stress?

CHAPTER REVIEW SECTION

KEY WORDS

adrenal cortex: Outer portion of adrenal gland that produces steroid hormones.

adrenal medulla: Core of the adrenal gland; secretes epinephrine and norepinephrine into the blood following sympathetic activation.

endocrine gland: A gland that secretes hormones into the blood.

glucagon (GLOO-ka-gon):   Hormone secreted by cells of the pancreatic islets; increases blood glucose concentrations.

hormone: A compound secreted by one cell that travels through the circulatory system to affect the activities of specific cells in another portion of the body.

hypophyseal (hī-po-FI-sē-al) **portal system:**   Network of vessels that carry blood from capillaries in the hypothalamus to capillaries in the anterior pituitary gland

hypothalamus: The region of the brain involved with the unconscious regulation of organ functions, emotions, drives, and the coordination of nervous and endocrine functions.

insulin: Hormone secreted by the cells of the pancreatic islets; causes a reduction in blood glucose concentrations.

negative feedback: Corrective mechanism that opposes or negates a variation from normal limits.

pancreas: Digestive organ containing exocrine and endocrine tissues; exocrine portion secretes pancreatic juice, endocrine portion secretes the hormones insulin and glucagon.

pituitary gland: The hypophysis, or "master gland," situated in the seat of the sphenoid bone and connected to the hypothalamus; secretes eight different hormones.

steroid: A ring-shaped lipid structurally related to cholesterol.

STUDY OUTLINE

INTRODUCTION

1. In general, the nervous system performs short-term "crisis management," whereas the **endocrine system** regulates longer-term, ongoing body processes.

SYSTEM BRIEF

1. *Endocrine cells* release chemicals called **hormones** that alter the metabolic activities of many different tissues and organs simultaneously. *(Figure 10-1, Table 10-1)*

HORMONES

CHEMICAL MAKEUP

1. Hormones can be divided into two groups based on chemical structure: **amino acid–based** and **lipid-based**.

2. Amino acid–based hormones range in size from single amino acid molecules to large proteins.

3. Lipid-based hormones include **steroid hormones** (built from cholesterol molecules) and **prostaglandins** (derived from fatty acids.)

ACTIONS ON CELLS

4. Hormones exert their effects by modifying the activities of **target cells** (cells that are sensitive to that particular hormone). *(Figure 10-2)*

5. Hormones alter a target cell by changing the *types*, *activities*, or *quantities* of its important enzymes and structural proteins.

CONTROL OF HORMONE SECRETION

6. The simplest control of endocrine secretions involves the direct negative feedback of changes in the extracellular fluid on the endocrine cells.

7. The most complex control of secretion involves the hypothalamus. The hypothalamus regulates the activities of the nervous and endocrine systems by three mechanisms: (1) Its autonomic centers exert direct neural control over the endocrine cells of the adrenal medullae; (2) it acts as an endocrine organ itself by releasing hormones into the circulation; (3) it secretes **regulatory hormones** that control the activities of endocrine cells in the pituitary gland.

MAJOR ENDOCRINE GLANDS

THE PITUITARY GLAND

1. The pituitary gland, or **hypophysis**, releases eight important protein hormones. *(Figure 10-3)*

2. The hypothalamus releases regulatory factors into the *hypophyseal portal system*, which carries them to target cells in the anterior pituitary.

3. The rate of regulatory hormone secretion by the hypothalamus is regulated through negative feedback mechanisms. *(Figure 10-3)*

4. The six hormones of the **anterior pituitary** include (1) **thyroid-stimulating hormone (TSH)**, which triggers the release of thyroid hormones; (2) **adrenocorticotropic hormone (ACTH)**, which stimulates the release of **glucocorticoids** by the adrenal gland; (3) **follicle-stimulating hormone (FSH)**, which stimulates **estrogen** secretion and egg development in women and sperm production in men; (4) **luteinizing hormone (LH)**, which causes ovulation and **progestin** production in women and **androgen** production in men; (5) **prolactin (PRL)**, which stimulates the development of the mammary glands and the production of milk; and (6) **growth hormone (GH)**, which stimulates cell growth and replication. *(Figure 10-3; Table 10-1)*

5. The **posterior pituitary** secretes **antidiuretic hormone (ADH)** and **oxytocin**. ADH decreases the amount of water lost at the kidneys. In women, oxytocin stimulates smooth muscle cells in the uterus and contractile cells in the mammary glands. In men, it stimulates prostatic smooth muscle contractions. *(Figure 10-3; Table 10-1)*

THE THYROID GLAND

6. The thyroid gland lies near the **thyroid cartilage** of the larynx and consists of two lobes. *(Figure 10-4)*

7. The thyroid gland contains numerous **thyroid follicles.** Thyroid follicles primarily release iodine-containing **thyroxine** hormone.

8. Thyroxine increases the rate of cellular metabolism.

9. The thyroid follicles also produce **calcitonin (CT),** which helps regulate calcium ion concentrations in body fluids.

THE PARATHYROID GLANDS

10. Four parathyroid glands are embedded in the posterior surface of the thyroid gland. They produce **parathyroid hormone (PTH)** in response to lower than normal concentrations of calcium ions. Together with the thyroid gland, the parathyroid glands maintain calcium ion levels within relatively narrow limits. *(Figure 10-4)*

THE THYMUS

11. The thymus produces several hormones called **thymosins,** which play a role in developing and maintaining normal immune defenses.

THE ADRENAL GLAND

12. A single **adrenal gland** lies above each kidney. The adrenal gland is made up of an outer **adrenal cortex** layer and an inner **medulla.**

13. The adrenal cortex manufactures steroid hormones called *corticosteroids*. The cortex produces (1) **glucocorticoids (GCs)**, the hormones that affect glucose metabolism; (2) **mineralocorticoids (MCs),** principally **aldosterone**, which regulates sodium ion, potassium ion, and water losses at the kidneys, sweat glands, digestive tract, and salivary glands; and (3) *androgens* of uncertain significance.

14. The adrenal medulla produces **epinephrine** and **norepinephrine.**

THE PANCREAS

15. The **pancreas** contains both exocrine and endocrine cells. The **exocrine pancreas** secretes an enzyme-rich fluid that travels to the digestive tract. Cells of the **endocrine pancreas** group in clusters called **pancreatic islets** (*islets of Langerhans*) and produce the hormones **glucagon** and **insulin**. *(Figure 10-5)*

16. Insulin lowers blood glucose by increasing the rate of glucose uptake and utilization; glucagon raises blood glucose by increasing the rates of glycogen breakdown and glucose manufacture in the liver.

THE REPRODUCTIVE ORGANS

17. The *interstitial cells* of the male testis produce **androgens** (steroid hormones). The androgen **testosterone** is the most important sex hormone in the male.

18. In women, ova develop in *follicles*; follicle cells surrounding the eggs produce **estrogens**. After ovulation, the follicle cells reorganize and release a mixture of estrogens and **progesterone**. If pregnancy occurs, the *placenta* functions as an endocrine organ.

THE PINEAL GLAND

19. The pineal gland synthesize **melatonin.** Melatonin appears to (1) slow the maturation of sperm, eggs, and reproductive organs and (2) establish daily 24-hour rhythms.

OTHER HORMONE SOURCES

THE KIDNEYS

1. Endocrine cells in the kidneys produce three hormones that regulate calcium metabolism, blood volume, and blood pressure.

2. **Calcitriol** stimulates calcium and phosphate ion absorption along the digestive tract.

3. **Erythropoietin (EPO)** stimulates red blood cell production by the bone marrow.

4. *Renin* release leads to the formation of **angiotensin II**, the hormone that stimulates the adrenal production of aldosterone.

THE HEART

5. Specialized muscle cells in the heart produce **atrial natriuretic peptide (ANP)**, which lowers blood pressure and/or blood volume.

THE DIGESTIVE SYSTEM

6. In addition to the pancreas, the lining of the digestive tract produces endocrine secretions that are essential to the normal breakdown and absorption of food.

THE ADIPOSE TISSUE

7. Adipose (fatty) tissue secretes *leptin*, a weight-control hormone.

HORMONES AND STRESS

1. **Stress** is any condition within the body that threatens homeostasis. The body's general response to stress of different causes is similar. Stress causes the sympathetic division of the ANS to be activated, and then, if necessary, glucocorticoids to be released. If conditions of stress continue for long periods and corrective actions to restore homeostasis are not taken, organ systems fail and death results.

REVIEW QUESTIONS

MATCHING

Match each item in Column A with the most closely related item in Column B. Use letters for answers in the spaces provided.

	Column A	Column B
H	1. thyroid gland	a. islets of Langerhans
E	2. pineal gland	b. size reduced after puberty
G	3. adrenal medullae	c. atrial natriuretic peptide
L	4. parathyroid gland	d. increased cell growth and division
B	5. thymus gland	e. melatonin
K	6. adrenal cortex	f. hypophysis
C	7. heart	g. secretes epinephrine and norepinephrine
A	8. endocrine pancreas	h. thyroxine
J	9. gonadotropins	i. secretes regulatory hormones
I	10. hypothalamus	j. FSH and LH
F	11. pituitary gland	k. secretes androgens, mineralocorticoids, and glucocorticoids
D	12. growth hormone	l. stimulated by low calcium levels

MULTIPLE CHOICE

13. Cells of different tissues and organs respond to the same hormone if they have the same kind of ___C___ molecules.
    (a) receptor
    (b) target
    (c) DNA
    (d) protein

14. ___D___ lowers the level of glucose in the blood by aiding cells to take glucose in.
    (a) calcitonin
    (b) glucagon
    (c) insulin
    (d) growth hormone

15. Which of the following hormones causes ovulation in women? ___A___
    (a) progesterone
    (b) estrogen
    (c) FSH
    (d) LH

16. Steroid hormones are produced from ___C___.
    (a) amino acids
    (b) cholesterol molecules
    (c) fatty acids
    (d) proteins

17. The hormone that reduces the loss of sodium and water by the kidneys is ___B___.
    (a) parathyroid hormone (PTH)
    (b) thyroxine
    (c) aldosterone
    (d) oxytocin

18. Milk production by the mammary glands is stimulated by ___B___.
    (a) prolactin
    (b) estrogen
    (c) progesterone
    (d) FSH

19. The hormone that increases the rate of cell growth and cell division is ___A___.
    (a) insulin
    (b) testosterone
    (c) glucagon
    (d) growth hormone

20. One of a group of hormones that has an anti-inflammatory effect is ___D___.
    (a) aldosterone
    (b) cortisol
    (c) epinephrine
    (d) thyroxine

TRUE/FALSE

___T___ 21. Atrial natriuretic peptide (ANP) is a hormone released by heart cells in response to low blood pressure.

___T___ 22. Prostaglandins are hormones built from amino acid molecules.

___V___ 23. The hormone-producing cells of the pancreas make up the islets of Langerhans.

24. The anterior pituitary stores hormones produced by the hypothalamus.
25. Blood glucose levels are increased by the action of glucagon.
26. Secondary sex characteristics are determined by testosterone in males and by estrogen in females.

SHORT ESSAY

27. What is the primary difference in the way the nervous and endocrine systems communicate with their target cells?
28. How can a hormone modify the activities of its target cells?
29. What effects do calcitonin and parathyroid hormone have on blood calcium levels?
30. Julie is pregnant and is not receiving any prenatal care. She has a poor diet consisting mostly of fast food. She drinks no milk, preferring colas instead. How will this situation affect Julie's level of parathyroid hormone?

✔ ANSWERS TO CONCEPT CHECK QUESTIONS

(p. 275)   **1.** Hormones affect the workings of a target cell by changing *the identities*, *activities*, or *quantities* of its important enzymes and structural proteins. **2.** The regulatory hormones secreted by the hypothalamus regulate the secretions of endocrine cells in the anterior pituitary gland. One class of regulatory hormones, the releasing hormones (RH), stimulates the production of pituitary hormones; the other class, the inhibiting hormones (IH), prevents the synthesis and secretion of pituitary hormones.

(p. 277)   **1.** The pituitary gland releases six hormones from its anterior portion and two from the posterior portion. Many of the pituitary's hormones stimulate or "turn on" other endocrine glands. As a result, the pituitary is called the "master" endocrine gland. **2.** Dehydration would cause an increase in the concentration of ions in the blood. In response, ADH would be released from the posterior pituitary gland. ADH reduces the amount of water lost at the kidneys and constricts blood vessels to increase blood pressure.

(p. 279)   **1.** The manufacture of thyroxine requires the element iodine. **2.** Calcium concentration in the blood is regulated by the thyroid and parathyroid glands. Calcitonin produced by the thyroid reduces blood calcium levels, and parathyroid hormone produced by the parathyroid glands causes calcium levels to rise in the blood.

(p. 282)   **1.** One of the functions of cortisol is to decrease the cellular use of glucose while increasing glucose availability by promoting the breakdown of glycogen and the conversion of amino acids to carbohydrates. The net result is an increase in blood glucose levels. **2.** Insulin increases the conversion of glucose into glycogen within skeletal muscle and liver cells. Glucagon stimulates the conversion of glycogen into glucose in the liver. Insulin reduces blood glucose levels, and glucagon increases blood glucose levels. **3.** Gonads of both sexes secrete steroid hormones. The testes secrete androgen hormones, such as testosterone, and the ovaries secrete estrogen and progesterone. These hormones are involved in the production of gametes and establishing secondary sex characteristics. **4.** The pineal gland receives nerve impulses from the optic tracts, and its secretion of melatonin is influenced by light–dark cycles. Increased amounts of light inhibit the production of and release of melatonin from the pineal gland.

(p. 282)   **1.** EPO stimulates the production of red blood cells by the bone marrow. The increase in red blood cells improves the transport of oxygen to all body tissues. **2.** Atrial natriuretic peptide (ANP) is released by special cardiac muscle cells when they are excessively stretched. ANP lowers blood volume by increasing the amount of water and sodium lost at the kidneys and reducing the sensation of thirst.

(p. 283)   **1.** Glucocorticoids act by maintaining adequate levels of glucose in the blood, primarily for use by the nervous tissue of the brain and spinal cord. At the same time, however, these secretions have side effects that decrease the immune response and increase the chances of infection.

Section Two
CLINICAL LABORATORY PROCEDURES

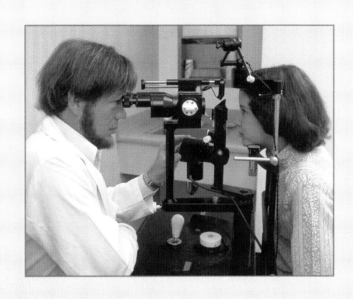

MEDICAL ASSISTANT ROLE DELINEATION CHART

Highlight indicates material covered in this chapter

ADMINISTRATIVE

ADMINISTRATIVE PROCEDURES

- Perform basic clerical functions
- Schedule, coordinate, and monitor appointments
- Schedule inpatient/-outpatient admissions and procedures
- Understand and apply third party guidelines
- Obtain reimbursement through accurate claims submission
- Monitor third-party reimbursement
- Perform medical transcription
- Understand and adhere to managed care policies and procedures
- *Negotiate managed care contracts (adv)*

PRACTICE FINANCES

- Perform procedural and diagnostic coding
- Apply bookkeeping principles
- Document and maintain accounting and banking records
- Manage accounts receivable
- Manage accounts payable
- Process payroll
- *Develop and maintain fee schedules (adv)*
- *Manage renewals of business and professional insurance policies (adv)*
- *Manage personal benefits and maintain records (adv)*

CLINICAL

FUNDAMENTAL PRINCIPLES

- Apply principles of aseptic technique and infection control
- Comply with quality assurance practices
- Screen and follow up patient test results

DIAGNOSTIC ORDERS

- Collect and process specimens
- Perform diagnostic tests

PATIENT CARE

- Adhere to established triage procedures
- Obtain patient history and vital signs
- Prepare and maintain examination and treatment areas

- Prepare patient for examinations, procedures, and treatments
- Assist with examinations, procedures, and treatments
- Prepare and administer medications and immunizations
- Maintain medication and immunization records
- Recognize and respond to emergencies
- Coordinate patient care information with other health care providers

GENERAL (TRANSDISCIPLINARY)

PROFESSIONALISM

- Project a professional manner and image
- Adhere to ethical principles
- Demonstrate initiative and responsibility
- Work as a team member
- Manage time efficiently
- Prioritize and perform multiple tasks
- Adapt to change
- Promote the CMA credential
- Enhance skills through continuing education

COMMUNICATION SKILLS

- Treat all patients with compassion and empathy
- Recognize and respect cultural diversity
- Adapt communications to individual's ability to understand
- Use professional telephone technique
- Use effective and correct verbal and written communications
- Recognize and respond to verbal and non-verbal communications
- Use medical terminology appropriately
- Receive, organize, prioritize, and transmit information
- Serve as liaison
  Promote the practice through positive public relations

LEGAL CONCEPTS

- Maintain confidentiality
- Practice within the scope of education, training, and personal capabilities
- Prepare and maintain medical records
- Document accurately
- Use appropriate guidelines when releasing information
- Follow employer's established policies dealing with the health care contract
- Follow federal, state, and local legal guidelines
- Maintain awareness of federal and state health care legislation and regulations
- Maintain and dispose of regulated substances in compliance with government guidelines
- Comply with established risk management and safety procedures
- Recognize professional credentialing criteria
- Participate in the development and maintenance of personnel, policy, and procedure manuals
- *Develop and maintain personnel, policy, and procedure manuals (adv)*

INSTRUCTION

- Instruct individuals according to their needs
- Explain office policies and procedures
- Teach methods of health promotion and disease prevention
- Locate community resources and disseminate information
- *Orient and train personnel (adv)*
- *Develop educational materials (adv)*
- *Conduct continuing education activities (adv)*

OPERATIONAL FUNCTIONS

- Maintain supply inventory
- Evaluate and recommend equipment and supplies
- Apply computer techniques to support office operations
- *Supervise personnel (adv)*
- *Interview and recommend job applicants (adv)*
- *Negotiate leases and prices for equipment and supply contracts (adv)*

SOURCE: Reprinted by permission of the American Association of Medical Assistants from the AAMA Role Delineation Study: Occupational Analysis of the Medical Assisting Profession.

ASSISTING WITH MEDICAL SPECIALTIES

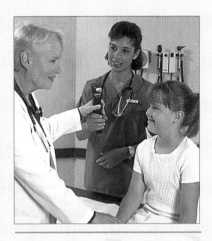

OBJECTIVES

After completing this chapter, you should:

- Define and spell the glossary terms for this chapter.
- Prepare patients for examinations and diagnostic procedures.
- Assist the physician with examinations and treatments.
- Perform selected diagnostic tests.
- Instruct patients with special procedures.
- Follow-up patient's test results.
- Document special procedures accurately.

CLINICAL PERFORMANCE COMPETENCIES

After completing this chapter, you should perform the following tasks:

- Prepare a set-up for a PAP test.
- Explain how to perform a breast self-examination and a testicular self-examination.
- Assist the physician with a diagnostic examination.
- Obtain a wound culture using proper technique.

Glossary

gynecology   The branch of medicine that deals with diseases and disorders of the female reproductive system.

malaise   Discomfort, uneasiness which is often indicative of an infection.

metastasize   Cancerous cells or tumors that spread to another location or organ.

▶ CARDIOVASCULAR SYSTEM

A study of the cardiovascular or circulatory system is called cardiology. This system includes the heart and blood vessels. The symptoms of cardiovascular disease and disorders are varied due to the wide variety of precipitating causes (for example, poor circulation, defective heart valves, conduction defect, blood clots in the heart layers or blood vessels). The most common symptoms of cardiovascular disorders are

- Chest pain (crushing type of pain)
- Cyanosis (bluish skin color due to lack of oxygen in the tissues)
- Diaphoresis (excessive sweating)
- Dyspnea (difficult breathing)
- Edema
- Irregular heartbeat

Disorders of the cardiovascular system are described in Table 6. Diagnostic procedures and tests related to the cardiovascular system are listed in Table 7. (See Appendix C)

▶ ENDOCRINE SYSTEM

Endocrinology is the study of the endocrine system. This glandular system secretes hormones directly into the bloodstream. The organs of the endocrine system are of two types of glands: exocrine glands which secrete through a duct or another organ and endocrine glands which produce internal secretions.

The endocrine glands include two adrenal glands, two ovaries in the female, two sets of parathyroid glands, the pancreas (islets of Langerhans), two testes in the male, the pituitary gland, thymus gland, and thyroid gland. The endocrine glands work together as a whole to affect the entire body. Disorders of the endocrine system are discussed in Table 8. Table 9 lists procedures and tests relating to the endocrine system. (See Appendix C)

▶ GASTROINTESTINAL SYSTEM

The gastrointestinal or digestive system includes mouth, esophagus, stomach, small and large intestine and the accessory organs liver, gallbladder, and pancreas. This system stores and digests food, eliminates waste, and utilizes nutrients. Table 10 describes common disorders and pathology of the digestive system. Table 11 lists procedures and tests relating to the digestive system. (See Appendix C)

SIGMOIDOSCOPY

The sigmoidoscopy, also called proctoscopic or proctosigmoidoscopic examination, is an examination of the interior of the sigmoid colon for diagnostic purposes. This is a useful procedure to assist in the detection of cancer of the colon, polyps, ulcerations, and other disorders of the lower intestinal tract.

The sigmoidoscope, a flexible, metal or plastic instrument with a light source and magnification lens, is used for the sigmoidoscopy. A newer type of flexible sigmoidoscope allows the physician to see further into the colon and view the mucous membranes of the intestines (Figure 11-1). Figure 11-2 pictures a proctoscopic examination table and Figure 11-3 a sigmoidoscope kit.

An obturator is inserted into the sigmoidoscope to guide it into the rectum. The tip of the obturator must be well lubricated to allow for easier insertion. Once into the rectum the physician removes the obturator, or guide, and can then see into the colon through the sigmoidoscope.

Preparation for this examination is important. Patients should be told to empty their bowel and bladder before coming in for the procedure. The physician will usually have the patient take a commercially-prepared enema 2 hours before the examination. They should be advised to drink plenty of clear liquids and eat sparingly the day before the exam. Some physicians will request the patient to refrain from eating raw fruits and vegetables, grains, and dairy products a few days prior to the exam so the colon will be easier to visualize. In some cases a cleansing enema may have to be administered in the physician's office if the patient's bowel is not clear enough. It is critical that every attempt is made to ensure the patient follows the instructions for the bowel preparation since an improperly prepared bowel may result in a reschedule of the procedure.

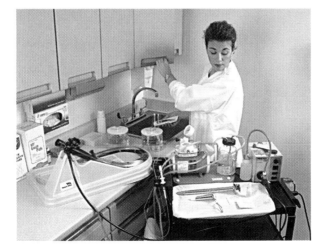

FIGURE 11-1

Sigmoidoscope in cold chemical sterilizer.

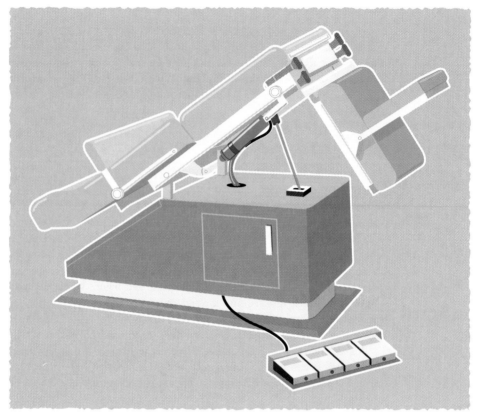

FIGURE 11-2

Proctoscopic examination table.

This procedure can be uncomfortable for patients. The procedure is made easier for patients if they are instructed to concentrate on breathing deeply through the mouth while trying to relax the abdominal muscles. During the procedure the intestinal wall is stretched as the instrument passes through and air may be introduced to distend the wall for easier visualization. This causes the patient to have an urge to defecate and may even be painful for the patient. The procedure only lasts a few minutes, however the patient will need encouragement throughout the procedure.

The physician may take several biopsy samples during the procedure. The patient should sign an informed consent form for both the procedure and any biopsy of materials.

PROCEDURE: Assisting with a Proctosigmoidoscopy

Terminal Performance
Competency: Student will assist the physician during the proctosigmoidoscopic examination by positioning the patient, handling all equipment, biopsy material, and providing support for the patient throughout the procedure without error.

Equipment and Supplies
Sigmoidoscope with obturator, flexible or inflexible (metal or plastic)
Anoscope
Rectal speculum
Insufflator
Suction equipment
Sterile specimen container with preservative
Sterile biopsy forceps
Cotton applicators (long)
Lubricating jelly
Basin of water
Patient drape
Gloves
Patient gown
Patient drape
Small towel or examination table pad
Tissue
Biohazard waste container

Procedural Steps
1. Wash hands.
2. Prepare equipment and supplies. Check all lights and light bulbs in equipment. Prepare a basin of warm water to receive used instruments. Test suction equipment. Place obturator within the sigmoidoscope.
3. Label specimen container with patient's name, address, date, source of specimen, and ID number.
4. Identify patient and explain procedure. Make sure the patient has followed the enema and diet instructions. Check to make sure the consent form has been signed.
5. Ask patient to undress and put on a patient gown.
6. Assist patient into the Sims', lateral, or knee-chest position. Some physicians may use a special proctologic table that will tilt the patient into the correct knee-chest position.
   Rationale: In the knee-chest position, the abdominal contents and organs move forward and away from the pelvic area which makes it easier to insert the sigmoidoscope.

7. Drape the patient and place a towel or disposable exam pad under the perineal area.
8. Place lubricant on the physician's gloved fingers for a digital examination.
9. Place metal scope in basin of warm water to warm it before insertion into patient.
10. Lubricate the tip of the scope.
11. Attach the inflation bulb (for air inflation during the procedure) and attach the light source. Turn the scope on just before the physician is ready to use it. **Rationale:** The scope tip becomes warm/hot if turned on too soon and may harm the patient.
12. Remind the patient to take deep breaths and relax the abdominal muscles.
13. Assist the physician by handling instruments and equipment such as suction, cotton tipped applicators, as they are needed. Place used equipment, including suction tubing, into basin of water.
14. Assist with biopsy by holding open specimen containers to receive specimen, while maintaining sterility of container.
15. Clean around patient's anal opening with tissue. Discard in biohazard waste container.
16. Remove gloves and wash hands.
17. Assist patient to slowly sit up.
    Rationale: Sitting up too quickly from the Sims' position can result in dizziness.
18. Ask patient to dress and provide assistance as needed.
19. Apply gloves and clean equipment and room.
20. Remove gloves and document procedure. The physician will document the results of the procedure.

Charting Example
2/14/XX   9:00 AM Assisted patient with sigmoidoscopic examination. Biopsy sent to lab. No dizziness or discomfort noted after procedure. M. King, CMA

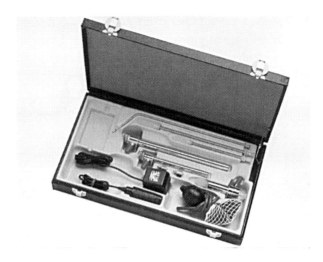

FIGURE 11-3

Sigmoidoscope kit from Welch-Allyn.

▶ LYMPHATIC (IMMUNE) SYSTEM

The lymphatic system, consisting of lymph glands, ducts, and nodes, tonsils, thymus gland, and spleen, are the basis of the body's defense system. This system protects the body against the invasion of foreign microorganisms. It works in conjunction with the circulatory system to purify the blood and drain fluids throughout the body.

In some diseases, such as acquired immune deficiency syndrome (AIDS), the body has lost its natural ability to fight off infection. Table 12 describes common disorders and pathology related to the lymphatic system. Table 13 lists procedures and tests related to the lymphatic system. (See Appendix C)

▶ MUSCULOSKELETAL SYSTEM

The study of the musculoskeletal system of bones and muscles is called orthopedics. Disorders of the musculoskeletal system are discussed in Table 14. Table 15 lists procedure and diagnostic tests relating to the musculoskeletal system. (See Appendix C)

▶ NERVOUS SYSTEM

The study of the nervous system is neurology. This system consists of the brain, nerves, and spinal cord. Table 16 describes disorders and diseases of the nervous system. Table 17 discusses procedures and tests relating to the nervous system. (See Appendix C)

▶ REPRODUCTIVE SYSTEMS

Gynecology is the branch of medicine that deals with disorders and diseases of the female reproductive system. The female reproductive system consists of the uterus, two fallopian tubes, two ovaries, the vagina, and the mammary glands. The practice of gynecology is closely related to the medical specialty of obstetrics, which is the branch of medicine concerned with the management of women during pregnancy, childbirth, and the period of time immediately after childbirth the puerperium (Figures 11-4 A and B). A gynecologist may also be an obstetrician.

FEMALE REPRODUCTIVE SYSTEM

An examination of the female reproductive organs will include a breast examination and a pelvic examination to determine the condition of both the external and the internal organs of reproduction. In addition a Papanicolaou (PAP) test may be performed for the early detection of precancerous or early cancer of the cervix and endometrium of the uterus.

The Breast Examination

The physician will generally begin by examining the patient's breasts. The patient lies in the supine position for this examination and is generally asked to place the hand on the side of the breast being examined behind her head. This allows the physician to examine the lymph nodes under that axilla. The physician palpates the breast using his or her finger tips in a circular fashion around all of the breast tissue to search for lumps, tenderness, or inflammation. In addition, any dimpling or puckering of the skin around the breast and nipple is noted. The nipples are checked for cracking, bleeding, or discharge.

The physician will advise the patient to perform a breast self-exam every month, a week after the menstrual period. The medical assistant may have the responsibility of explaining the correct procedure for the breast self-exam. The American Cancer Society also advises a monthly self-exam of both breasts. Women who have reached menopause should examine their breasts on the same day each month. If the woman notes any abnormality during an examination she should call her physician for an appointment and not wait for another month to see if the abnormality disappears. Figure 11-5 demonstrates the correct procedure for a breast self-examination and Figure 11-6 illustrates a medical assistant using a prosthetic teaching breast to instruct a patient on breast self-examination. The guidelines and procedure for instructing a woman on performing a breast self-examination are important elements in patient education.

The American Cancer Society recommends that:

1. Women between the ages of 20 and 39 have a breast examination performed by a physician every three years; women over 40 should have one every year.
2. Women between 40 and 49 who are without any symptoms of breast cancer should have a mammogram every 1-2 years; women over 50 should have a yearly mammogram.

Guidelines: Performing a Breast Self-Examination

1. Breast examinations should be performed at the same time each month, preferably 7-10 days after the menses.
2. Examine the breasts in three positions: before a mirror, lying down, and in a warm shower.
3. Keeping the fingers flat and using the pads of the three middle fingers, use a circular motion starting at the 12 o'clock position and moving around the breast clockwise. Then use an up and down motion, and then move from the nipple outward covering the entire breast. In this manner all of the breast tissue will be examined.

Hollister™

Initial Pregnancy Profile

Hollister Maternal/Newborn Record System

To order call: **1.800.323.4060** Re-order No **5701**

Patient's Name: *Beth Riley*

ID. No.: *358-62-9847*

34 Grove St.

Libertyville, IL. 60048

History Since LMP

Pregnancy Complications (✓)

1. Vaginal Bleeding ☐
2. Abdominal or Epigastric Pain ☐
3. Headache/Dizziness ☐
4. Change in Vision ☐
5. Hyperemesis ☐
6. Urinary Complaint ☐
7. Febrile Episode ☐
8. Rash with Viral Illness ☐
9. Physical Trauma or Surgery ☐
10. Other ______ ☐

Exposure To Environmental Teratogens

11. HIV, CMV, HSV, Syphilis ☐
12. Rubella, Varicella ☐
13. PKU ☐
14. Encephalitis ☐
15. Occupational Chemicals ☐ (Heavy Metal, Organic Solvent, etc.)
16. Radiation ☐
17. Toxoplasmosis ☐
18. Tuberculosis ☐
19. Other ______ ☐

Check and detail all positive findings below. Use reference numbers.

20. Advised abstention during pregnancy.

Substance Use

20. Alcohol ☑
    type *wine*
    amt/day *5oz/occas.*
21. Tobacco ☐
    type ______
    amt/day ______
22. Non-Prescribed Drugs ☐
    type ______
    amt/day ______
23. Prescribed Drugs ☐
    type ______
    amt/day ______
    type ______
    amt/day ______
    type ______
    amt/day ______
24. Street Drugs ☐
    type ______
    amt/day ______
    type ______
    amt/day ______

Physical Assessment

Height	Weight	Pregravid Weight	B.P.	Pulse
5'7"	*140*	*135*	*114/72*	*68*

System	Normal	Abnormal
25. Skin	☑	☐
26. Neurologic	☑	☐
27. Extremities	☑	☐
28. HEENT/Fundi	☑	☐
29. Mouth/Teeth	☑	☐
30. Neck/Thyroid	☑	☐
31. Breasts/Nipples	☑	☐
32. Cardiovascular	☑	☐
33. Respiratory	☑	☐
34. Abdomen	☑	☐
35. Gastrointestinal	☑	☐
36. Urinary	☑	☐
37. Other ______	☐	☐
Pelvic Examination		
38. Vulva	☑	☐
39. Vagina	☑	☐
40. Cervix	☑	☐
41. Uterus Size *6* Wks	☐	☑
42. Adnexa	☑	☐
43. Rectum	☑	☐

Check and detail abnormal findings below. Use reference numbers.

41. Previously diagnosed

Bicornuate uterus

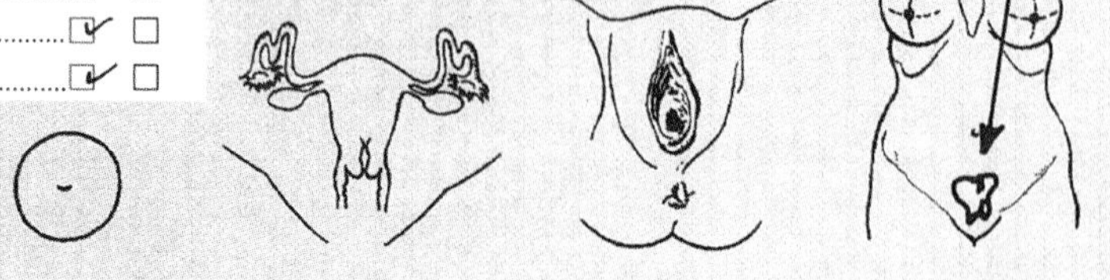

44. Pelvic Type
    ☑ Gynecoid ☐ Anthropoid
    ☐ Android ☐ Platypelloid
45. Measurements
    ☑ Adequate ☐ Inadequate
    ☐ Borderline
46. Diagonal Conjugate Reached
    ☑ Yes ☐ No
    ____ cms
47. Ischial Spines
    ☑ Average ☐ Prominent
    ☐ Blunt
48. Intertuberous Diameter *10* cms
49. Sacrum
    ☑ Concave ☐ Anterior
    ☐ Straight
50. Coccyx
    ☑ Moveable ☐ Malpositioned
    ☐ Fixed
51. Pubic Arch
    ☑ Normal ☐ Narrow
    ☐ Wide

M Brown MD
Examined by

Date *11 / 8 / 95*

Hollister Incorporated, 2000 Hollister Drive, Libertyville, Illinois 60048

INITIAL PREGNANCY PROFILE FORM #5701 696

FIGURE 11-4 A AND B

Initial Pregnancy Profile. (continued)

Hollister™

Initial Lifestyle Profile

Hollister Maternal/Newborn Record System

To order call: 1.800.323.4060 Re-order No. 5702

Patient's Name: Beth Riley

ID. No.: 358-62-9847

34 Grove St.

Libertyville, IL. 60048

Nutritional Assessment

24 Hour Diet History — Usual Pattern: ☑ Yes ☐ No

Nutritional Status: ☑ Well-nourished ☐ Obese ☐ Malnourished ☐ Other ______

Eating Disorder: ☑ None ☐ Anorexia ☐ Bulimia ☐ Pica

Breakfast	Lunch	Dinner	Snacks
cereal c̄ milk	grilled cheese sand.	spaghetti c̄ meatball	yogurt
banana	fruit	tossed salad	fruit
	veg. soup	garlic toast	nuts
Fluids: coffee 8oz.	Fluids: Milk 8oz	Fluids: Milk 8oz	Fluids: Soft drink c̄ caffeine/H_2O

	No	Yes	
Special Diet (i.e. veg, diab...)	☑	☐	
Food Intolerance/Allergies	☑	☐	
Vitamin/Mineral Supplement	☑	☐	
Other ______	☐	☐	

	No	Yes	Frequency/Amount
Artificial Sweeteners	☑	☐	
Caffeine	☐	☑	1 coffee/occas. tea
Excessive Vitamin Intake	☑	☐	
Raw Meat/Fish	☑	☐	

Activity Assessment

	No	Yes	Comments
1. Job Outside Home	☐	☑	1. RN, works 12hr. shifts
2. Work at Home	☐	☑	2. Home maintenance, childcare 2+4 yr. olds.
3. Frequent Travel	☑	☐	
4. Commute > 2 hrs per day	☑	☐	
5. Exercise	☐	☑	5. Walks 4mi. 3x/wk
6. Leisure Activities	☐	☑	6. Reading, sewing
7. Other ______	☐	☐	

Sexuality Assessment

8. Partners ☐ None ☑ One ☐ Many
9. Physical Changes ☑ None
   Identify ______
10. Psychological Changes ☑ None
    Identify ______
11. Other ______

Psychosocial Assessment

Emotional Status: ☑ Happy ☐ Ambivalent ☐ Concerned ☐ Depressed ☐ Angry ☐ Other ______

Basic Needs Met	Yes	No
12. Housing	☑	☐
13. Clothing	☑	☐
14. Food	☑	☐
15. Finances	☑	☐
16. Transportation	☑	☐
Social Support		
17. Biological Father Involved	☑	☐
18. Others Available	☑	☐
Adaptation to Pregnancy		
19. Planned Pregnancy	☑	☐
20. Lifestyle Modifications	☐	☑
Life Stress		
21. Physical Abuse	☐	☑
22. Emotional Abuse	☐	☑
23. Major Change	☐	☑
24. Serious Illness or Death	☐	☑
25. Other ______	☐	☐

26. Feels she has adequate experience.

18. Maternal parents + siblings live in area.

Education Assessment

	Yes	No
26. Learning Needs	☐	☑
27. Interest/Motivation	☑	☐
28. Ability to Read/Communicate	☑	☐
29. Access to Information	☑	☐
30. Other ______	☐	☐
Preferred Learning Methods		
31. One-on-One Instruction	☑	☐
32. Group Instruction	☐	☑
33. Written Information	☑	☐
34. Audio/Video Information	☐	☑
35. Demonstration/Practice	☑	☐
36. Other ______	☐	☐

Personal/Cultural/Religious Customs Affecting Care and/or Learning

☐ None ☑ Identify ______

Initial Lifestyle Risk Status

☑ **No Risk Factors Noted**

☐ **At Risk (Identify)**

Signature: J. Smith RNC Date: 12.16.95

Hollister Incorporated, 2000 Hollister Drive, Libertyville, Illinois 60048

INITIAL LIFESTYLE PROFILE FORM #5702 696

FIGURE 11-4 A AND B

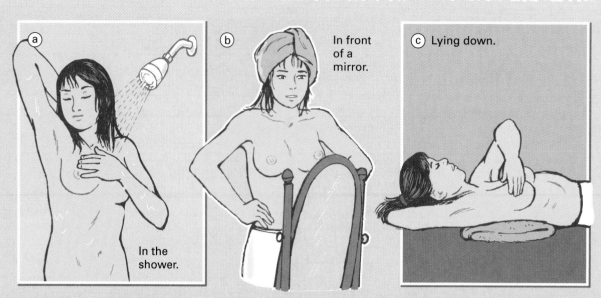

(a) In the shower.

Raise one arm. With fingers flat, touch every part of each breast, gently feeling for a lump or thickening. Use the right hand to examine the left breast, and the left hand to examine the right breast.

(b) In front of a mirror.

With arms at your sides, and then with arms raised above your head, look carefully for changes in the size, shape, and contour of each breast. Look for puckering, dimpling, or changes in skin texture.
Gently squeeze both nipples and look for discharge.

(c) Lying down.

Place a towel or pillow under the right shoulder and the right hand behind the head. Examine the right breast with your left hand.

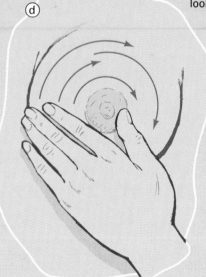

(d)

Fingers flat, press gently in small circles, starting at the outermost top edge of your breast and spiraling in toward the nipple. Examine every part of the breast. Repeat with left breast.

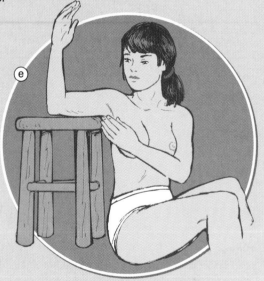

(e)

With the arm resting on a firm surface, use the same circular motion to examine the underarm area. This is breast tissue, too.

This self-examination is not a substitute for periodic examinations by a qualified physician.

FIGURE 11-5

Correct procedure for a breast self-examination.

PROCEDURE: Instructing a Patient on Breast Self-Examination

Equipment and Supplies

Breast Model, if available

Pamphlets on breast self-examination

Procedural Steps

1. Wash hands.

2. Assemble equipment.

3. Identify patient and explain the necessity for performing the procedure correctly in three different positions each month. Use the breast model to explain the correct application of fingertips.

4. **Before a mirror:**

   a. Inspect the breasts for any irregularity in shape while arms are at the side of the body.

   b. Raise the arms overhead and look for contour changes in each breast.

   c. Look for swelling, dimpling of the skin, lumps, or changes in the nipples, such as retracting or discharge.

   d. With palms resting on hips, flex check muscles to observe for any obvious differences in breasts. *Note:* the left and right breasts on most women do not match exactly.

Lying Down:

a. To examine the right breast place a pillow or rolled towel behind the right shoulder with the right hand.

b. Using the left hand with fingers flat, gently press the breast tissue using small circular motions starting at the top of the breast in the 12 o'clock position. Cover all the breast tissue feeling for lumps or any abnormal changes in breast tissue. Gently squeeze the nipple of each breast between thumb and index finger to note lumps or discharge.

c. Repeat the procedure for the left breast.

In the Shower:

a. Using the flat fingertips check breast tissue and underarm tissue when skin is wet. *Rationale:* Hands will move easily over the softened wet skin.

5. Report any abnormalities to the physician.

Charting Example

2/14/XX   2:00 PM   Breast self-exam explained to patient using breast model.

M. King, CMA

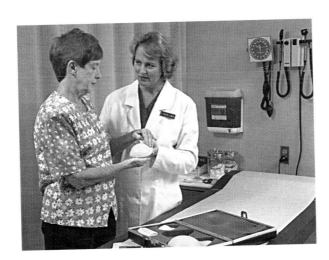

FIGURE 11-6

Medical assistant using a prosthetic teaching breast to instruct a patient on breast self-examination.

The Pelvic Examination

The gynecologic examination, or pelvic exam, is generally included as part of a routine physical examination for the female. It may also be conducted alone in order to diagnose a problem relating specifically to the female reproductive organ. The medical assistant is usually present to assist with a gynecologic examination. Figure 11-7 illustrates the speculum and the manual examination for women. The patient may need reassurance that the procedure is painless, especially if it is the first gynecologic examination the woman has had.

Figure 11-8 displays instruments used for a PAP smear and Figure 11-9 A and B shows an Andwin Safetex One PAP Smear Kit and a PAP smear. The colposcope (gyne) used to ID abnormal tissue is shown in Figure 11-10. See the procedures for assisting with a pelvic examination and a PAP test.

Table 22 describes common disorders and pathology of the reproductive system. Procedures and diagnostic tests relating to the female reproductive system are described in Table 23. (See Appendix A)

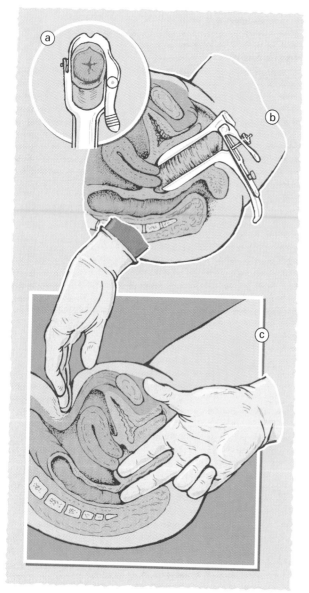

FIGURE 11-7 A AND B

Speculum examination and manual examination for woman.

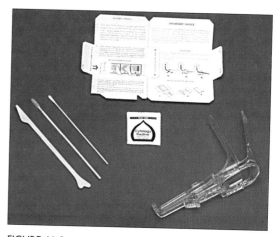

FIGURE 11-8

Instruments needed for a PAP smear.

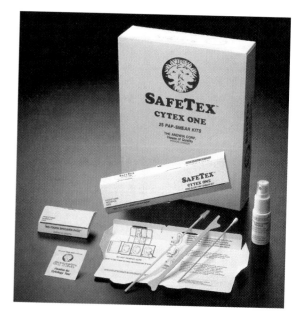

FIGURE 11-9A

Andwin Safetex One PAP Smear Kit.

FIGURE 11-9B

Preparing PAP smear.

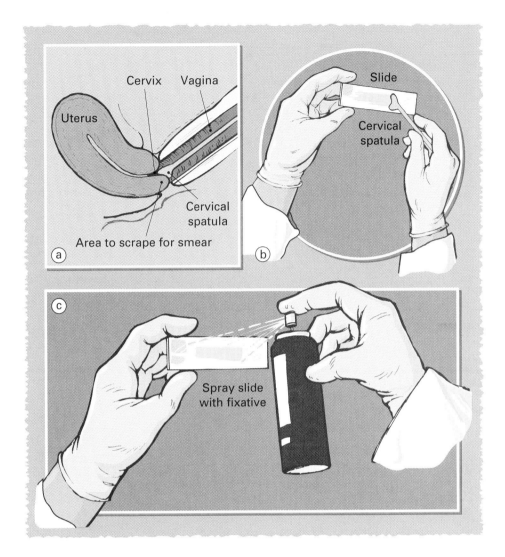

Cervix   Vagina

Uterus

Cervical
spatula

Area to scrape for smear

a

Slide

Cervical
spatula

b

c

Spray slide
with fixative

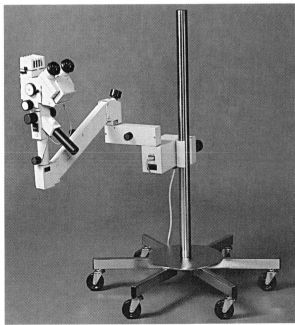

FIGURE 11-10

Seiler Colposcope 121.

PROCEDURE: Assisting With a Pelvic Examination and PAP Test

Terminal Performance
Competency: Student will set-up and assist with a gynecologic examination including collection of PAP smear without error.

Equipment and Supplies
Vaginal speculum
Water-soluble lubricant
Cotton-tipped applicator
Patient drape
PAP smear materials: cervical spatula, glass slides, fixative spray or liquid, identification label
Laboratory request form
Cleansing tissue
Gloves
Container for contaminated vaginal speculum
Goose-neck lamp
Biohazard waste container

Procedural Steps
1. Wash hands.
2. Assemble equipment.
3. Label slides and complete the laboratory form.
4. Identify patient and explain procedure.
5. Direct the patient to the bathroom to empty her bladder.
6. Request patient to remove clothing from the waist down and use drape to cover herself.
7. Position the patient into the dorsal lithotomy position with her buttocks at the edge of the table and feet in the stirrups. Expose the genitalia by moving the drape away from this area while it still covers the legs.
8. Adjust goose-neck lamp and place physician's stool in proper position at end of examination table.
9. Assist the physician with procedure:
   a. Apply gloves.
   b. Hand gloves and equipment to physician as needed. Place lubricant onto the speculum as the physician holds it.
   c. Hold the microscopic slide as the physician places the smear on the slide.
   d. Spray fixative on the slide.
   e. Place the slide into container with label.
10. Hold the receptacle as the physician places the contaminated speculum into it. Set the container into the sink for later cleaning.
11. Apply lubricant to the physician's gloved fingers in preparation for the manual examination.
12. Properly dispose of gloves into hazardous waste container and wash hands.
13. Assist the patient to sit up by (1) helping her move back on the table, (2) taking her feet out of the stirrups, and (3) helping her to a sitting position.

Note: The physician will chart the procedure.

MALE REPRODUCTIVE SYSTEM

The male reproductive system is a combination of reproduction and urinary systems. The major male organs of reproduction are located outside the body in the scrotum and penis. The scrotum (scrotal sac) contains two testes and the seminal ducts. The penis contains the urethra which carries both urine and sperm to the outside of the body. The internal organs of reproduction are the seminal vesicles, ejaculatory duct, and the prostate gland. Common disorders of the male reproductive system are described in Table 24.

The Testicular Examination

Procedures and diagnostic tests relating to the male reproductive system are described in Table 25. (See Appendix C) See Figure 11-11 A-D for an explanation of testicular self-examination for the male patient.

SEXUALLY TRANSMITTED DISEASES

Both genders—male and female—are susceptible to sexually transmitted diseases if they are sexually active. Table 26 contains a description of some of the more common diseases.

There are many genetic disorders that one or both parents can pass on to their child. Table 27 contains a description of several. (See Appendix C)

▶ RESPIRATORY SYSTEM

The respiratory system consists of the nose, pharynx, larynx (voicebox), trachea, bronchi, and lungs. This branch of medicine is called pulmonary medicine. A description of disorders and pathology of the respiratory system is in Table 28. Table 29 describes procedures and diagnostic tests relating to the respiratory system. (See Appendix C)

▶ URINARY SYSTEM

The organs of the urinary system are the bladder, two kidneys, two ureters which are the tubes that carry urine from the kidneys to the bladder, and one urethra which carries the urine from the bladder to the outside of the body. Table 30 describes the disorders and diseases of the urinary system. Procedures and diagnostic tests relating to the urinary system are described in Table 31. (See Appendix C)

FIGURE 11-11 (A)–(D)

(a) Male reproductive system. (b) Begin by examining the testicles. Roll the testicle gently between the thumb and fingers while applying very slight pressure while attempting to feel any hard, painless lumps. (c) Next examine the cord behind each testicle (the epididymis). This may be tender and is the location of most non-cancerous conditions. (d) Continue the examination by gently feeling the tube that runs up from the epididymis (the vas). The vas is normally a smooth, firm movable tube.

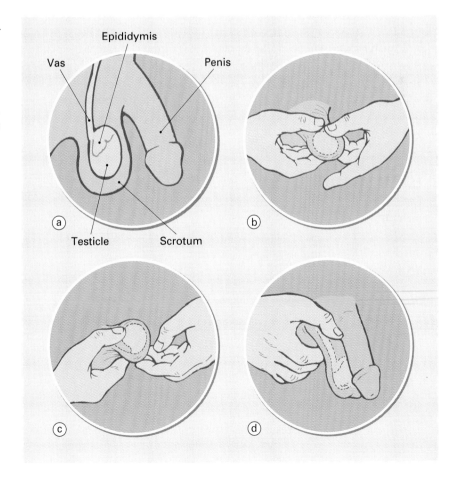

LEGAL AND ETHICAL ISSUES

Many of the procedures discussed in this chapter require written consent either from the patient or the parents, if the patient is a child. Careful explanation of the benefits and risks associated with all treatments should be explained by the physician. The medical assistant needs to reinforce the physician's explanation and determine if the patient has understood the explanation.

The patient has a right to privacy and confidentiality during the examination process. Doors should be closed during any examination or procedure and patients, including children, should be draped to protect their modesty. The examination of infants and children carries an additional safety risk since they are unable to protect themselves. The medical assistant must never leave an infant or child unattended.

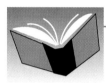

PATIENT EDUCATION

Many patients are not ready either physically or emotionally to fully understand their medical diagnosis. The medical assistant will need to be able to clearly explain in simple language any terms that are confusing to the patient. All follow-up instructions regarding further treatment, appointments, medications, and mobility need to be explained and documented.

The medical assistant will need to utilize many teaching methods to facilitate the patient's comprehension of their diagnosis and treatment plan. Many patients will not be able to understand the medical terminology relating to their illness. Drawing charts for medication dosages, writing instructions for home care and appointment schedules, and asking the patient to repeat what the physician has told them are all effective learning aids.

Summary

The topics presented in this chapter represent a variety of medical specialty areas. No physician's practice will include all of them. Since the profession of medical assisting is for the multi-skilled individual, he or she is expected to have a general knowledge of medicine.

Much of the clinical role of the medical assistant involves assisting with procedures relating to the body systems including: digestive, musculoskeletal (orthopedics), reproductive, urinary, respiratory, integumentary, endocrine, lymphatic, cardiovascular, and special senses. No matter what the task involves, the trademark of a good medical assistant should be careful, caring attention to detail.

Competency Review

1. Define and spell the glossary terms for this chapter.
2. Develop a teaching plan for a patient with diabetes mellitus.
3. Develop a brochure instructing female patients how to do a breast self-examination and male patients a testicular self-examination.
4. Describe the set-up for a PAP smear. What is the medical assistant's responsibility for assisting with this procedure?

References

American Cancer Society. *Cancer Facts for Women*. Publication no. 2007, April 1992.

Anderson, K., and Anderson, L. *Mosby's Pocket Dictionary of Medicine, Nursing, & Allied Health*. Chicago: Mosby, 1994.

Andrews, L, Fullerton, J., Holtsman., and Motulsky, M. *Assessing Genetic Risks*. Washington DC: National Academy Press, 1994.

Badash, S. and Chesbro, D. *Introduction to Health Occupations*. Upper Saddle River, NJ: Brady/Prentice Hall, 1997.

Clayman, C., *The Human Body*. New York: Dorling Kindersley, 1995.

DeSando, M., "How Perfect Is Your 20/20 Vision? *PMA*. November/December, 1992.

Fiesta, J. "The Physical Exam." *RN*. 54:11, 1991.

Fremgen, B., *Medical Terminology*. Upper Saddle River, NJ: Brady/Prentice Hall, 1997.

Greenberg, A. editor, *Primer on Kidney Disease*. New York: Academic Press, 1994.

Heller, M., and Krebs, C. *Delmar's Clinical Handbook for Health Care Professionals*. New York: Delmar, 1997.

Potter, P., and Perry, A. *Fundamentals of Nursing—Concepts, Process and Practice*, 3rd ed. St. Louis: Mosby Year Book, 1993.

Seidel, H. *Mosby's Guide to Physical Examination*. St. Louis: Mosby-Year Book, 1991.

Straasinger, S. *Urinalysis & Body Fluids*. Philadelphia: F.A. Davis, 1994.

Taber's Cyclopedic Medical Dictionary, 18th ed. Philadelphia: F.A. Davis, 1997.

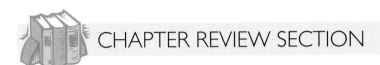

CHAPTER REVIEW SECTION

FILL IN THE BLANK (Refer to text appendix for tables.)

1. Sigmoidoscopy is the examination of the _____ of the _____ _____.

2. The study of the circulatory system is called _____.

3. _____ _____ _____ is a pathological condition of the heart in which there is a reduced outflow of blood from the left side of the heart.

4. Phlebitis is an inflammation of a _____.

5. A disease that involves a defect in the cell-mediated immunity system is _____ _____ _____.

6. _____ is a malignant tumor of the lymph nodes and tissue.

7. A cyst found at the end of long bones is a _____ _____.

MULTIPLE CHOICE (The student may refer to the appendix for assistance with these questions.)

1. Bradycardia is
   (A) an abnormally slow heartbeat
   (B) an abnormally fast heartbeat
   (C) thickening or hardening of the walls of the arteries of the heart
   (D) an abnormal dilation of a blood vessel due to a congenital weakness or defect in the wall of the vessel
   (E) abnormal quivering or contractions of the heart

2. Swollen and distended veins are
   (A) ischemia
   (B) infarct
   (C) thrombophlebitis
   (D) thrombus
   (E) varicose

3. A surgical procedure of altering the structure of a vessel by dilating it using a balloon inside the vessel is
   (A) angiography
   (B) angioplasty
   (C) cardiac catheterization
   (D) aneurysmectomy
   (E) cardiorrhaphy

4. A chronic disorder of carbohydrate metabolism which results in hyperglycemia and glycosuria is
   (A) Cushing's syndrome
   (B) diabetes insipidus
   (C) diabetes mellitus
   (D) Grave's disease
   (E) Hashimoto's disease

5. Surgical removal of the thyroid gland is
   (A) thymectomy
   (B) thyroidotomy
   (C) thymotomy
   (D) thyroidectomy
   (E) thyroparathyroidectomy

6. Medical term for indigestion is
   (A) gastritis
   (B) dyspepsia
   (C) emesis
   (D) regurgitation
   (E) halitosis

7. Crushing of gallstones in the common bile duct is
   (A) colectomy
   (B) cholecystectomy
   (C) choledocholithotripsy
   (D) cholecystogram
   (E) choledocholithotomy

8. Virus that is believed to be the cause of infectious mononucleosis is
   (A) Epstein-Barr
   (B) Hodgkin's
   (C) Paget's
   (D) Bell's
   (E) Rhomberg

9. Softening of the bones caused by a deficiency of phosphorus or calcium is
   (A) osteoarthritis
   (B) osteomalacia
   (C) osteomyelitis
   (D) osteoporosis
   (E) osteosarcoma

10. Surgically cutting into a joint is
    (A) arthrodesis
    (B) arthroplasty
    (C) arthrography
    (D) arthrocentesis
    (E) arthrotomy

11. Painful condition in which the trigeminal nerve is affected by pressure or degeneration is
    (A) tic douloureaux
    (B) shingles
    (C) pica
    (D) spina bifida
    (E) transient ischemic attack

MATCHING
A.

1. Intrauterine device

2. Doppler ultrasound

3. Pelvic ultrasonography

4. Tubal ligation

a. Device inserted into the uterus for purpose of contraception

b. Surgical tying off of the fallopian tube to prevent conception

c. Using an instrument placed externally over the uterus to detect the presence of fibroid tumors to outline the shape of the fetus

d. Use of ultrasound waves to produce an image of organ or fetus

B.

1. Hematuria

2. Enuresis

3. Anuria

4. Nocturia

5. Pyuria

a. pus in the urine

b. absence of urine

c. excessive urination at night

d. bed wetting

e. blood in the urine

SHORT ANSWER

1. List the most common symptoms of cardiovascular disorders.

    a. _____

    b. _____

    c. _____

    d. _____

    e. _____

    f. _____

2. Name and describe 10 tests relating to the endocrine system.

   a. _____

   b. _____

   c. _____

   d. _____

   e. _____

   f. _____

   g. _____

   h. _____

   i. _____

   j. _____

3. Describe the equipment and procedure for a proctosigmoidoscopy.

   _____

   _____

   _____

   _____

   _____

   _____

   _____

   _____

   _____

   _____

4. List the steps in a breast self-examination.

   a. _____

   b. _____

   c. _____

5. List the most common sexually transmitted diseases.

   a. _____

   b. _____

   c. _____

   d. _____

   e. _____

   f. _____

   g. _____

   h. _____

   i. _____

   j. _____

6. Discuss the disorders, procedures, and tests relating to the cardiovascular system.

_____

_____

_____

_____

7. Discuss the disorders, procedures, and tests relating to the endocrine system.

_____

_____

_____

_____

8. Discuss the disorders, procedures, and tests relating to the digestive system.

_____

_____

_____

_____

9. Discuss the disorders, procedures, and tests relating to the urinary system.

_____

_____

_____

_____

10. Discuss the disorders, procedures, and tests relating to the lymphatic system.

_____

_____

_____

_____

11. Discuss the disorders, procedures, and tests relating to the musculoskeletal system.

_____

_____

_____

_____

12. Discuss the disorders, procedures, and tests relating to the reproductive system.

FEMALE	MALE

13. Discuss the disorders, procedures, and tests relating to the respiratory system.

_____

_____

_____

_____

_____

_____

CASE STUDY

Jane Adams, a medical assistant in Dr. Taylor's endocrinology practice, is taking the medical history of Karen Joy, an obese middle-aged woman with diabetes mellitus. She takes 50 units of NPH insulin/day. She has hypertension due to her diabetic condition. Her previous physician treated her for an infection of the kidneys two months ago. She also sees an ophthalmologist for eye problems that she has developed since her diabetes.

Karen hands Jane a copy of her medical history from her previous physician. The record states she has had the following conditions, tests, and procedures.

Conditions:
diabetes mellitus
nephritis
hypertension (secondary)
diabetic retinopathy

Tests:
glucose tolerance test
glycosolated hemoglobin
glaucoma screening
intravenous pyelogram (IVP)

Surgical Procedure:
Laser treatment for diabetic retinopathy

1. Using correct medical terms, chart her presenting symptoms.

2. Define each of the procedures and conditions listed on her medical record. (You may need to use a medical dictionary.)

PROBLEM SOLVING

Karen Joy, the patient in the above case study, opens her purse to take out her insurance card for the medical assistant, Jane. Jane notices several bottles of over-the-counter medications, diet pills, and candy bars in Karen's purse.

1. What, if anything, should Jane say to Karen about what she sees in the purse?

2. Does Jane have a responsibility to report her findings to the physician?

3. What should Jane chart, if anything, regarding her observations of the contents of Karen's purse?

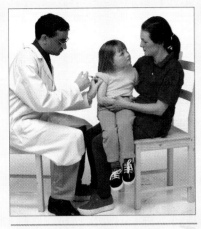
(Courtesy of Dorling Kindersley.)

12

PEDIATRICS

OBJECTIVES

After completing this chapter, you should be able to:

- Identify and spell chapter medical terminology.

- Define the medical assistant's role in a pediatric specialty office.

- Discuss different physical and developmental factors relating to the age of the child.

- Describe different techniques used for positioning and securing the child for examination and treatment.

- Discuss diseases common to the pediatric patient.

- Discuss common childhood contagious diseases.

- List recommended immunizations and possible side effects.

- List and describe different treatments.

- List and describe diagnostic procedures used in the pediatric patient.

SKILLS PERFORMANCE

After completing this chapter, you should be able to:

- perform and record measurements of height, weight, head, and chest circumference.

- perform urine collection with a pediatric urine collection bag.

- document immunizations that are stored and administered.

Glossary

Clinical

MEDICAL TERMINOLOGY

Acyanotic—no blue tint noticed in the skin.

Cyanotic—skin takes on a blue tint which indicates reduced oxygen content of blood

Pediatrician—physician who specializes in treating children from birth to age 20.

phenylketonuria (PKU)—a recessive hereditary disease caused by the lack of an enzyme, phenylaline hydroxylase, which results in severe mental retardation in children if not detected and treated soon after birth.

Prognosis—prediction of the course and outcome of a disease.

Administrative

ABBREVIATIONS

CSF—cerebrospinal fluid

FAS—Fetal Alcohol Syndrome

HCT—hematocrit test

hgb—hemoglobin test

MMR—measles-mumps-rubella vaccine

N/V–nausea and vomiting

PDA—patent ductus arteriosus

ROM—range of motion

VIS—vaccination information sheet

VSD—ventricular septal defect

▶ INTRODUCTION

The *pediatrician* is a physician who specializes in treating children from birth to age 20. A primary care physician may also include care of the pediatric patients in his or her practice. A pediatric practice involves wellness and illness. Early care is important for disease prevention, evaluation of growth and development, and disease diagnosis. Visits are categorized as well child or sick child. A well-child visit is health maintenance, including routine inoculations. A sick-child visit is for assessing disease symptoms and treatment. Additional visits may be required for school check-ups as well as any sports or camp check-ups.

▶ PEDIATRIC MEDICAL ASSISTANT'S ROLE

As a medical assistant in a pediatric office, you will perform many tasks. You will:

- obtain the child's health history,
- obtain the child's developmental history,
- take and record vital signs,
- measure growth and record,
- assist parents in undressing the child, if necessary,
- assist the physician during the physical examination and treatment,
- help the parents restrain the child, if necessary,
- obtain a urine specimen, and
- administer medications, injections, and immunizations.

Children, ages zero through 20 years of age, go through many changes over time. A child's ability to understand medical care and treatment is based on developmental, mental, and emotional growth levels.

As an MA, you must be sensitive to emotions, such as fear, mistrust, and embarrassment. Respect the parent's or guardian's instinct and observations. Use them as a valuable tool. Presenting symptoms may be subtle. Listen to the parent or guardian. His or her finely tuned understanding of the child can provide vital clues, such as a noticeable loss of appetite, changes in fussiness or irritability, changes in sleep habits, changes in the child's cry, and changes in mental alertness and energy levels. Just because a parent or guardian is seriously concerned and anxious, avoid labeling him or her as neurotic, overanxious, or overbearing.

A parent or guardian should be allowed and encouraged to stay with the child unless a parent's or guardian's presence hinders effective care. When it is necessary, the parent or guardian may be asked to leave or escorted from the room.

Another factor to consider is how big and threatening you may look to the child. Whenever possible, it is good practice to get down to the child's eye level when talking with him or her. Sitting in a chair while obtaining history is helpful.

NEVER take a child from the parent. When weighing a child, ask the parent place the child on the scales and stand beside the scales reassuring the child. When the child can be held during a portion of the examination, encourage the parent to hold the child. Show the parent how to hold the child during the examination.

NEVER tell a child "This will not hurt," when a potentially painful procedure is about to be done. Always be truthful with the child. Reassure the parent or guardian about the procedure.

Work with the child and the parent or guardian when a child feels uncomfortable and threatened when clothing needs to be removed. Provide covering for the child in the form of a drape, gown, or sheet. Many times the child will have a security blanket with him or her; this is a excellent source of comfort. Let the child keep the blanket or any other security item, such as a stuffed animal or doll.

▶ PHYSICAL, DEVELOPMENTAL, AND EMOTIONAL GROWTH FACTORS

Each child progresses through a sequence, or series of stages, of the growth process (*see* **Figures 12–1** through **12–7**).

Factors that influence physical growth include:

- heredity,
- racial and ethnic characteristics,
- sex,
- environment (prenatal and postnatal), and
- hormonal balance.

Some prenatal factors that a mother can experience that can cause harm and delays in normal physical growth of a child are:

- contracting rubella,
- using drugs,
- ingesting alcohol,
- smoking,
- sustaining a physical injury, and
- having a poor diet.

Illnesses or injury during childhood may also affect the progression of "normal" development.

Certain physical, developmental, and emotional growth stages have been found to be common to specific age groups (*see* **Table 12–2**).

NORMAL OR EXPECTED CHILD DEVELOPMENT

Infant:

- Begins to smile at six weeks.
- Rolls from stomach to back at ten weeks.
- Gains strength to raise head from a supine position.
- Begins to recognize sounds and make associations.
- Sits without support at six to eight months.
- Begins to crawl, stand, and take steps at eight to 12 months.
- Begins to develop language skills with simple words.

Toddler:

- Strength improves or develops to include climbing and running.
- Coordination develops (including manual dexterity) and improves.
- Continues to process information through senses.
- Continues to develop communication and speech skills.
- Begins to develop small motor skills.
- Begins development of finger dexterity.
- Begins to develop independence.

TABLE 12–1 General Physical, Developmental, and Emotional Growth Stages Names

• From conception to birth— fetus or embryo	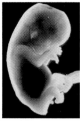 FIGURE 12–1 *(Courtesy of Photo Researchers.)*
• Birth to four weeks— neonate or newborn	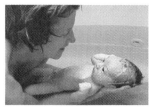 FIGURE 12–2 *(Courtesy of Prentice-Hall, Inc.)*
• Four weeks to one year—infant	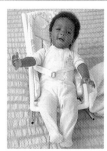 FIGURE 12–3

- One to three years—toddler

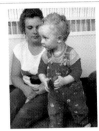

FIGURE 12–4 *(Courtesy of Prentice-Hall, Inc.)*

- Three to six years—preschool
(early childhood)

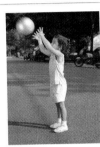

FIGURE 12–5 *(Courtesy of Prentice-Hall, Inc.)*

- Six to 12 years or puberty—
school age (late childhood)

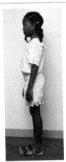

FIGURE 12–6

- 12 years or puberty to beginning
of adult life—adolescence

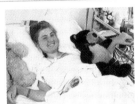

FIGURE 12–7 *(Courtesy of Prentice-Hall, Inc.)*

Preschooler:
- Begins to mimic older children and adults.
- Gains independence.
- Enhances communication techniques.
- Talks in simple, complete sentences.
- Can dress and undress self.

School-age:
- Eye and body coordination improves.
- Makes choices.
- Feels guilt and shame.
- Can experience emotional withdrawal or shyness.

Preadolescent or teen years:
- Develops secondary sex characteristics.
- Strives for independence.
- Experiences puberty and self-image changes.

Stages of Emotional or Personality Development
- Infancy: birth to one year—Sense of Trust
- Toddler: one to three years—Sense of Autonomy
- Preschool: three to six years—Sense of Initiative
- School age: six to twelve years—Sense of Industry
- Adolescence: 12 years—Sense of Identity
- Late adolescence—Sense of intimacy

Summary Growth Development

Measuring growth and keeping growth records for each patient is important. The physician uses growth patterns to observe normal physical development or diagnose diseases. Growth charts are usually a part of a child's medical file and are updated with weight and height on each visit. Recommended charts for growth record keeping are developed by the National Center for Health Statistics (NCHS) along with the Center for Disease Control and Prevention's (CDC's) National Center for Chronic Disease Prevention and Health Promotion. Charts are colored with a blue background for boys and pink background for girls. Charts are specific for age groups of the children as well as length-for-age and weight-for-age percentiles; head circumference-for-age and weight-for-length percentiles; body-mass-index-for-age percentiles and weight-for-stature percentiles. The age groups are birth to 36 months and two to 20 years.

▶ GROWTH MEASUREMENT

Growth is measured to evaluate the child for normal developmental patterns. When growth patterns are abnormal, further assessment and diagnostic testing are performed to determine the cause.

▶ COMMON PEDIATRIC TREATMENTS

Inoculations and well-baby or child checks account for many of the visits to the pediatric office (*see* **Table 12–2** and **FOR THE RECORD: ROUTINE VISITS—WELL-BABY CHECKS** following). A common complaint during well-baby check is that the infant has a diaper rash that has not responded to regular treatment. Non-responsive diaper rash may have a fungal origin and require the prescription medication. Also, frequent diaper changing, gentle cleansing of the skin, and avoiding rubbing the dry, irritated perianal skin is recommended. After washing, patting the skin dry gently or using a hair dryer **ONLY** on a cool setting will help ease the discomfort of the condition. The medication treats the fungal infection. If oral thrush, a possible parallel condition, is also present, a prescription for an oral suspension to coat the white patchy mucous membranes of the mouth is prescribed.

Candida albicans is a fungus that can result from an immunodeficiency-related disease or from over use of antibiotics. The young, and sometimes older, infant can display signs of oral thrush or a rash of the perianal area that will not resolve without medication.

One of the most common medical conditions experienced by infants and toddlers is *otitis media* (ear inflammation). These children experience pain and may pull at their ear or sit with the head held to one side.

The condition responsible for the most lost school time is asthma. Asthma usually is the result of an allergic response. The children experience shortness of breath (SOB) and usually wheeze.

PROCEDURE 12-1:   Perform and Record Measurements of Height or Length, Weight, and Head and Chest Circumference

Procedure Theory:

Recording a newborn's length, weight, and head circumference shows the infant's growth status. An infant can move quickly and suddenly. Watch the infant from the periphery of your vision. Keep a hand within reach of the infant to prevent accidental falls when weighing or measuring. It is important for you to do the measurements quickly.

A platform scale is used to weigh an infant. Cover it with a paper protector. The protector prevents cross-contamination between patients. Balance the scale with the protector in place. Set the scale to "0" before the weight is taken. Infants are generally weighed without clothing or diaper as standard office policy.

Measuring the length of the infant requires the help of the parent or guardian. Some exam tables are equipped with length scales, or the exam table is marked. Ask the parent or guardian to hold the infant's head at the "zero" mark. With the legs straightened, hold the infant's feet at right angle to the exam table to make a mark or hold the infant's feet to the board of the length scale.

Length is measured to approximately two years of age. When a child can stand on the *stadiometer* (device used to measure height) with minor help from the parent, the exam table is no longer used.

Use a plastic or paper tape measure at the greatest round distance of the head to measure head circumference. Head circumference is measured during the first three years of life.

Infant chest circumference is not routinely measured, except when respiratory or cardiac abnormalities are suspected.

DO NOT use a cloth measuring tape because it can stretch and measurements would not be accurate.

Procedure Materials:
- Plastic or paper tape measure
- Infant or platform scale
- Stadiometer
- Growth charts
- Patient chart
- Black ink pen

Procedure Competency:

With the necessary materials, you will be able to measure length (height), weight, and head and/or chest circumference correctly within 15 minutes.

1. Wash your hands completely. Gather equipment and supplies.
2. Identify the parent or guardian with the child and guide them to the treatment area.
3. Remove all clothing, except the diaper before weighing.
4. Remove the diaper and dispose.
5. Weigh the child on the platform scale (*see* **Figure 12–8**).
6. Record the weight on the growth charts and/or progress notes within the child's chart.
7. Diaper the child.
8. Wash hands.
9. Move or ask the parent or guardian to move the child to exam table.
10. Measure the length of the child (*see* **Figure 12–9**).
11. Record the height on the growth charts and/or progress notes within the child's chart.
12. Measure the child's head circumference (*see* **Figure 12–10**).
13. Record the head circumference on the growth charts and/or progress notes within the child's chart.
14. Measure the child's chest circumference, if necessary (*see* **Figure 12–11**).
15. Record the chest circumference on the growth charts and/or progress notes within the child's chart.
16. Tell the physician that the child is ready.
17. After the physician has examined the child, tell the parent or guardian to redress the child.
18. Dispose of disposables.
19. Clean the room.
20. Wash hands.
21. Prepare room for next patient.

Procedure Patient Education:

Tell the parent or guardian about the purpose of growth measurements. Encourage him or her to ask questions.

Procedure Charting Example

09/23/XX   9:00 A.M. Wt. 15lbs 9 oz, Ht 26 in., head circumference 42 cm. Results given to physician for evaluation. Signature, CMA or RMA

FIGURE 12–8

Infant being weighed on a platform scale.
(Courtesy of Phototake.)

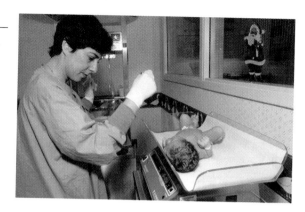

FIGURE 12–9

Photo of an infant being measured on an examination table.
(Courtesy of Prentice-Hall, Inc.)

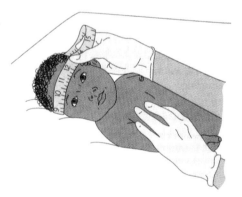

FIGURE 12–10

Photo of an infant's head being measured for circumference.
(Courtesy of Prentice-Hall, Inc.)

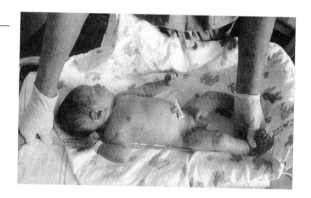

FIGURE 12–11

Photo of an infant's chest being measured for circumference.
(Courtesy of Prentice-Hall, Inc.)

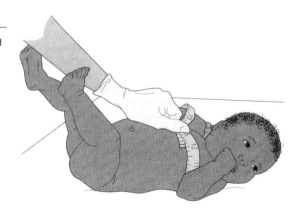

For the Record: New Information on Autism

Autism is a disorder with symptoms of diminished language, social, and emotional development. The child is described as *introverted* (withdrawn from reality). There is no appropriate social interaction with family and other caregivers. Recent research findings from the University of California suggest abnormally rapid brain growth during infancy as a clue for early diagnosis and treatment. Usually, autism is rarely diagnosed before two or three years of age. Researchers studied head circumference measurements in the medical records of autistic children and discovered the linking information.

TABLE 12–2   Well-Child Visit Schedule

First Year of Life	Second Year of Life	After Two Years of Age
2 weeks	15 months	Annually
1 month	18 months	
2 months		
4 months		Include preschool check
6 months		
9 months		
12 months (one year)		

For the Record: Routine Visits—Well-Baby Checks

During routine visits and well-baby checks, certain tests are performed. Each office will have procedures that may include the following:

- measuring weight and height,
- measuring head and chest circumference,
- taking temperature, pulse, respiration and on older children, blood pressure,
- testing range of motion (ROM) of limbs, head, and neck,
- testing pupil reaction,
- checking ears, nose, and throat,
- checking cardiac and respiratory status, and
- palpitating the abdomen.

Depending on age, other assessments include:

- *ambulation* (walking or moving about freely),
- *gait* (way of walking)
- *scoliosis* (curvature of the spine),
- musculoskeletal abnormalities in feet and legs, and
- dental eruptions.

For the Record: Administering Liquid Medications

A physician may prescribe a liquid medications to given to a child. These require special care. A child's body uses and excretes medications differently than the adult or elderly person. Because pediatric dosages are different, the medical and other clinical staff must calculate and double-check for calculation accuracy.

A parent or guardian should be instructed about need to use the dropper supplied with the medication or a medication spoon. A parent or guardian is often tempted to use a household teaspoon or tablespoon to measure the liquid medication. Tell him or her that it is vital that the medication is measured with the spoons or cups supplied by the pharmacist or the manufacturer. For example, it is common to give a child an over-the-counter (OTC) medication, such as acetaminophen. This medication can be administer by drops or liquid. Giving 5 ml of acetaminophen drops on a regular schedule or 150mg/kg could be toxic for the child causing liver damage and even death. Instruct parents to read and follow directions carefully.

► COMMON CONTAGIOUS DISEASES OF CHILDHOOD

Common contagious diseases of childhood are now experienced much less than 50 years ago due to routine preventive inoculations. These diseases include chickenpox (herpes varicella) (*see* Figure 12–16), measles (rubeola) (*see* Figure 12–17), Rubella (German measles), mumps (parotitis) (see Figure 12–18), whooping cough (pertussis), polio, and diptheria. Smallpox, once thought of as being extinct from the world, is now considered as a possible terrorist threat (*see* FOR THE RECORD: SMALL POX following). Recent additions to the routine vaccinations include hepatitis B and

For the Record: Positioning and Securing the Child for Examination and Treatment

As an MA, you will be responsible for positioning and securing the child for an examination or procedure. When possible, involve the parent. Show the parent how to hold and restrain the child and then help the parent to do so.

Ear Examination:
Position 1 (See Figure 12–12):

- Ask the parent or guardian to hold the child or infant upright against his or her body.
- The child's or infant's arms and legs should be tucked in under the parent's arms.
- The child's or infant's head should be turned to the side and held firmly against the parent's or guardian's chest.
- Turn the child's or infant's head and continue holding as the physician examines the other ear.

Position 2 (See Figure 12–13):

- Lay the child on the exam table.
- Ask the parent or guardian to hold both of the child's or infant's arms against the child's or infant's head grasping the hands together above the head.

- Someone else may need to hold the child's or infant's body down, gently, against the exam table.
- Turn the child's or infant's head from side to side, gently, for the physician to examine each ear.

NOTE: Position 2 is also used for examining the eyes, nose, and throat.

Mummy Restraint Method:
This procedure is used when it is not possible for the parent or guardian to hold the child.

1. Fold a large sheet in half.
2. Lay the sheet across the exam table.
3. Ask the parent or guardian to place the child on the sheet.
4. Place the child's arms at his or her sides with hands open and palms against the body (*see* Figure 12–15A).
5. Wrap the sheet from one side and place the end under the child (*see* Figure 12–15B).
6. Wrap the other end of the sheet around the child from the opposite side and secure under the child (*see* Figure 12–15C).

Adaptations of the securing of the sheet and exposure of an arm or leg may be necessary for the procedure. This is only done when it is necessary for the child to be completely restrained.

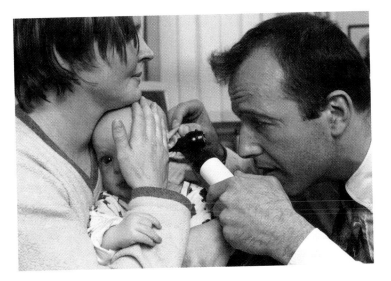

FIGURE 12–12

Photo of an infant in Position 1
(Courtesy of Photoresearchers)

FIGURE 12–13

Photo of an infant in Position 2
(Courtesy of Taxi/Getty Images, Inc.)

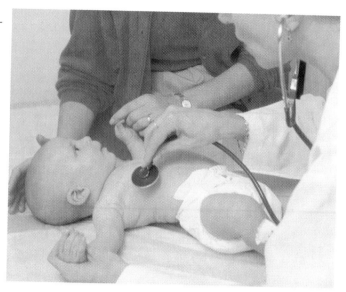

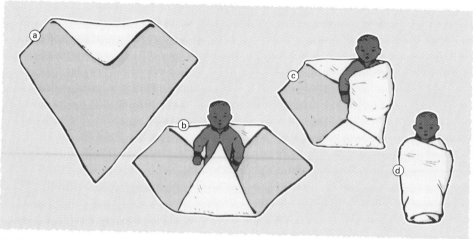

FIGURE 12–14A

Examples of baby wrap for self-containment

FIGURE 12–14B

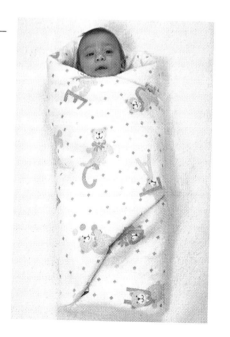

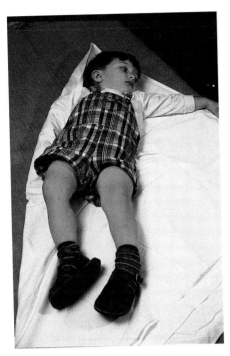
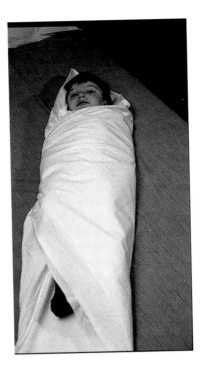
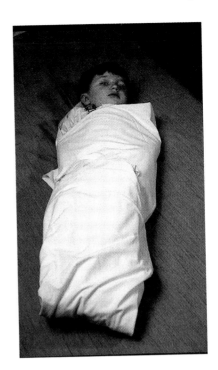

FIGURE 12–15A   B   C

Steps in applying a mummy restraint.

For the Record: Circumcision

A procedure that usually is conducted in the hospital shortly after birth is circumcision. During this procedure, the foreskin on an infant boy is surgically removed. Presurgical diagnosis is *phimosis* (the foreskin can not be pushed back over the glans penis). What traditionally was a routine procedure on most male babies is now an informed decision of the parents.

Tradition of the Jewish faith mandates the male infant to be circumcised on the seventh day of life. This is a celebration for the family. The rabbi routinely performs the procedure as part of a religious ceremony. The medical office may become involved should an infection or other complication develop post operatively.

Haemophilus b (HiB). Booster injections are suggested according to the American Academy of Pediatrics' schedule. Epidemics of childhood contagious diseases have a tendency to occur in college students when there has been a laxity in booster injections.

▶ IMMUNIZATIONS, PATIENT RECORDS AND OFFICE RECORDS

Potency of immunizations is maintained by correct refrigerator or freezer temperature of vaccines as stated by the manufacturer's directions. Transporting is done by placing vaccines inside an insulated cold container with cold packs. The vaccines are put on the front passenger seat of the vehicle for safety. Upon delivery, immediately move the vaccines to the freezer or refrigerator as required. Refrigerator storage must be maintained between 35° and 46°F with the safest temperatures between 41° and 46°F when refrigerator door openings are frequently. Freezer temperatures should be kept below 5°F. Logs are kept of twice daily refrigerator and freezer temperature checks. It is mandatory that the office policy keep a month's stock ahead of vaccine supply and have a pre-arranged back up plan for emergencies without power for the refrigerator or freezer stored vaccine materials. The emergency plan may include an emergency generator or storage at a hospital, fire station or other facility.

For the Record: Small Pox

An English physician, Edward Jenner, 1749–1823, first used the word virus. Jenner developed a smallpox vaccination in 1796 to immunize individuals against cowpox. The weakened dose of vaccine stimulates the creation of antibodies that will attack a specific invading microorganism.

As a result of Jenner's pioneering work in the field of immunization, smallpox became the first contagious disease to be eradicated by vaccination practices. Recent information about the storage of the smallpox virus in laboratories around the world has raised concern about use of the virus as a bioterrorism weapon.

FIGURE 12–16

Child with chicken pox
(Courtesy of Phototake.)

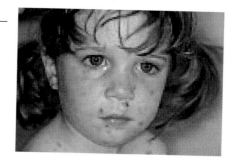

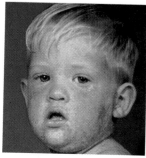
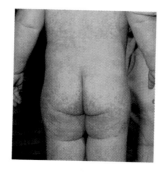

FIGURE 12–17

Child with measles

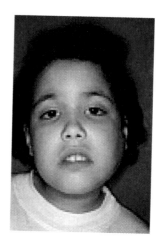

FIGURE 12–18

Child with mumps
(Courtesy of Phototake.)

Recommended Childhood and Adolescent Immunization Schedule
United States · July–December 2004

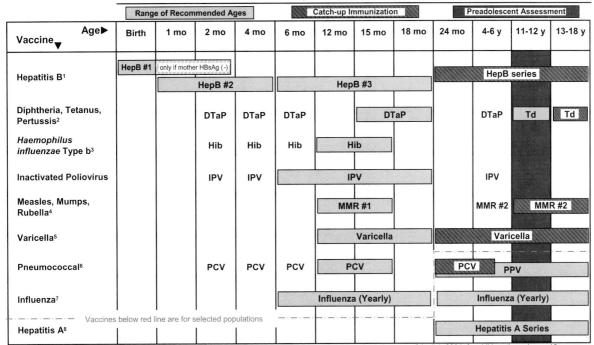

Age▶ Vaccine▼	Birth	1 mo	2 mo	4 mo	6 mo	12 mo	15 mo	18 mo	24 mo	4-6 y	11-12 y	13-18 y
Hepatitis B[1]	HepB #1	only if mother HBsAg (-)								HepB series		
		HepB #2			HepB #3							
Diphtheria, Tetanus, Pertussis[2]			DTaP	DTaP	DTaP		DTaP			DTaP	Td	Td
Haemophilus influenzae Type b[3]			Hib	Hib	Hib	Hib						
Inactivated Poliovirus			IPV	IPV		IPV				IPV		
Measles, Mumps, Rubella[4]						MMR #1				MMR #2	MMR #2	
Varicella[5]						Varicella				Varicella		
Pneumococcal[6]			PCV	PCV	PCV	PCV			PCV	PPV		
Influenza[7]					Influenza (Yearly)				Influenza (Yearly)			
Hepatitis A[8]										Hepatitis A Series		

Range of Recommended Ages · Catch-up Immunization · Preadolescent Assessment

Vaccines below red line are for selected populations

This schedule indicates the recommended ages for routine administration of currently licensed childhood vaccines, as of April 1, 2004, for children through age 18 years. Any dose not given at the recommended age should be given at any subsequent visit when indicated and feasible. ▨Indicates age groups that warrant special effort to administer those vaccines not previously given. Additional vaccines may be licensed and recommended during the year. Licensed combination vaccines may be used whenever any components of the combination are indicated and the vaccineís other components are not contraindicated. Providers should consult the manufacturers' package inserts for detailed recommendations. Clinically significant adverse events that follow immunization should be reported to the Vaccine Adverse Event Reporting System (VAERS). Guidance about how to obtain and complete a VAERS form can be found on the Internet: www.vaers.org or by calling 800-822-7967.

1. Hepatitis B (HepB) vaccine. All infants should receive the first dose of hepatitis B vaccine soon after birth and before hospital discharge; the first dose may also be given by age 2 months if the infantís mother is hepatitis B surface antigen (HBsAg) negative. Only monovalent HepB can be used for the birth dose. Monovalent or combination vaccine containing HepB may be used to complete the series. Four doses of vaccine may be administered when a birth dose is given. The second dose should be given at least 4 weeks after the first dose, except for combination vaccines which cannot be administered before age 6 weeks. The third dose should be given at least 16 weeks after the first dose and at least 8 weeks after the second dose. The last dose in the vaccination series (third or fourth dose) should not be administered before age 24 weeks.

Infants born to HBsAg-positive mothers should receive HepB and 0.5 mL of Hepatitis B Immune Globulin (HBIG) within 12 hours of birth at separate sites. The second dose is recommended at age 1–2 months. The last dose in the immunization series should not be administered before age 24 weeks. These infants should be tested for HBsAg and antibody to HBsAg (anti-HBs) at age 9–15 months.

Infants born to mothers whose HBsAg status is unknown should receive the first dose of the HepB series within 12 hours of birth. Maternal blood should be drawn as soon as possible to determine the mother's HBsAg status; if the HBsAg test is positive, the infant should receive HBIG as soon as possible (no later than age 1 week). The second dose is recommended at age 1–2 months. The last dose in the immunization series should not be administered before age 24 weeks.

2. Diphtheria and tetanus toxoids and acellular pertussis (DTaP) vaccine. The fourth dose of DTaP may be administered as early as age 12 months, provided 6 months have elapsed since the third dose and the child is unlikely to return at age 15–18 months. The final dose in the series should be given at age ≥4 years. **Tetanus and diphtheria toxoids (Td)** is recommended at age 11–12 years if at least 5 years have elapsed since the last dose of tetanus and diphtheria toxoid-containing vaccine. Subsequent routine Td boosters are recommended every 10 years.

3. *Haemophilus influenzae* type b (Hib) conjugate vaccine. Three Hib conjugate vaccines are licensed for infant use. If PRP-OMP (PedvaxHIB or ComVax [Merck]) is administered at ages 2 and 4 months, a dose at age 6 months is not required. DTaP/Hib combination products should not be used for primary immunization in infants at ages 2, 4 or 6 months but can be used as boosters following any Hib vaccine. The final dose in the series should be given at age ≥12 months.

4. Measles, mumps, and rubella vaccine (MMR). The second dose of MMR is recommended routinely at age 4–6 years but may be administered during any visit, provided at least 4 weeks have elapsed since the first dose and both doses are administered beginning at or after age 12 months. Those who have not previously received the second dose should complete the schedule by the visit at age 11–12 years.

5. Varicella vaccine. Varicella vaccine is recommended at any visit at or after age 12 months for susceptible children (i.e., those who lack a reliable history of chickenpox). Susceptible persons age ≥13 years should receive 2 doses, given at least 4 weeks apart.

6. Pneumococcal vaccine. The heptavalent **pneumococcal conjugate vaccine (PCV)** is recommended for all children age 2–23 months. It is also recommended for certain children age 24–59 months. The final dose in the series should be given at age >12 months. **Pneumococcal polysaccharide vaccine (PPV)** is recommended in addition to PCV for certain high-risk groups. See *MMWR* 2000;49(RR-9):1-35.

7. Influenza vaccine. Influenza vaccine is recommended annually for children aged ≥6 months with certain risk factors (including but not limited to asthma, cardiac disease, sickle cell disease, HIV, and diabetes), healthcare workers, and other persons (including household members) in close contact with persons in groups at high risk (see *MMWR* 2004;53;[RR-6]:1-40) and can be administered to all others wishing to obtain immunity. In addition, healthy children aged 6–23 months and close contacts of healthy children aged 0–23 months are recommended to receive influenza vaccine, because children in this age group are at substantially increased risk for influenza-related hospitalizations. For healthy persons aged 5–49 years, the intranasally administered live, attenuated influenza vaccine (LAIV) is an acceptable alternative to the intramuscular trivalent inactivated influenza vaccine (TIV). See *MMWR* 2003;53;[RR-6]:1-40. Children receiving TIV should be administered a dosage appropriate for their age (0.25 mL if 6–35 months or 0.5 mL if ≥3 years). Children aged ≤8 years who are receiving influenza vaccine for the first time should receive 2 doses (separated by at least 4 weeks for TIV and at least 6 weeks for LAIV).

8. Hepatitis A vaccine. Hepatitis A vaccine is recommended for children and adolescents in selected states and regions and for certain high-risk groups; consult your local public health authority. Children and adolescents in these states, regions, and high-risk groups who have not been immunized against hepatitis A can begin the hepatitis A immunization series during any visit. The 2 doses in the series should be administered at least 6 months apart. See *MMWR* 1999;48(RR-12):1-37.

For additional information about vaccines, including precautions and contraindications for immunization and vaccine shortages, please visit the National Immunization Program Web site at www.cdc.gov/nip/ or call the National Immunization Information Hotline at 800-232-2522 (English) or 800-232-0233 (Spanish).

Approved by the Advisory Committee on Immunization Practices (www.cdc.gov/nip/acip), the American Academy of Pediatrics (www.aap.org), and the American Academy of Family Physicians (www.aafp.org).

FIGURE 12–19

Recommended Childhood and Adolescent Immunization Schedule, 2004 www.cdc.gov

TABLE 12–3 Common Preventable Contagious Diseases

Disease	Patient Symptoms	Diagnosis	Type of Vaccine
CHICKENPOX It is caused by a highly contagious virus—*herpes varicella*. Spread by droplets from respiratory tract or direct contact with the blisters. The virus can become reactivated later in life as *herpes zoster* (shingles).	Blister-like vesicles over body starting at head and moving downward	Patient presenting symptoms	**Varicella virus vaccine live.**
DIPHTHERIA It is caused by contagious, droplets from respiratory system. May damage heart or central nervous system (CNS)	False membrane develops in the throat interfering with breathing	Patient presenting symptoms	**Diphtheria-pertussis-tetanus (DPT).**
HAEMOPHILUS INFLUENZA MENINGITIS It occurs mostly in children under age five. It causes acute respiratory infections and meningitis.	Fever Nausea and vomiting (N/V) Loss of appetite Irritability Headache Bulging fontanelles Stupor Seizures Pneumonia Meningitis Septic arthritis	Patient presenting symptoms	**Haemophilus B conjugate vaccine (HiB).**
HEPATITIS B It is caused by a virus It is spread by blood and body fluids. It can possibly cause death.	Jaundice Anorexia N/V Joint pain Flu-like symptoms Liver damage Liver failure	Patient presenting symptoms Blood studies	**Hepatitis B vaccine (recombinant).**
MEASLES (RUBEOLA) It is caused by a virus. The virus is spread by air born droplets	Fine rash over the body Fever Malaise Eye problems Otitis Pneumonia Encephalitis	Patient presenting symptoms	**Measles-mumps-rubella (MMR) vaccine.**
RUBELLA (GERMAN MEASLES) It is caused by a virus. It is spread by direct contact with infected persons and nasal or oral secretions. It can cause birth defects in an unborn child when pregnant mother contracts the disease.	Fine rash over body Fever	Patient presenting symptoms	**MMR.** Immunity confirmed with rubella titer.

Disease	Patient Symptoms	Diagnosis	Type of Vaccine
MUMPS (INFECTIOUS PAROTITIS) It is caused by a virus It is spread by direct contact with salivary secretions of an infected person. Male sterility is possible when it is contracted as an adult	Swollen parotid glands Fever Diarrhea Malaise Difficulty swallowing	Patient presenting symptoms	**MMR.**
PERTUSSIS (WHOOPING COUGH) Contagious, spread by direct contact or droplet from infected person's respiratory tract Complications include pneumonia, atelectasis, otitis, or convulsions	Dry, harsh cough with spasms Fever Dyspnea	Patient presenting symptoms	**DPT injections (series of three).**
POLIOMYELITIS It is caused by one of three polio viruses. It enters the body through the mouth. It is transmitted in the feces of infected individuals. Respiratory system is affected by paralysis and muscle atrophy follows. Post-polio syndrome may occur as late as 30 years post infection.	Fever Malaise Headache Paralysis N/V	Patient presenting symptoms	**Trivalent live oral form, (Sabin)** **Inactivated poliovirus vaccine (Salk), given under the skin.**
SMALLPOX It is caused by a virus. Once thought to be eradicated from the earth. Now may be used as a terrorist weapon. Most often fatal.	Pustule-like blisters on the skin.	Patient presenting symptoms	**Smallpox vaccine.**
TETANUS It is caused by *Clostridium tetani* entering the body through a puncture wound or open skin. CNS can become involved resulting in death if not treated aggressively.	Headaches Fever Muscle spasms	Patient presenting symptoms	**Tetanus diphtheria (Td) or DPT vaccines.** **Tetanus antitoxin.** **Tetanus toxoid.**

► COMMON PATHOLOGY AND DISEASES

Respiratory conditions are common with children. Two respiratory diseases that are of major concern are respiratory *syncytial* (fusion of human cells) virus (RSV) pneumonia and cystic fibrosis. RSV starts as a mild upper respiratory infection. It progresses downward into the lungs and pneumonia develops. Symptoms include fever, coughing, dyspnea and lethargy. Contact with respiratory secretions of an infected person is the usual source of the infection. Microscopic exam of secretions obtained by a nasal *lavage* (washing out of a cavity) confirms the presence of the virus. *Hydration* (fluid intake) of the child is important and supplemental oxygen may be required. Fever is treated with antipyretics.

PROCEDURE 12-2: Perform Documentation of Immunizations—Stored and Administered

Review the information from the vaccine package insert, or from other sources, such as the *Physician's Desk Reference* (*PDR*), or CDC. Know the purpose of the medication; precautions; potential side effects or adverse reactions; correct route for administration; and procedure for storage. The National Childhood Vaccine Injury Act, 1988 requires that benefit and risk information about immunizations be given to a parent or legal guardian, and that consent to proceed be given by the parent or legal guardian before the child is vaccinated (*see* **Figure 12–19**).

Encourage the parent to stay and help during administering the vaccine. Discourage the parent or guardian from making comments that infer the medical staff is bad because of giving the painful injection. Trust is an important part of the child's visit.

Before any immunizations, it is important to gather medical history from the parent or guardian. Ask the parent or guardian about any known allergies, any recent illness, and general medical history. The physician reviews the information obtained from the parent and from his or her assessment before immunizations are given. Due to the cost of vaccinations, it is fairly common for a physician to refer patients to the Public Health Department for free or low-cost vaccinations.

After the immunization has been given, record the information in the child's chart and immunization record. Include in the child's immunization record the date and your or a staff member's initials giving the immunization. It may also include the physician's name and number. The child's chart information includes date and time of immunization, lot number and expiration date, manufacturer, product name, injection site and/or route given, and your signature or other staff member administering the vaccination.

Procedure Materials:
- Vaccine Information Sheets
- Vaccination dosage
- Sterile gloves
- Patient chart
- Black ink pen

Procedure Competency:
With the necessary materials, you will be able to provide the parent or guardian instruction and give childhood immunizations correctly within 45 minutes.

1. Wash your hands completely. Gather equipment and supplies.
2. Identify the parent or guardian with the child and guide them to the treatment area.
3. Ask the parent or guardian questions about the child's recent health or if there is medical history that would exclude the child temporarily or permanently from any of the immunizations.
4. Provide Vaccine Information Sheets for each immunization to be given.
5. Take and record vital signs.
6. After physician has seen patient, wash hands
7. Put on sterile gloves.
8. Administer immunizations (*see* **Figure 12–21**).
9. Dispose of sharps or biohazardous materials into the appropriate materials containers.
10. Wash hands.
11. Document on child's record for parents or guardians and on the child's chart.

Procedure Patient Education:
Educate the parent or guardian about possible side effects of each immunization. Instruct the parent or guardian to give the child antipyretics and analgesics as directed by the physician. This is to provide comfort to the child during the first day or two after the immunizations. Instruct the parent or guardian to call the physician during office hours or the emergency room after hours for any symptoms that are worsening or of concern.

Procedure Charting Example
08/20/XX   8:00 A.M. Child seen for 12-month well-child visit. Mother stated that insurance has paid maximum benefits for immunizations and cannot afford immunizations. Physician gave phone number of local public health department for free immunizations. Signature, CMA or RMA

MEASLES MUMPS & RUBELLA VACCINES

W H A T   Y O U   N E E D   T O   K N O W

1 Why get vaccinated?

Measles, mumps, and rubella are serious diseases.

Measles

- Measles virus causes rash, cough, runny nose, eye irritation, and fever.
- It can lead to ear infection, pneumonia, seizures (jerking and staring), brain damage, and death.

Mumps

- Mumps virus causes fever, headache, and swollen glands.
- It can lead to deafness, meningitis (infection of the brain and spinal cord covering), painful swelling of the testicles or ovaries, and, rarely, death.

Rubella (German Measles)

- Rubella virus causes rash, mild fever, and arthritis (mostly in women).
- If a woman gets rubella while she is pregnant, she could have a miscarriage or her baby could be born with serious birth defects.

You or your child could catch these diseases by being around someone who has them. They spread from person to person through the air.

Measles, mumps, and rubella (MMR) vaccine can prevent these diseases.

Most children who get their MMR shots will not get these diseases. Many more children would get them if we stopped vaccinating.

2 Who should get MMR vaccine and when?

Children should get 2 doses of MMR vaccine:

✓ The first at **12-15 months** of age
✓ and the second at **4-6 years** of age.

These are the recommended ages. But children can get the second dose at any age, as long as it is at least 28 days after the first dose.

Some **adults** should also get MMR vaccine:
Generally, anyone 18 years of age or older, who was born after 1956, should get at least one dose of MMR vaccine, unless they can show that they have had either the vaccines or the diseases.

Ask your doctor or nurse for more information.

MMR vaccine may be given at the same time as other vaccines.

3 Some people should not get MMR vaccine or should wait

- People should not get MMR vaccine who have ever had a life-threatening allergic reaction to **gelatin**, the antibiotic **neomycin**, or to **a previous dose of MMR vaccine**.

- People who are moderately or severely ill at the time the shot is scheduled should usually wait until they recover before getting MMR vaccine.

- Pregnant women should wait to get MMR vaccine until after they have given birth. Women should avoid getting pregnant for 4 weeks after getting MMR vaccine.

- Some people should check with their doctor about whether they should get MMR vaccine, including anyone who:
  - Has HIV/AIDS, or another disease that affects the immune system
  - Is being treated with drugs that affect the immune system, such as steroids, for 2 weeks or longer.
  - Has any kind of cancer
  - Is taking cancer treatment with x-rays or drugs
  - Has ever had a low platelet count (a blood disorder)

Over . . .

4 What are the risks from MMR vaccine?

A vaccine, like any medicine, is capable of causing serious problems, such as severe allergic reactions. The risk of MMR vaccine causing serious harm, or death, is extremely small.

Getting MMR vaccine is much safer than getting any of these three diseases.

Most people who get MMR vaccine do not have any problems with it.

Mild Problems

- Fever (up to 1 person out of 6)
- Mild rash (about 1 person out of 20)
- Swelling of glands in the cheeks or neck (rare)

If these problems occur, it is usually within 7-12 days after the shot. They occur less often after the second dose.

Moderate Problems

- Seizure (jerking or staring) caused by fever (about 1 out of 3,000 doses)
- Temporary pain and stiffness in the joints, mostly in teenage or adult women (up to 1 out of 4)
- Temporary low platelet count, which can cause a bleeding disorder (about 1 out of 30,000 doses)

Severe Problems (Very Rare)

- Serious allergic reaction (less than 1 out of a million doses)
- Several other severe problems have been known to occur after a child gets MMR vaccine. But this happens so rarely, experts cannot be sure whether they are caused by the vaccine or not. These include:
  - Deafness
  - Long-term seizures, coma, or lowered consciousness
  - Permanent brain damage

5 What if there is a moderate or severe reaction?

What should I look for?

Any unusual conditions, such as a serious allergic reaction, high fever or behavior changes. Signs of a

What should I do?

- Call a doctor, or get the person to a doctor right away.
- Tell your doctor what happened, the date and time it happened, and when the vaccination was given.
- Ask your doctor, nurse, or health department to file a Vaccine Adverse Event Reporting System (VAERS) form. Or call VAERS yourself at **1-800-822-7967** or visit their website at http://www.vaers.org

6 The National Vaccine Injury Compensation Program

In the rare event that you or your child has a serious reaction to a vaccine, a federal program has been created to help you pay for the care of those who have been harmed.

For details about the National Vaccine Injury Compensation Program, call **1-800-338-2382** or visit the program's website at http://www.hrsa.gov/osp/vicp

7 How can I learn more?

- Ask your doctor or nurse. They can give you the vaccine package insert or suggest other sources of information.

- Call your local or state health department's immunization program.

- Contact the Centers for Disease Control and Prevention (CDC):
  - Call **1-800-232-2522** (English)
  - Call **1-800-232-0233** (Español)
  - Visit the National Immunization Program's website at http://www.cdc.gov/nip

U.S. DEPARTMENT OF HEALTH & HUMAN SERVICES
Centers for Disease Control and Prevention
National Immunization Program

Vaccine Information Statement
MMR (1/15/03)   42 U.S.C. § 300aa-26

FIGURE 12–20

Sample Vaccination Information Sheet

Cystic fibrosis, a genetic metabolic disorder, involves a chronic dysfunction of the exocrine glands. A thick, sticky mucus secretion is produced by the glands blocking the ducts. Tissues most frequently affected include the lungs, digestive system (particularly the pancreas), and the sweat glands.

Other serious childhood conditions are neural tube defects, congenital heart conditions, and blood disorders. Treatment is required immediately for most of these conditions.

NEURAL TUBE DEFECTS

Neural tube defects are congenital disorders that occur when an embryo's neural tube fails to close during development. Spinal fusion disorders are *spina bifida occulta* (*see* **Figure 12–22**), meningocele, and myelomeningocele (*see* **Figure 12–23**). Cranial fusion disorders are hydrocephalis (*see* **Figure 12–24**), micrencephaly, and anencephaly (*see* **Figure 12–25**).

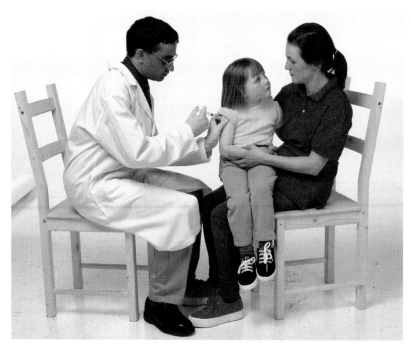

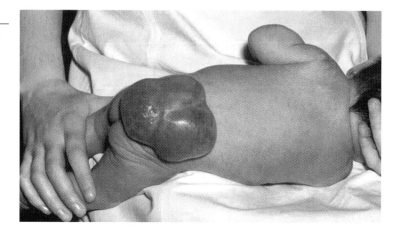

FIGURE 12–21

Photo of a child receiving an immunization
(Courtesy of Dorling Kindersley.)

FIGURE 12–22

Photo of a child with spina bifida occulta
(Courtesy of Photoresearchers.)

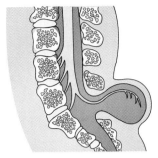

FIGURE 12–23

Myelomeningocele
(Courtesy of LifeART/Lippincott Williams and Wilkins.)

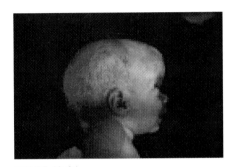

FIGURE 12–24

Photo of a child hydrocephalis
(Courtesy of Phototake.)

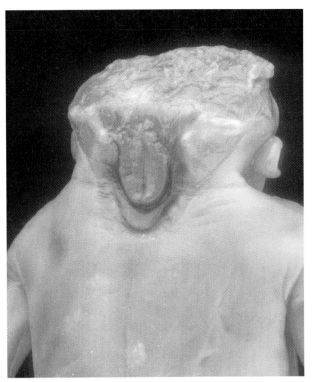

FIGURE 12–25

Photo of a child anencephaly
(Courtesy of P. Barber/Custom Medical Stock Photo.)

TABLE 12–4   Congenital Neurological Disorders

Disorder	Patient Symptoms	Diagnosis	Treatment
SPINA BIFIDA OCCULTA A condition resulting in the failure of neural tube to close. Usually, it is located in the lumbar region with no displacement or insult to the spinal cord.	Dimpling or depression of skin over affected lumbar region, often with a tuft of hair over the site	Patient presenting symptoms	**No intervention.** Close observation for any signs of neurological symptoms.
MENINGOCELE It is a congenital hernia that results in the *meninges* (membranes) protruding through a defect in the skull or spinal column. If surgery is successful, the prognosis is good.	Apparent bulging over the spinal column, usually in the lumbar region.	Patient presenting symptoms Imaging studies	**Surgery.** *Recommended to close the opening in the vertebral column.*
MYELOMENINGOCELE It is a form of *spina bifida* resulting in a portion of the spinal cord and membranes protruding. Many of these children require intense physical care and often do not survive into teen years.	Deformity in lumbar region of spinal column Paralysis possible Loss of bowel and bladder function possible	Patient presenting symptoms	**Surgery.** Recommended to protect the exposed spinal nerves and cord. **Supportive care.** Recommended for any paralysis or bowel and bladder dysfunction.

Disorder	Patient Symptoms	Diagnosis	Treatment
HYDROCEPHALIS It is an accumulation (buildup) of the *cerebrospinal fluid* (CSF) within the brain and skull. This may be the result of developmental error, trauma, infection, or blood clot developing during or shortly after delivery. If surgery is performed before any permanent neurological damage, the child has a good prognosis. Continual observation for neurological symptoms is necessary. They signal reduced or impaired functioning of the shunt.	Enlargement of the skull with bulging *fontanelles* (soft spots)	Patient presenting symptoms	**Surgery.** Recommended to insert a shunt that will drain excess fluid into the circulatory system.
MICRENCEPHALY It is an abnormally small brain. Most of these children die in infancy.	Small head	Patient presenting symptoms Imaging studies	**Supportive.**
ANENCEPHALY The child's cranial vault is missing and very little cerebral tissue is present. Most of these children are stillborn or die during the neonatal period.	Posterior cranial vault is small or absent	Patient presenting symptoms Imaging studies	**Supportive.**

CONGENITAL HEART CONDITIONS

Congenital heart conditions are easily identified at birth or before birth by prenatal ultrasound examinations. Some of the congenital heart conditions occur due to failure of fetal circulation conversion to normal cardiac circulation after birth. Others are caused by developmental anomalies. There are two classes of congenital heart conditions, *acyanotic* (no bluish skin tint) and *cyanotic* (bluish skin tint).

TABLE 12–5   Congenital Heart Conditions

Condition	Patient Symptoms	Diagnosis	Treatment
ACYANOTIC ***VENTRICULAR SEPTAL DEFECT (VSD)*** It is an opening in septum between the right and left ventricle resulting in shunting of blood from left to right side of heart.	Heart murmur Increased heart rate Increased respiratory rate Failure to gain weight Restlessness Irritability	Patient presenting symptoms	**Surgery.** Recommended to repair or patching of ventricular septum.
PATENT DUCTUS ARTERIOSUS (PDA) It is the failure of the ductus arteriosus to close after birth resulting in shunting of oxygenated blood to lungs. If medication or surgery is prompt, prognosis is good.	Heart murmur Growth retarded Signs of heart failure	Patient presenting symptoms	**Antiprostaglandin.** Prescribed to inhibit prostaglandin synthesis. **Surgery.** Recommended to close the patent ductus arteriosus.

Condition	Patient Symptoms	Diagnosis	Treatment
COARCTATION OF THE AORTA A portion of the aorta is narrowed restricting blood flow from the left ventricle. If surgery is performed promptly, the prognosis is fair.	Left ventricular failure Pulmonary *edema* (swelling) Decreased pulse in legs Rapid heart rate Dyspnea	Patient presenting symptoms	**Surgery.** Recommended to remove the coarctation.
ATRIAL SEPTAL DEFECT It is an opening in the atrial septal wall. If surgery is performed promptly, the prognosis is good.	Fatigue SOB Respiratory infections.	Patient presenting symptoms	**Surgery.** Recommended to repair the wall.
CYANOTIC DEFECTS **TETRALOGY OF FALLOT** It is a combination of ventricular septal defect, pulmonary stenosis, displacement of the aorta to the right, and right ventricular hypertrophy. If surgery is prompt and successful, the prognosis is fair.	Cyanotic–"Blue baby" Hypoxia Tachycardia Tachypnea, Dyspnea Seizures	Patient presenting symptoms	**Surgery.** Recommended immediately to correct the defect.
TRANSPOSITION OF THE GREAT ARTERIES Aorta and pulmonary artery are reversed as they exit the heart. If surgery is immediate, the prognosis is variable.	Cyanosis Tachypnea Heart failure	Patient presenting symptoms Imaging studies	**Prostaglandins.** Prescribed to keep the ductus arteriosus open until surgery. **Surgery.** Recommended to repair the defect.

BLOOD DISORDERS

Blood disorders include anemia, leukemia, and lead poisoning.

TABLE 12–6   Blood Disorders

Disorder	Patient Symptoms	Diagnosis	Treatment
ANEMIA Although anemia can have a number of causes, commonly in children, it is caused by a lack of iron. Breast milk may have low iron, depending on if the mother did not take a supplement. Older children often develop anemia from a poor diet.	Pale skin Weakness Fatigue SOB	Patient presenting symptoms Physical examination Hemoglobin (hgb) test Hematocrit (HCT) test	**Fortified formula.** Recommended for infants. **Iron supplements.** Prescribed for prenatal care. **Proper diet.** Recommended for older children. Egg yolks and fortified cereals are good sources. **Vitamin and mineral supplements.** Recommended for older children. *(continued)*

TABLE 12–6   (continued)

Disorder	Patient Symptoms	Diagnosis	Treatment
LEUKEMIA			
It is an abnormal increase in white blood cells. With treatment, prognosis is variable.	Tired Aching Infection Enlarged lymph nodes	Patient presenting symptoms Blood studies Lymph biopsy	**Chemotherapy.** **Bone-marrow transplant.**
LEAD POISONING			
It is disorder caused by lead found in the environment. It can affect a child's physical and mental development. Sources include: • lead-based paint, • water from lead pipes, • lead salts in certain foods, • ceramic food containers painted with lead-based paint, • food grown in contaminated soil, • playing in contaminated soil or sand, and • older vinyl mini-blinds. Leaded gasoline emissions and seepage are a main cause of soil and sand contamination. Neurological damage can not be reversed.	Loss of appetite Vomiting Irritability Difficulty walking Stumbling Anemia Weakness Colic Peripheral neuritis Possible mental retardation Headache Stupor Convulsions Coma	Patient presenting symptoms Environmental history Blood studies Urine studies	**Remove the source.** **Chelating agents.** Prescribed to remove lead from the blood. **Supportive treatment.**

OTHER CONDITIONS

A fetal alcohol syndrome (FAS) baby is often growth retarded, including height, weight, and mental capacity. A few days after birth, the baby suffers from alcohol withdrawal. Any neurological damage cannot be reversed, so most treatment involves supportive care. A crack baby is very irritable and also may have growth retardation. Any of these children may have severe emotional and behavioral problems in life.

For the Record: Tape Test for Worm/Egg Collection

A classic sign of roundworm and pinworm infestation is a child scratching the *anus* (rectal area). A positive test is the stool collection followed by microscopic examination for *ova* (eggs).

An easy method of collecting the worms is to place scotch type tape across the rectum when the child goes to bed. The worms have a tendency to migrate to the anus. They become trapped on the tape adhesive. Removal of the tape in the early morning reveals the worms.

Another method of confirming an infestation is to take a flashlight and shine the light on the child's anus in the dark. Many times the worms can be seen around the anus.

Treatment involves a physician prescribing an antihelmintic regimen for the entire family and laundering all bedding in hot water and, if possible, in bleach.

A common digestive disease in children is helminth infestation. Toxocariasis (roundworm) and enterobiasis (pinworm) infestations are caused by the transfer of larvae by children's unclean hands and nails to the mouth. In both cases, the larvae are swallowed and hatch in the intestines. Roundworm infestation can cause symptoms of cough, fever, nausea and vomiting, weight loss, or *hepatomegaly* (enlargement of the liver).

▶ DIAGNOSTIC PROCEDURES

Diagnostic procedures that may be performed in the medical office include urinalysis, strep screens, hemoglobin and hematocrit, and obtaining cultures for culture and sensitivity (C&S). The physician may order blood drawn for a blood lead level and/or theophyline level. It is possible that some physicians may perform a lumbar puncture on a child with a fever of unknown origin.

Urine samples are performed on the pediatric patient to obtain laboratory data regarding the presence of blood, glucose, acetone, bilirubin, protein, drugs or hormones, microorganisms. Also, samples are used to determine specific gravity and pH of the urine. Because the newborn, infant, or toddler pediatric patient cannot physically or mentally follow directions to urinate into a sterile specimen container, a urine collection bag is applied often by you or catheterization by the physician is done.

▶ PREVIEW FOR CERTIFICATION

- The pediatric practice offers an MA a variety of tasks. The office and medical procedures include obtaining and recording the child's health and developmental history; take and record vital signs; measure and record growth; assist the parents or guardian and the physician with the child; obtain a urine specimen; and administer medications, injections, and immunizations.
- An important role for the MA is to be aware of the needs and concerns of the parent or guardian and the child. Fear, mistrust, anxiety, and embarrassment are all common emotions. Listening can provide valuable information about the child.
- Children, ages 0–20 years of age, go through many physical, developmental, mental and emotional changes related to various age-related categories.
- Growth measurement is usually a part of a child's file. This is vital information because it can show normal and abnormal growth.
- While inoculations and well-baby and child checks are a major part of office visits, diaper rash, thrush, ear inflammation, and asthma are also common.

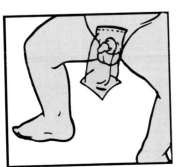 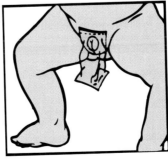

FIGURE 12–26

Drawing of a child with a urine collection bag

(Courtesy of Prentice-Hall, Inc)

- Common contagious diseases are control more now by preventive inoculations. Diseases include chicken pox, measles, German measles, mumps, whooping cough, polio, and diptheria. Also, vaccinations for hepatitis B and Haemophilus b have been added.
- Serious respiratory conditions, RSV and cystic fibrosis, require immediate care.
- Neural tube disorders are congenital. They occur when the embryo's neural tube fails to close. There are two categories—spinal and cranial fusion. There is no cure.
- Acyanotic and cyanotic are the two classifications of congenital heart disorders.
- Anemia, leukemia, and lead poisoning are all serious blood disorders.
- Fetal alcohol syndrome and crack babies are more likely to have retarded growth and neurological damage. Often they experience severe emotional and behavioral problems later in life.
- Diagnostic procedures that may be performed include strep screens, urinalysis, hemoglobin and hematocrit and obtaining cultures for C&S.

PROCEDURE 12-3:   Perform Urine Collection with a Pediatric Urine Collection Bag

Procedure Theory:

When you collect a urine sample with a collection bag, it is important for the specimen to be a recent urination. A fresh specimen provides more accurate information for correct diagnosis and treatment. For example, if the specimen is old, it may contain additional bacterial growth above what may have been present at the time of urination. Transport the specimen immediately to the laboratory for correct storage if it is not processed immediately.

Skin cleansing is important to obtain accurate information relating to microorganisms present in the urine. Microorganisms on the skin may contaminate the urine specimen. To contain the urine specimen in the collection bag, it is important to have a wrinkle-free seal when the adhesive is removed from the tabs and placed on the skin. The wrinkle-free seal becomes more important in the pediatric patient with *oliguria* (scanty urine production). The smallest urine specimen may be the only specimen available for urine diagnostic testing.

Procedure Materials:

- Urine collection bag for newborn or pediatric patient
- Sterile gloves
- Sterile container
- Container label
- Laboratory requisition form
- Cotton balls
- Prepackaged sterile cleansing swabs or towelettes
- Patient chart
- Black ink pen

Procedure Competency:

With the necessary materials, you will be to collect a urine specimen within 40 minutes correctly using the urine collection bag method.

1. Wash your hands completely. Gather equipment and supplies.
2. Identify the parent or guardian with the child and guide them to the treatment area.
3. Explain procedure to the parent or guardian with child.
4. Put on sterile gloves.
5. Remove diaper and dispose.
6. Wipe the genital area with sterile towelettes or cleansing swabs. For boy infants, wipe circular around and away from the urinary meatus. For girl infants, wipe from the clitoris toward the rectal area. Repeat the wipe with a separate towelette or cleansing swab a second and third time to cleanse the area immediately surrounding the urinary meatus and then cleanse the wider surrounding area.
7. Dry cleansed area with dry cotton balls.
8. Remove adhesive tabs and apply to genital area skin securely without gaps between tabs and skin (*see* **Figure 12–26**).
9. Diaper the child.
10. Wash hands.
11. Instruct parent or guardian to encourage the infant or toddler to drink or nurse.
12. Recheck diaper every 20 minutes until specimen is obtained in urine collection bag.
13. Wash hands.

(*continues*)

PROCEDURE 12-3:   Perform Urine Collection with a Pediatric Urine Collection Bag (continued)

14. Put on sterile gloves.
15. Remove the urine collection bag.
16. Place the bagged urine specimen into the sterile cup and cover the container tightly.
17. Diaper the infant or toddler.
18. Remove gloves.
19. Wash hands.
20. Prepare container label and laboratory requisition.
21. Transport or arrange for transporting to the laboratory.
22. Document the procedure in the child's chart.
23. Dispose of biohazardous materials in the proper containers.
24. Clean the area.
25. Wash hands.

Procedure Patient Education:

Give instructions to the parent or guardian to increase fluids for stimulation of urine production. It may be necessary to explain that the urine collection bag for the urine specimen is preferred, but the physician may choose to catheterize the patient. When a parent or guardian is very or extremely anxious, it is often wise to avoid explaining too many details. Tell the parent or guardian only the information needed to help him or her understand and assist the child through the medical evaluation process.

Procedure Charting Example

09/27/XX   2:35 P.M. One year old female child with history of 101 fever for two days with fussiness. Mother states child is fussy, not drinking, and urine is darker than normal. Urine collection bag applied per physician order and office procedure. Signature, CMA or RMA

09/27/XX   3:15 P.M. Urine collection bag removed and placed in sterile urine container. Urine is dark yellow and smells strong. Laboratory requisition sent with labeled urine specimen. Signature, CMA or RMA

► VITAL SIGNS

HEART RATE

The apical heart rate is preferred in children. To count the rate, place the stethoscope on the anterior chest at the fifth intercostal space in a midclavicular position. Each "lub-dub" sound is one beat. Count the beats for 1 full minute. While auscultating the heart rate, note whether the rhythm is regular or irregular.

Pulse rates may be checked at sites other than the apex, for example, the carotid, brachial, radial, femoral, and dorsal pedis sites. Compare the distal and proximal pulses for strength. Compare the upper and lower pulses for strength. Also record whether the pulse is normal, bounding (very strong), or thready (weak).

The range of normal heart rates based on age is listed in Table 12–7.

RESPIRATORY RATE

The procedure for measuring a child's respiratory rate is essentially the same as for an adult. However, keep in mind these points:

- Since a child's respirations are diaphragmatic, observe abdominal movement to count respirations.
- Abdominal movement in a child will be irregular.

The range of normal respiratory rates based on age is listed in Table 12–8. Count breaths for 1 full minute.

BLOOD PRESSURE

Blood pressure measurement for the child is basically the same as for an adult. Whether manual or electronic equipment is being used, the size of the blood pressure cuff is determined by the size of the child's arm or leg. Generally, the width of the bladder cuff is two thirds of the length of the long bone of the extremity on which the blood pressure is taken. The length of the bladder should be about three-fourths the circumference of the extremity and should not overlap (Fig. 12–27). If the bladder is too small, the pressure will be falsely high; if it is too large, the pressure will be falsely low.

If electronic equipment is being used, place the cuff around the desired extremity and activate the equipment according to the manufacturer's recommendations.

If a manual cuff is being used, wrap the cuff around the desired extremity. Close the air escape valve. Palpate for the pulse, and place the stethoscope over the pulse area (Fig. 12–28). Pump the cuff with the bulb until the mercury rises and no beat is auscultated; continue pumping until the mercury rises another 20–30 mm. Slowly release the air through the valve at 2–3 mm/sec while watching the falling column of mercury. Note the number at which the first return of a pulse is heard; this is the systolic pressure. Continue releasing the air to determine the diastolic pressure:

TABLE 12–7   Range of Normal Heart Rate in Children, Birth to 14 years

Age	Range (beats/min)
Newborn	100–170
6 mo–1 yr	90–130
3 yr	80–120
5 yr	70–110
10–14 yr	60–100

Blood pressure cuffs are available in various types and sizes for pediatric patients.

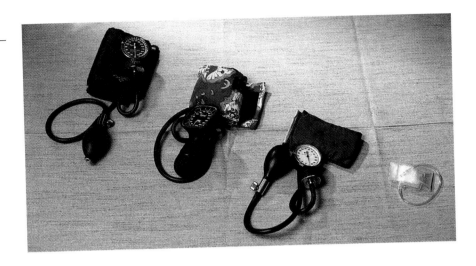

TABLE 12–8   **Range of Normal Respiratory Rates in Children, Birth to 17 Years**

Age	Range (breaths/min)
Newborn	30–80
6 mo	24–36
1 yr	20–40
3 yr	20–30
6 yr	16–22
10 yr	16–20
17 yr	12–20

FIGURE 12–28

Measuring blood pressure with a manual cuff.

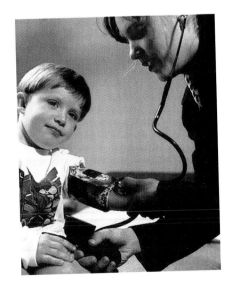

If the child is younger than 12 years, a muffled sound will be heard and is recorded at the diastolic pressure; if the child is older than 12 years, all sound will disappear at the diastolic pressure. Blood pressure is read as systolic over diastolic pressure (Table 12–9).

If the pulse cannot be auscultated, blood pressure can still be measured by touch. Wrap the cuff around the desired extremity, close the air valve, and palpate for the pulse. Keeping your fingers on

TABLE 12–9   Median Systolic and Diastolic Blood Pressure Values for Children of Different Ages*

Age	Systolic (mm Hg)	Diastolic (mm Hg)
Newborn	73	55
1 mo	86	52
6 mo	90	53
1 yr	90	56
3 yr	92	55
6 yr	96	57
9 yr	100	61
12 yr	107	64
15 yr	114	65
18 yr	121	70

*Readings show 50th percentile.

Note: Children who are in the 95th percentile for blood pressure for their age, gender, and height should be referred for hypertensive workup. See the following references for these standards: Joint National Committee on Prevention, Detection, Evaluation and Treatment of High Blood Pressure and the National High Blood Pressure Education Program Coordinating Committee. (1997). The sixth report of the Joint National Committee on Prevention, Detection, Evaluation, and Treatment of High Blood Pressure. *Archives of Internal Medicine, 157,* 2413–2443; and National High Blood Pressure Program Working Group on Hypertension Control in Children and Adolescents. (1996). Update on the 1987 task force report on high blood pressure in children and adolescents: A working group report from the National High Blood Pressure Education Program. *Pediatrics, 98*(4), 649–658.

Adapted from the Normal Blood Pressure Readings for Boys from the Second Task Force on Blood Pressure Control in Children, National Heart, Lung, and Blood Institute (1987), Bethesda, MD. Normal blood pressure readings for girls are very similar to those for boys at all age

the pulse, pump the cuff with the bulb until the pulse is no longer felt. Slowly open the air valve, watching the column of mercury, and note the number at which the pulse is again palpated. This is the palpated systolic blood pressure read as the number over "P."

Systolic pressure can also be measured by using Doppler ultrasonography (Fig. 12–29). With this technique, the frequency of ultrasonic waves is reflected by movement of the surface of the blood vessels, which differs slightly from that of other structures in the same area. Pressure is recorded as the number over "D."

BODY TEMPERATURE

Body temperature can be measured on two scales: Fahrenheit or centigrade. If an electronic thermometer is being used, follow the manufacturer's guidelines. There is no documented "universal" agreement on the length of time that a mercury thermometer should be kept in place. Follow the

Home and Community Care Considerations

Ask parents what type of thermometer they use at home and provide instruction in its correct use. Often parents do not know how to shake down a mercury thermometer, resulting in faulty readings. They may not know for how long to insert the thermometer or how to clean and store it after use. Nurses in schools and day-care centers should asses the knowledge of the care providers in these settings and provide teaching as needed.

FIGURE 12–29

Measuring blood pressure using Doppler ultrasonography.

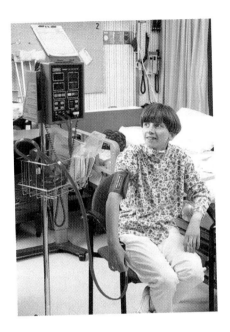

guidelines of your institution. General recommendations usually list 3–5 minutes for oral, 2–5 minutes for rectal, and 6–8 minutes for axillary.

The four routes for measuring body temperature are tympanic, oral, rectal, and axillary.

Tympanic Route

The tympanic route (Fig. 12–30) is a convenient and fast method for taking temperatures in infants and children.

Make sure the thermometer tip is aimed toward the tympanic membrane to ensure accuracy. Always use a clean probe tip for each child.

If you are using the child's right ear, hold the thermometer in your right hand. For the child's left ear, hold the thermometer in your left hand.

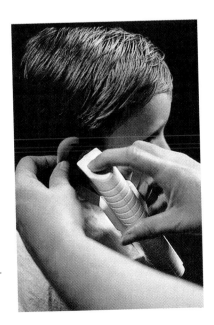
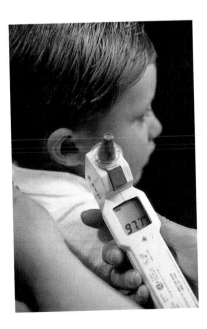

FIGURE 12–30

A. Position for inserting thermometer when tympanic route is used. **B.** Digital readout of temperature appears within 1 minute.

▶ ASSESSING BODY TEMPERATURE USING THE TYMPANIC ROUTE

Selected Equipment
Thermometer (electronic)

PROCEDURE

Child Younger Than 1 Year

- Place the infant in a supine position on a flat surface.
- Stabilize the infant's head.
- Turn the infant's head 90 degrees for easy access.
- Pull the pinna of the ear straight back and downward.
- Approach the ear from behind to direct the tip of the probe anteriorly.
- Place the probe in the ear as far as possible to seal the canal.
- Turn on the scanner.
- Leave the probe in the ear according to the manufacturer's recommendations.
- Remove the probe. Read and record the temperature.

Child Older Than 1 Year

- Have the parent hold the child on his or her lap, keeping the child's head against his or her chest for support. The child's arms and legs may need to be held.
- Pull the pinna back and up in children over about 3 years or back and downward under that age.
- Place the probe and continue as described above for the child younger than 1 year.
- Read and record the temperature.

Oral Route
The oral route may be used for the child over 3 years of age. (An electronic nonbreakable probe is preferred.)

▶ ASSESSING BODY TEMPERATURE USING THE ORAL ROUTE

Selected Equipment
Thermometer (glass with oral bulb—usually blue tipped) or electronic thermometer with sheath

Procedure—Clean Gloves
- Place the oral probe or an electronic thermometer (with protective sheath) or the glass thermometer under the tongue and have the child close his or her mouth.
- If electronic equipment is being used, turn on the scanner and follow the manufacturer's recommendations. It will sound a tone or beep when finished. Remove the probe.
- If you are using a glass thermometer, keep it in place for approximately 3–5 minutes; then read the temperature based on the column of mercury.
- Read and record the temperature.

Rectal Route
The rectal route should be used only when no other route is possible. It is not recommended because of the potential for rectal perforation and because most children view this as an intrusive procedure. The rectal temperature is one degree higher than the oral temperature.

ASSESSING BODY TEMPERATURE USING THE RECTAL ROUTE

Selected Equipment
Thermometer (electronic or rectal—with stubby bulb and usually red tipped) or electronic
thermometer with sheath
Protective sheath for glass thermometer
Water-soluble lubricant

Procedure—*Clean Gloves*
- Place the infant or child prone on a bed or the parent's lap; turn the older child on the side.
- Cover the tip of the rectal probe of an electronic thermometer (with protective sheath) or the glass thermometer (with protective sheath) with a water-soluble lubricant.
- For the infant, place the tip ¼ to ½ inch into the rectum.
- For the child, place the tip 1 inch into the rectum.
- If electronic equipment is being used, turn on the scanner and follow the manufacturer's recommendations. It will sound a tone or beep when finished. Remove the probe.
- If you are using a glass thermometer, hold the thermometer in place for 2–5 minutes.
- Read and record the temperature.

Axillary Route
The axillary route (Fig. 12–31) is often used for children who are seizure-prone, unconscious, or immunosuppressed, or who have a structural abnormality that precludes an alternate route. It may be used in settings such as schools where the least invasive route is desired. The axillary temperature is one degree lower than the oral temperature. Current research indicates that this method is not as accurate as other methods in identifying children with fevers.

ASSESSING BODY TEMPERATURE USING THE AXILLARY ROUTE

Selected Equipment
Thermometer (glass with any bulb) or electronic thermometer with sheath

Procedure
- The probe with sheath (on electronic model) or the thermometer (rectal or oral) is held in place in the axilla, with the child's arm pressed close to his or her side.
- If you are using an electronic probe, wait for the tone before removing it to read the temperature. If you are using a glass thermometer, keep it in place for approximately 6–8 minutes before reading it.
- Read and record the temperature.

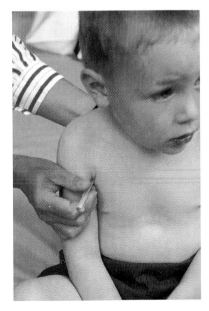

FIGURE 12–31

Measuring the axillary temperature.

▶ PHYSICAL GROWTH CHARTS

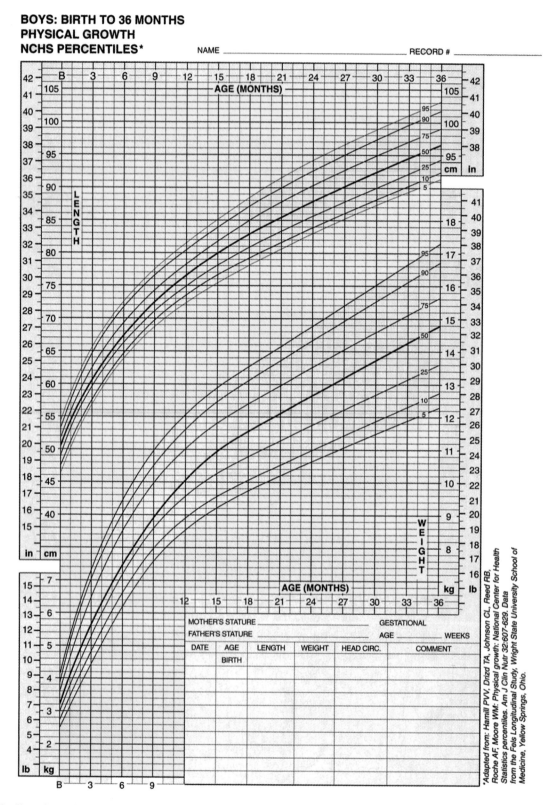

FIGURE A–I   Physical growth percentiles for length and weight—boys; birth to 36 months.
From NCHS Growth Charts, copyright © 1982 Ross Laboratories. Reprinted with permission of Ross Laboratories, Columbus OH 43216.

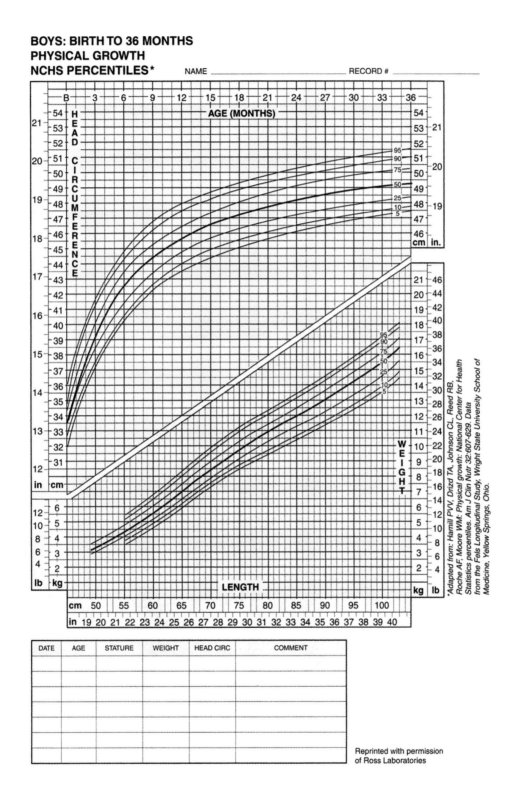

FIGURE A–2   Physical growth percentiles for head circumference, length, and weight—boys; birth to 36 months.
From NCHS Growth Charts, copyright © 1982 Ross Laboratories. Reprinted with permission of Ross Laboratories, Columbus OH 43216.

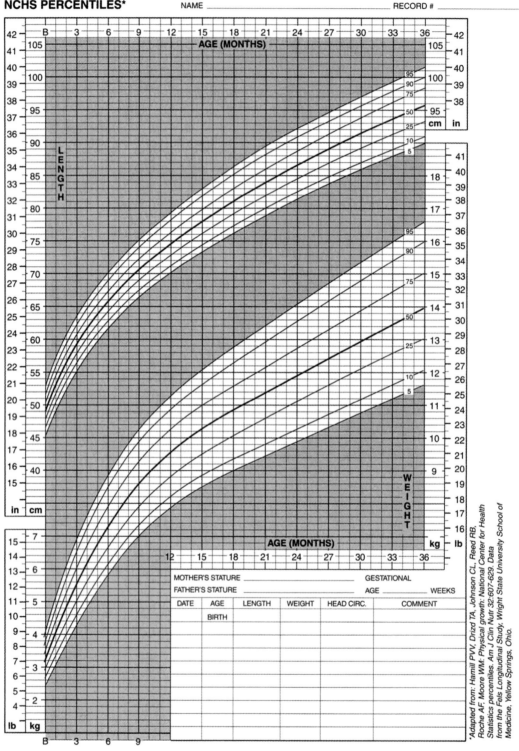

FIGURE A–3   Physical growth percentiles for length and weight—girls; birth to 36 months.
From NCHS Growth Charts, copyright © 1982 Ross Laboratories. Reprinted with permission of Ross Laboratories, Columbus OH 43216.

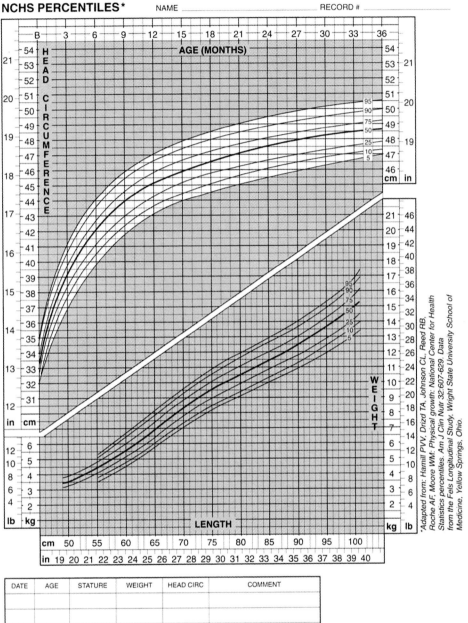

FIGURE A–4   Physical growth percentiles for head circumference, length, and weight—girls; birth to 36 months.
From NCHS Growth Charts, copyright © 1982 Ross Laboratories. Reprinted with permission of Ross Laboratories, Columbus OH 43216.

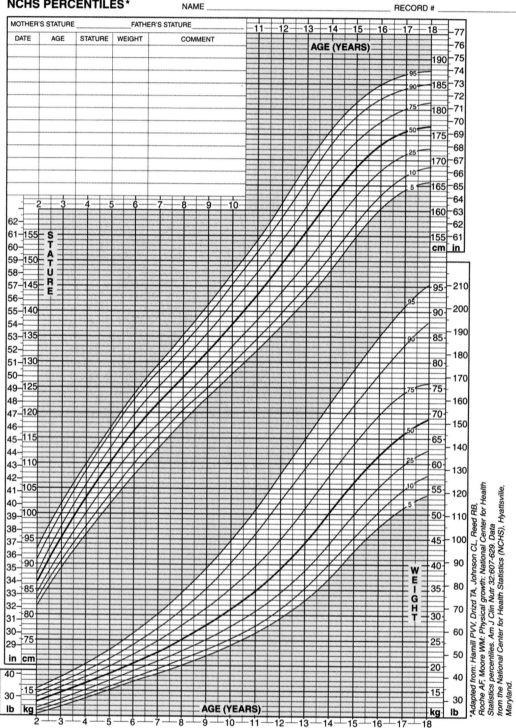

FIGURE A–5   Physical growth percentiles for stature and weight according to age—boys: 2 to 18 years.
From NCHS Growth Charts, copyright © 1982 Ross Laboratories. Reprinted with permission of Ross Laboratories, Columbus OH 43216.

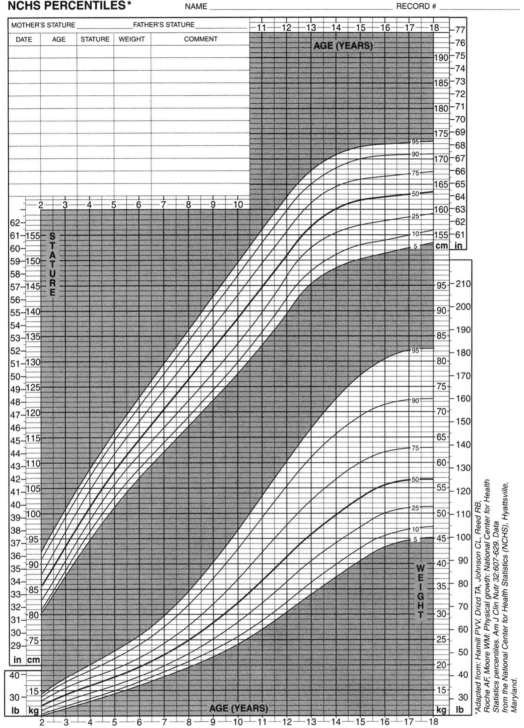

FIGURE A–6   Physical growth percentiles for stature and weight according to age—girls: 2 to 18 years.
From NCHS Growth Charts, copyright © 1982 Ross Laboratories. Reprinted with permission of Ross Laboratories, Columbus OH 43216.

▶ ADMINISTRATION OF MEDICATION

Administering medications to children presents a number of challenges: deciding which drugs to use, determining dosage, choosing methods and sites, and taking into account implications based on the child's development.

Although the drug and the dosage are determined by the prescriber, it is imperative that the nurse observe the "Five Rights" of medication administration (Table 12–10) before any medication is given.

Explain all procedures or treatments to the child and parents, based on the child's developmental stage and the level of understanding of both parties. Answer all questions before giving the medication. Identify any known drug allergies.

When a medication is given, record the name of the drug, the route, the date and time, and, if appropriate, the site. It is often necessary to record the response to the medication, including desired effects and undesired side effects. This is especially important with medications for pain control and those for treatment of an acute problem such as respiratory difficulty.

TABLE 12–10   "Five Rights" of Medication Administration

1. Right medication

- Compare the name of the drug on the medication sheet with the name of the drug on the label of the drug container three times. Check the container's expiration date.
- Know the action of the drug.
- Identify the potential side effects of the drug.
- Use the pharmacy, hospital, or other drug formulary as a reference for medications with which you are unfamiliar.

2. Right patient

- Verify the name on the medication sheet against the name on the child's identification band. When in a setting with no name band (eg, clinic), verify the child's name with the child and parent by asking them to state the name.

3. Right time

- When ordered for a specific time, a medication should be given within 20–30 minutes of that time.
- For prn medications, check the last time the dose was given as well as the total 24-hour dose the child has received to verify that the child can receive another dose at this time.

4. Right route of administration

- Always use the ordered route for administration of a medication. If a change is needed (such as a change from oral medication when a child is vomiting), check with the prescriber to get an order for a change in route.

5. Right dose

- Calculate the ordered dose based on the child's weight in kilograms.
- If in doubt about what constitutes an appropriate dose, compare to the pharmacy, hospital, or other drug formulary guidelines for recommended dose.
- Question the order if the dose is outside of recommended amounts.

Sample Documentation

September 6, 1998, 1400 hours: 250 mg (1 mL) ceftriaxone injected into the right deltoid. No redness, swelling noted. September 6, 1998, 1420 hours: No reaction to medication noted at this time. Vital signs stable (see flowsheet). Patient discharged to home with instructions to return immediately if he has difficulty breathing or the area becomes red, painful, or swollen.

▶ ORAL MEDICATION

Children younger than 5 years of age usually have difficulty swallowing tablets and capsules. For this reason, most medications for pediatric use are also available in the form of elixirs, syrups, or suspensions. If a medication is available only in tablet or capsule form, it may need to be crushed before being administered. Be sure not to crush medications with enteric coating. Remember to wear clean gloves if your hands might come in contact with the child's saliva.

▶ ADMINISTERING AN ORAL MEDICATION

Preparation
- Measure the medication accurately to ensure that the dose is correct.
- If the oral medication is liquid (especially if less than 5 mL), it should be measured in a syringe or calibrated small medicine cup or dropper. A specially designed medication bottle may also be used (Fig. 12–32).
- Choose the appropriate device from those available to administer an oral liquid medication (Fig. 12–32).
- If a tablet or pill needs to be crushed, place it in a mortar or between two paper medicine cups and crush it with a pestle. Once the tablet or pill has been pulverized, mix the powdered medication with a small amount of flavored substance such as juice, applesauce, or jelly to disguise any unpleasant flavor.

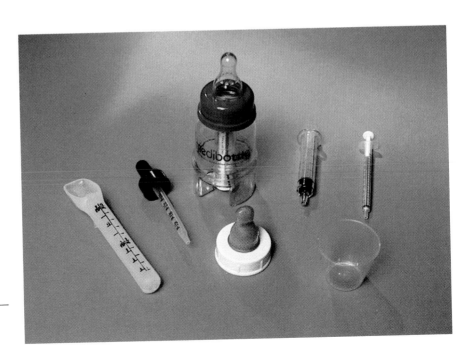

FIGURE 12–32

Oral medications can be administered with various types of equipment, depending on the child's age.

FIGURE 12–33

This father needs to administer a medication to his daughter at home. He has been instructed how to hold her and administer the dose safely and effectively.

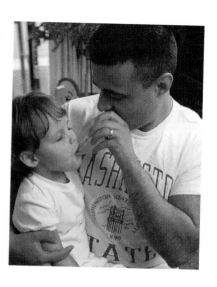

Selected Equipment

Medicine cup, syringe, or other device for administering medication
Medication

Procedure

Infant

- A syringe or dropper provides the best control.
- Place small amounts of liquid along the side of the infant's mouth. To prevent aspiration or spitting out, wait for the infant to swallow before giving more.
- *Alternative method:* Have the infant suck the liquid through a nipple.

Toddler or Young Child

- Place the child firmly on your lap or the parent's lap in a sitting or modified supine position (Fig. 12–33).
- Administer the medication slowly with a syringe or small medicine cup.

▶ INTRAMUSCULAR INJECTION

The site of the intramuscular injection (Fig. 12–34) depends on the age of the child, the amount of muscle mass, and the density and volume of medication to be administered. Young infants may not tolerate volumes greater than 0.5 mL in a single site, whereas older infants or small children may be able to tolerate 1 mL per site. As the child grows, greater volumes can be administered. Remember: The larger the volume of medication, the larger the muscle to be used. If possible, avoid areas that involve major blood vessels or nerves.

The preferred site for the infant is the vastus lateralis muscle (Fig. 12–35), which lies along the mid-anterior lateral aspect of the thigh. After the child has been walking for 1 year, the dorsogluteal site can be used. However, since that muscle is poorly developed, it is not the ideal choice for a child less than 5 years old.

For the older child and adolescent, the sites are the same as for the adult: the vastus lateralis, deltoid, and ventrogluteal muscles.

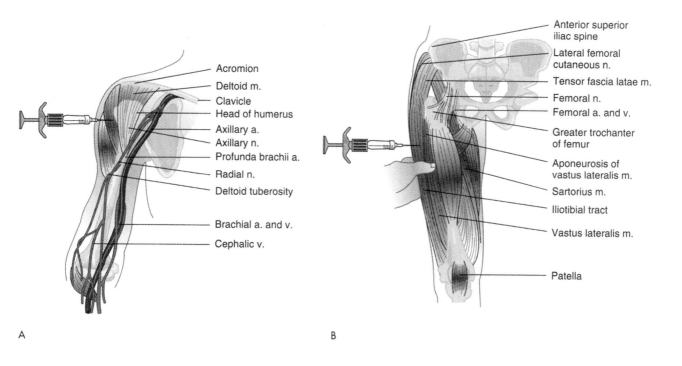

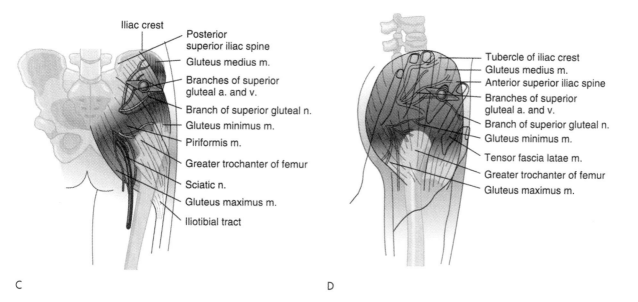

FIGURE 12–34

Intramuscular injection sites. **A,** Deltoid. **B,** Vastus lateralis. **C,** Dosogluteal. **D,** Ventrogluteal.
Redrawn and modified from Bindler, R., & Howry, L. (1997). Pediatric drugs and nursing implications (2nd ed., pp. 39–42). Stamford, CT: Appleton & Lange.

FIGURE 12–35

In infants, the vastus lateralis muscle is preferred for intramuscular injections.

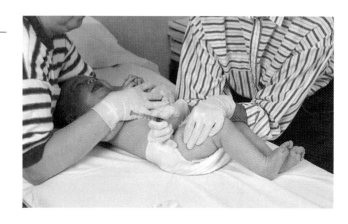

▶ ADMINISTERING AN INTRAMUSCULAR INJECTION

Preparation

- Select the syringe size according to the volume and dose of medication to be delivered. The needle must be long enough to penetrate the subcutaneous tissue and enter the muscle. Needles with a length of 0.5–1 inch (25 to 21 gauge) are recommended for infants and children.
- Choose the appropriate site (see the preceding discussion).

Selected Equipment
Syringe filled with medication

Procedure—*Clean Gloves*

- Have a nurse, an assistant, or the parent restrain the child during the injection (Fig. 12–36).
- Locate the site. Clean with alcohol using an outward circular motion.
- Grasp the muscle between your thumb and fingers for stabilization.
- Remove the cap from the syringe. Insert the needle quickly at a 90-degree angle. Pull back the plunger.
- If no blood is aspirated, inject the medication, withdraw the needle, massage the area with a gauze pad (alcohol will sting), and return the child to a position of comfort.
- Do not recap the needle. Discard it in a puncture-resistant container according to standard precaution recommendations.

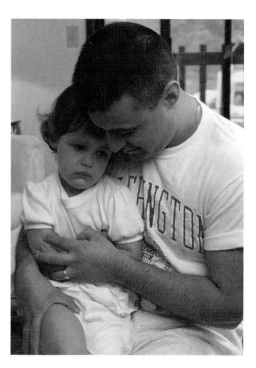

FIGURE 12–36

The child should be restrained by the parent or an assistant during intramuscular injection.

▶ SUBCUTANEOUS INJECTION

The site of the subcutaneous injection depends on the age of the child. Usually the dorsum of the upper arm or the anterior thigh is used in newborns, infants, and toddlers. The upper arm is the most common site for older children.

▶ ADMINISTERING A SUBCUTANEOUS INJECTION

Preparation

- Select the syringe size based on the volume or dose of medication to be delivered. The needle must be just long enough to penetrate the subcutaneous tissue, which lies below the skin and fat surface and above the muscle. Needles with a length of ⅜ to ⅝ inch (26 to 25 gauge) are recommended for infants and children.
- Choose the appropriate site (see the preceding discussion).

Selected Equipment
Syringe filled with medication

Procedure—*Clean Gloves*

- Have a nurse, an assistant, or the parent restrain the child while the injection is being given.
- Locate the site. Clean with alcohol using an outward circular motion. Pinch the skin between your thumb and index finger.
- Remove the cap from the syringe. Insert the needle quickly at about a 45-degree angle. Release the skin and pull back the plunger.
- If no blood is aspirated, inject the medication, withdraw the needle at the angle at which it was inserted, massage the area with a gauze pad (alcohol will sting), and return the child to a position of comfort.
- Do not recap the needle. Discard it in a puncture-resistant container according to standard precaution recommendations.

▶ OPHTHALMIC MEDICATION

Young children fear having anything placed in their eyes, and special care is often needed to reduce the child's anxiety and promote cooperation during instillation of ophthalmic medications. An explanation of the procedure may help gain the child's cooperation. To prevent the transfer of pathogens to the eye, the medication and its dispensing port must be kept sterile.

▶ ADMINISTERING AN OPTHALMIC MEDICATION

Selected Equipment
Medication

Procedure—*Clean Gloves*

- Have a nurse, an assistant, or the parent restrain the child in a supine position with the child's head extended.
- Use your nondominant hand to pull the child's lower lid down while your other hand rests on the child's head (Fig. 12–37).
- Instill the drops or ointment into the conjunctival sac that has formed.

- *Alternative method:* Pull the lower lid out far enough to form a reservoir in which the medication can be instilled.
- After the medication has been instilled, close the child's eyelids to prevent leakage.
- Have the child lie quietly for a minimum of 30 seconds. Discourage the child from squeezing the eyes shut.
- Dry the inner canthus of the eye.
- Keep the child's head in the midline position to prevent the medication from contaminating the other eye.

▶ OTIC MEDICATION

Otic medications, which are available in liquid form, are placed in the external ear canal using a dropper. Otic drops are sometimes applied to soften cerumen, enabling it to be cleansed from the canal. The ear canal is not treated with sterile technique unless the tympanic membrane is ruptured and draining.

▶ ADMINISTERING AN OTIC MEDICATION

Selected Equipment
Medication
Cotton ball

Procedure—*Clean Gloves*
- Have a nurse, an assistant, or the parent restrain the child in a supine position with the head turned as appropriate for administration (Fig. 12–38).
- *For the child less than 3 years of age:* Gently pull the pinna straight back and downward to straighten the ear canal.
- *For the older child:* Pull the pinna back and upward.
- When the pinna is in the proper position, instill the drops into the ear.
- Keep the child in the same position for a few minutes. Gently rub the area just anterior to the ear to facilitate drainage of the medication into the ear canal. If desired, a cotton ball may be loosely placed in the ear to promote retention of the medication.

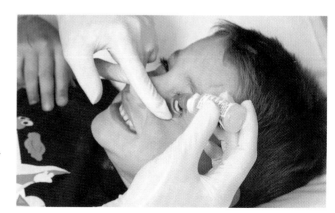

FIGURE 12–37

Administering on ophthalmic medication. The child is instructed to close the eyes and pretend to look up toward his head. The nurse then gently retracts the lower lid and inserts the medication.

FIGURE 12–38

Administering an otic medication.

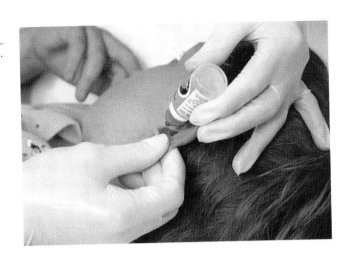

▶ NASAL MEDICATION

Medications instilled into the nares drain into the back of the mouth and throat, and may cause sensations of difficulty in breathing, tickling, or bad taste. After instillation of the drops, the child should be observed for choking or vomiting. Saline nose drops are sometimes given to young infants who have respiratory disorders to clear the nasal passages.

▶ ADMINISTERING A NASAL MEDICATION

Selected Equipment
Medication

Procedure—Clean Gloves
- Place the child in a supine position with the head hyperextended over the parent's lap or over the edge of the examination table or bed.
- Instill the drops into the nostrils.
- Keep the child in the same position for at least 5 minutes to allow the medication to contact the nasal mucosa.

▶ RECTAL MEDICATION

Rectal administration is sometimes used when the oral route is contraindicated. Although absorption is less reliable than with oral preparations, many medications, such as acetaminophen, aspirin, antimetics, analgesics, and sedatives, come in suppository form.

▶ ADMINISTERING A RECTAL MEDICATION

Selected Equipment
Water-soluble lubricant
Suppository

Preparation
If the suppository is to be halved, cut it lengthwise.

Procedure—*Clean Gloves*
- Have another nurse, an assistant, or the parent hold the child in a side-lying or (if small enough) a prone position on the parent's lap.
- Slightly lubricate the tapered tip of the suppository. Using either the index finger (in children over 3 years of age) or the little finger (in infants and toddlers), gently insert the suppository into the child's rectum, just beyond the internal sphincter.
- Hold the buttocks together for 5–10 minutes, until the urge to expel the medication has passed.

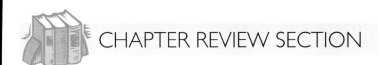

CHAPTER REVIEW SECTION

MULTIPLE CHOICE

1. Which of the following is an *acceptable* way to handle a anxious parent?
   (A) Show the parent how to hold the child during the exam.
   (B) Ask the parent to leave the room and calm down.
   (C) Take the child away from the parent, so you have control of the child.
   (D) Tell the child and parent that "It won't hurt."

2. When you weigh an infant, you must:
   (A) watch the infant because he or she can move suddenly.
   (B) swab the platform scale before using it.
   (C) set the platform scale to -.05.
   (D) leave the infant's diaper on for comfort.

3. Liquid acetaminophen drops can be administered:
   (A) only as directed.
   (B) in a 5ml dosage.
   (C) in a 6ml dosage.
   (D) in a 7ml dosage.

4. The "mummy" restraint method involves:
   (A) wrapping a sheet around a child.
   (B) the parent holding the child's hands on the child's chest.
   (C) using a board.
   (D) tucking the infant's arms and legs under the parent's arms.

5. Which one of the following is a spinal fusion disorder?
   (A) meningocele
   (B) cystic fibrosis
   (C) anencephaly
   (D) RSV

6. *Hydrocephalis* is treated by surgically:
   (A) inserting a shunt.
   (B) closing the opening.
   (C) protecting the exposed spinal cord.
   (D) repairing the septal wall.

7. Which one of the following is a cyanotic congenital heart condition?
   (A) transposition of the great arteries
   (B) patent ductus arteriosus
   (C) coarctation of the aorta
   (D) atrial septal defect

8. Anemia in an older child is *most* often caused by:
   (A) eating a poor diet.
   (B) taking supplements.
   (C) drinking too much soda.
   (D) exercising too little.

9. A urine specimen from a toddler must be:
    (A) recent for an accurate laboratory result.
    (B) obtained only by catheterization.
    (C) stored at room temperature.
    (D) done as soon as the child wakes in the morning.

10. Immediately after removing the urine collection bag, you must:
    (A) put the specimen into a sterile cup and seal.
    (B) put the specimen into a sterile cup, but leave unsealed.
    (C) take the bag to the laboratory sealed.
    (D) take the bag to the laboratory unsealed.

▶ EXTERNSHIP APPLICATION

A mother refuses the first immunization series for her child during the first well-child checkup. As a medical assistant, how do you respond?

Section Three
CERTIFICATION
EXAM PREPARATION

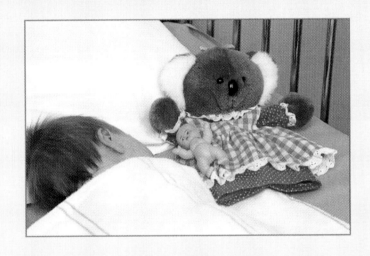

▶ CHAPTER 13, ASSISTING WITH MEDICAL SPECIALITIES

1. A discomforting uneasiness that is often a sign of infection is

(A) metastasis   (D) malaise
(B) acuity   (E) contagious
(C) benign

   (D) is correct. Malaise is a discomforting uneasiness that is often a sign of infection.
        It is noncontagious.
   (A) Metastasis occurs when cancerous cells or tumors spread to another location or organ.
   (B) Acuity is a sharpness. This term is usually associated with visual acuity.
   (C) Benign is a nonthreatening, noncancerous condition.
   (E) Contagious diseases are those that can be transmitted from one person to another.

2. The branch of medicine that deals with diseases and disorders of the female reproductive system is

(A) pediatrics   (D) nephrology
(B) gynecology   (E) neurology
(C) urology

   (B) is correct. Gynecology is the branch of medicine that deals with diseases and disorders of
        the female reproductive tract.
   (A) Pediatrics is the branch of medicine that involves the development, diagnosis, and treatment
        of disorders and diseases of children.
   (C) Urology is the branch of medicine that involves disorders and diseases of the urinary and
        male reproductive tract.
   (D) Nephrology is the branch of medicine that deals with the disorders and diseases of the kidney.
   (E) Neurology is the branch of medicine that treats the nonsurgical patient who has a disorder or
        disease of the nervous system.

3. A cardiovascular condition that results in death of tissue from lack of blood supply is a/an

(A) aneurysm   (D) infarct
(B) angioma   (E) Reynaud's phenomenon
(C) murmur

   (D) is correct. An infarct is a cardiovascular condition that results in death of tissue from lack of
        blood supply.
   (A) An aneurysm is an abnormal dilation of a blood vessel, usually an artery, due to a congenital
        weakness or defect in the wall of the vessel.
   (B) An angioma is a tumor, usually benign, consisting of blood vessels.
   (C) A murmur is a soft blowing or rasping sound heard upon auscultation of the heart.
   (E) Reynaud's phenomenon is intermittent attacks of pallor or cyanosis of the fingers or toes
        associated with cold or emotional distress.

4. The most common symptom/s of cardiovascular disorders is/are

   (A) edema and cyanosis
   (B) irregular heartbeat
   (C) diaphoresis and dyspnea

   (D) crushing chest pain
   (E) all of the above

   (E) is correct.

5. Dyspnea is difficulty

   (A) swallowing
   (B) urinating
   (C) breathing

   (D) performing a function
   (E) menstruating

   (C) is correct. Dyspnea is difficulty breathing.
   (A) Difficulty swallowing is called dysphagia.
   (B) Difficulty urinating is called dysuria.
   (D) Difficulty performing a function is called dysfunction.
   (E) Difficulty menstruating is called dysmenorrhea.

6. A tuberculin skin test is a

   (A) Mantoux test
   (B) tine test
   (C) culture for tuberculosis

   (D) A and B
   (E) none of the above

   (D) is correct. The Mantoux test is a tuberculosis antibody test using an interdermal injection. The tine test is a test for tuberculosis using a small multipuncture device.

7. What disease results in edema, slowed speech, enlarged facial features and tongue, drowsiness, and mental apathy?

   (A) myasthenia gravis
   (B) myxedema
   (C) von Recklinghausen's disease

   (D) Graves' disease
   (E) Cushing's syndrome

   (B) is correct. Myxedema is a disease that results in edema, slowed speech, enlarged facial features and tongue, drowsiness, and mental apathy.
   (A) Myasthenia gravis is a condition in which there is great muscular weakness and progressive fatigue.
   (C) von Recklinghausen's disease is an excessive production of parathyroid hormone, which results in degeneration of the bones.
   (D) Graves' disease results from an overactivity of the thyroid gland and can result in a crisis.
   (E) Cushing's syndrome is a set of symptoms, including weakness, edema, excessive hair growth, and osteoporosis, that is caused by hypersecretion of the adrenal cortex.

8. A procedure in which contrast medium is used to visualize the bile ducts is called

(A) endoscopic retrograde cholangiopancreatography (ERCP)
(B) cholecystogram
(C) intravenous cholangiogram
(D) peritoneoscopy laparoscopy
(E) choledocholithotripsy

    (C) is correct. An intravenous cholangiogram is a procedure in which contrast medium is used to visualize the bile ducts

    (A) Endoscopic retrograde cholangiopancreatography (ERCP) is the use of an endoscope to x-ray the bile and pancreatic ducts.

    (B) A cholecystogram is an x-ray taken to visualize the gallbladder as dye enters it.

    (D) A peritoneoscopy laparoscopy is a procedure in which an instrument or scope is passed into the abdominal wall through a small opening in order to examine the abdominal cavity for tumors and other conditions.

    (E) A choledocholithotripsy is using lithotripsy equipment to crush gallstones located in the common bile duct.

9. The crushing of a stone located within the gallbladder is called

(A) cholecystectomy
(B) proctoplasty
(C) colostomy
(D) cholelithotripsy
(E) lithotripsy

    (D) is correct. A cholelithotripsy is the crushing of a stone located within the gallbladder.

    (A) A cholecystectomy is surgical removal of the gallbladder.

    (B) A proctoplasty is plastic surgery of the anus or rectum.

    (C) A colostomy is the surgical creation of an opening of some portion of the colon through the abdominal wall to the outside surface.

    (E) Lithotripsy refers to crushing a kidney stone.

10. A musculoskeletal disorder in which a softening of bone occurs that may result from a deficiency in vitamin D is

(A) osteoporosis
(B) osteomalacia
(C) osteoarthritis
(D) talipes
(E) scoliosis

    (B) is correct. Osteomalacia is a musculoskeletal disorder in which a softening of bone occurs that may result from a deficiency in vitamin D.

    (A) Osteoporosis is a decrease in bone mass that results in a thinning and weakening of the bone with resulting fractures.

    (C) Osteoarthritis is a noninflammatory type of arthritis resulting in degeneration of the bones and joints.

    (D) Talipes is a congenital deformity of the foot.

    (E) Scoliosis is an abnormal lateral curvature of the spine.

11. Another name for hyperthyroidism is

   (A)   Graves' disease   **(D)**   Paget's disease
   (B)   goiter   **(E)**   Bright's disease
   (C)   Hashimoto's disease

   (A)   is correct. Graves' disease is another name for hyperthyroidism.
   (B)   A goiter is an enlargement of the thyroid gland.
   (C)   Hashimoto's disease is a chronic form of thyroiditis.
   (D)   Paget's disease is an inherited disease causing a progressive muscle weakness and atrophy.
   (E)   Bright's disease is an inflammatory kidney disease with proteinuria and hematuria.

12. Paget's disease is a/an

   (A)   deficiency in calcium and vitamin D
   (B)   metabolic disease of the bone characterized by deformity
   (C)   autoimmune disorder causing loss of muscle strength and paralysis
   (D)   inherited disease causing a progressive muscle weakness and deformity
   (E)   A and B

   (D)   is correct. Paget's disease is an inherited disease causing a progressive muscle weakness and atrophy.

13. Another name for Lou Gehrig's disease is

   (A)   cerebral palsy   **(D)**   Addison's disease
   (B)   Bell's palsy   **(E)**   Bright's disease
   (C)   amyotropic lateral sclerosis

   (C)   is correct. Lou Gehrig's disease is also called amyotropic lateral sclerosis. Lou Gehrig was a famous baseball player who had the disease.
   (A)   Cerebral palsy is a nonprogressive paralysis resulting from a defect or trauma at the time of birth.
   (B)   Bell's palsy is a one-sided facial paralysis caused by herpes simplex virus.
   (D)   Addison's disease results from a deficiency of adrenocortical hormones that results in skin pigmentation, generalized weakness, and weight loss.
   (E)   Bright's disease is an inflammatory degenerative kidney disease.

14. A mitral valve prolapse is a serious condition in which the mitral valve drops back into the

   (A)   left ventricle during diastole   **(D)**   left atrium during systole
   (B)   right ventricle during diastole **(E)**   none of the above
   (C)   right atrium during systole

   (D)   is correct. A mitral valve prolapse is a serious condition in which the mitral valve drops back into the left atrium during systole.

15. When giving an immunization to an infant or child, never administer within

   (A)   the flu season
   (B)   24 hours of a fever
   (C)   48 hours of a fever
   (D)   24 hours of another immunization
   (E)   none of the above

   (B)   is correct. When giving an immunization to an infant or child, never administer within 24 hours of a fever.

16. According to the American Cancer Society, women should examine both breasts

(A) weekly

(B) monthly

(C) bimonthly

(D) quarterly

(E) annually

    (B)   is correct. The American Cancer Society recommends that women examine their breasts monthly.

17. A hernia of the bladder that protrudes into the vagina is called a/an

(A) cystoscope

(B) condyloma

(C) colposcopy

(D) cystocele

(E) eclampsia

    (D)   is correct. A cystocele is a hernia of the bladder that protrudes into the vagina.

    (A)   A cystoscope is a lighted instrument used to visualize the urinary bladder.

    (B)   A condyloma is a wartlike skin growth usually found on the genitalia or in the anal area.

    (C)   A colposcopy is a visual examination of the cervix and vagina using a colposcope.

    (E)   Eclampsia is a condition during the 20th week of pregnancy and the first week of postpartum that results in convulsive seizures and coma.

18. A colposcopy is a/an

(A) examination of the female pelvic cavity using an endoscope

(B) exposing of tissues to high temperatures in order to destroy tissues

(C) visual examination of the bladder and vagina

(D) surgical removal of a core of cervical tissue

(E) examination of the urinary bladder using a lighted instrument

    (C)   is correct. Colposcopy is the visual examination of the bladder and vagina.

19. Facilitating the removal of secretions from the bronchi by placing the patient in a position that uses gravity to promote this is known as

(A) intermittent positive pressure breathing

(B) postural drainage

(C) endotracheal intubation

(D) hyperbaric oxygen therapy

(E) none of the above

    (B)   is correct. Postural drainage is the removal of secretions from the bronchi by placing the patient in a position that uses gravity to promote this.

    (A)   Intermittent positive pressure breathing (IPPB) is a method for assisting the breathing of patients by the use of increased pressure.

    (C)   Endotracheal intubation is placement of a tube through the mouth to create an airway.

    (D)   Hyperbaric oxygen therapy is the use of oxygen under great pressure to treat cases of carbon monoxide poisoning, smoke inhalation, and other conditions.

20. The newborn reflex that occurs when the infant turns his or her head in the direction of a stimulus is called the

(A) sucking reflex

(B) rooting reflex

(C) palmar grasp reflex

(D) China doll reflex

(E) Moro reflex

(B)   is correct. The rooting reflex is tested by stroking an infant's cheek. The infant with a normal response will turn toward the side that is stroked.

(A)   The sucking reflex is an automatic reflex at birth. The infant will suck nipples and other objects placed in his or her mouth.

(C)   The palmar grasp reflex occurs when the infant closes his or her hand as the palm is stroked.

(D)   The China doll reflex occurs when the infant is pulled into a sitting position. This will cause the infant's eyes to open and shoulders to tense as the infant tries to keep his or her head up.

(E)   The Moro reflex occurs when infants become startled. They will normally arch their back, throw back their head, extend their arms, and then quickly close (or flex) into a ball as though they were falling.

21. A test used to assess neonatal status is the

(A) Snellen test

(B) Apgar scale

(C) Moro reflex

(D) sucking reflex

(E) B, C, and D

(B)   is correct. The Apgar scale is used immediately after birth, and then 5 minutes later, to assess the status of the newborn. The infant (neonate) is rated in 5 categories (heart rate, respirations, body color, muscle tone, and reflex irritability) on a scale of 1 to 10. In addition, reflexes such as the Moro and sucking reflexes are tested.

APPENDICES

Appendix A

SYLLABUS AND CALENDARS

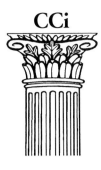

CORINTHIAN COLLEGES, INC.
Medical Assisting Program

MODULE F—ENDOCRINOLOGY AND REPRODUCTION

Syllabus and Topic Outline

Prerequisite: None

Module Length: 20 days

Date:

Instructor:

Time:

Module Description:

Module F covers general anatomy and physiology, including an overview of the study of biology and the various body structures and systems. This module also identifies and examines the basic structural components and functions of the skeletal, endocrine and reproductive systems. Students learn about child growth and development, and how heredity, cultural and the environmental aspects affect behavior. Students gain an understanding about assisting in a pediatrician's office and learn the important differences that are specific to the pediatric field. Some of the skills students learn in this area are height, weight, measurements and restraining techniques used for infants and children. They check vital signs, assist with diagnostic examinations and laboratory tests, instruct patients regarding health promotion practices, and perform certain invasive procedures. Students study essential medical terminology, build on their keyboarding and word processing skills, and become familiar with the self-directed job search process by learning all about how to become and learn from mentoring.

Module F is comprised of three sections:

Semester Credits

Theory	41 hours/ 2.73 credit units
Clinical/Lab	30 hours/ 1 credit unit
Computers	10 hours/ .33 credit units
Total:	81 hours / 4 credit units

Quarter Credits

Theory	40 hours/ 4 credit units
Clinical/Lab	30 hours/ 1.5 credit units
Computers	10 hours/ .5 credit units
Total:	80 hours / 6 credit units

Student must receive a grade of 70% or above to pass this module.

Module F Textbook:

Medical Assisting: Module F - Endocrinology and Reproduction; Corinthian Colleges, Inc., 2004

Reference Material:

Insurance Handbook for the Medical Office; 8th edition; Marilyn T. Fordney, W.B. Saunders, 2002.
Student Workbook for the Insurance Handbook for the Medical Office; 8th edition; Marilyn T. Fordney, W.B. Saunders, 2002.
Medical Transcribing: Techniques and Procedures; 5th edition; Diehl and Fordney, W.B. Saunders, 2003.
Microsoft Word 2000; Nita Rutkosky, EMC Paradigm Publishers, 2000.

Additional Reference material: Medical management software, Video series, Medical dictionary and Physicians Desk Reference

Instructional Methods:

Instructors for Module F will utilize lectures, classroom discussions, hands-on experiences, laboratory exercises, role playing, presentations, demonstrations, research and student assignments (depending on section requirements) to facilitate students' achievement of course objectives.

Grading:

The Clinical/Laboratory section grade will be determined as follows:

Hands-on practice and experiences	50%
Tests/quizzes	50%

The grade distribution for Module F is as follows:

Theory	30%
Clinical/Laboratory	40%
Computer/Keyboarding	30%
Total Module F Grade	100%

Attendance:

Students are expected to attend every class session. Make up work will be allowed only with instructor's approval. Refer to catalog for explanation of attendance policy.

Date of last Revision: August 2004

Objectives and Topic Outline:

Upon successful completion of this course the student will be able to:
1. Identify and define terms related to basic medical terminology, including prefixes, suffixes, word parts, abbreviations, and symbols. Define and spell the glossary terms for each chapter.
2. Differentiate between anatomy, physiology, cytology, histology and pathology
3. Apply the appropriate anatomical directional terminology to points of reference on the human body.
4. Identify the eight body cavities, locate each on an illustration of the body, and name the major body organs located with each cavity.
5. Identify the regions of the abdomen.
6. Describe the basic characteristics of the cell.
7. Explain what happens when cell mutation occurs.
8. Identify the patterns of inheritance and explain how they affect a trait.
9. Describe the ways molecules pass through cell membranes.
10. Explain DNA "fingerprinting."
11. Identify the distinguishing characteristics of each of the following genetic conditions: cleft lip, cleft palate, Down syndrome, spina bifida, Klinefelter's syndrome, talipes, and Turner's syndrome.
12. Identify and describe the main types of body tissue.
13. Identify the ten systems of the body.
14. Describe the functions of bones and the skeletal system
15. Compare the structure of compact and spongy bone
16. Discuss the processes by which bones develop and grow
17. Describe the effects of aging on the bones of the skeletal system
18. Identify the two divisions of the skeletal system and the bone groups in each division
19. Describe the three basic types of joints
20. Relate body movements to the action of specific joints
21. Identify the types of bone fractures and the characteristics of each
22. Outline the treatment of a fracture
23. Describe the healing process for a bone fracture
24. Identify common diagnostic examinations for the skeletal system
25. Identify common diseases and disorders of the skeletal system
26. Differentiate between sexual and asexual reproduction.
27. Describe the differentiation of reproductive organs.
28. Identify the female sex organs and describe their location and function.
29. Explain the interaction of pituitary hormones with the ovaries and other organs.
30. Identify the female secondary sex characteristics.

31. Describe the maturation and release of an ovum.
32. Compare the internal and external sexual organs of the male and female.
33. Describe the phases of the menstrual cycle and the purpose of menstruation.
34. Explain how fertilization occurs.
35. Identify the events occurring during each trimester of pregnancy as they relate to the woman and the embryo/fetus.
36. Identify the events that occur in the three stages of labor.
37. Identify reasons for practicing contraception.
38. Identify contraceptive methods, and give an indication of the relative effectiveness of each.
39. Identify the diagnostic tests for the female reproductive system.
40. Identify the diseases and disorders of the female reproductive system
41. Identify the sexually transmitted diseases, and describe the characteristics of each.
42. Identify the male sex organs and describe their location and function.
43. Describe male prenatal development
44. Explain the relationship between pituitary hormones and the function of the testes.
45. Identify the male secondary sex characteristics.
46. Describe the pathway of sperm from production to expulsion.
47. Identify the components of semen.
48. Describe the diseases and disorders of the male reproductive system.
49. Provide appropriate instruction to a female patient regarding a Pap test appointment and explain why it is necessary.
50. List and describe the necessary instruments and supplies needed for a Pap test and pelvic examination.
51. Demonstrate the female patient preparation and patient education for a Pap test and pelvic examination.
52. Demonstrate the proper technique for assisting with a Pap test and pelvic examination.
53. Correctly prepare the Pap test specimen for laboratory analysis.
54. Explain Breast self-examination (BSE) and instruct a patient in conducting BSE.
55. Identify patient education appropriate for female patients having a Pap test and pelvic examination.
56. Correctly instruct a patient in the preparation for a sigmoidoscopy and explain why it is necessary.
57. Identify and describe the instruments and equipment used for a sigmoidoscopy.
58. Explain how to properly assist with a sigmoidoscopy examination.
59. Identify patient education appropriate for patients having a sigmoidoscopy examination.
60. Provide appropriate patient instruction on how to administer an enema.
61. Correctly complete a health department request form for the PKU test and obtain a blood specimen.
62. Briefly describe the field of pediatrics
63. Explain the importance of incorporating age-appropriate behavior to communicate with pediatric patients.
64. Identify equipment used during a pediatric examination.
65. Distinguish between well child examinations and sick child examinations and identify functions performed in each.
66. Describe the different methods of administering medication specific to pediatric patients.
67. Transport an infant safely.
68. Describe different restraining techniques.
69. Identify normal ranges of pediatric vital signs
70. Explain the importance of preventive dental care and list specific preventive measures.
71. Identify common childhood injuries and safety precautions of each.
72. Recognize and describe the needs of each developmental stage of life.
73. Incorporate age-appropriate behaviors to enhance interaction with all patients of all ages.
74. Recognize normal developmental milestones in all stages of life.
75. Identify the various body system changes involved in the aging process and the implications for the medical assistant.
76. Describe special health risks of the elderly and implications for the medical assistant.
77. Describe common diseases and disorders that occur with age in various systems of the body.
78. List and explain the normal immunization schedule for adults and children.
79. Discuss the diseases that can be prevented with immunization.
80. Explain the importance of informing patients of the benefits and risks of immunization before administering.
81. Identify proper procedure for obtaining an informed consent
82. Document administration of a simulated medication and immunization in a patient's record.
83. Identify how to cite information given to parents about maintaining the immunization record.
84. List the two types of molecules that form the main groups of hormones

85. Explain the general action of hormones
86. Explain how endocrine organs are controlled by negative feedback
87. Discuss the location, hormones, and functions of the following endocrine glands and tissues: pituitary, thyroid, parathyroids, thymus, adrenals, pancreas, testes, ovaries and pineal gland
88. Briefly describe the functions of the hormones secreted by the kidneys, heart, digestive system, and adipose tissue
89. Explain how the endocrine system responds to stress
90. Identify the diagnostic examinations used to confirm diabetes, thyroid function, pregnancy, and Cushing's syndrome
91. Identify common diseases and disorders of the endocrine system.
92. Identify the role and responsibilities of a mentor and describe how a mentor can assist in achieving goals
93. Identify ways a person can find and work with a mentor
94. Identify how a person can become a mentor
95. Identify useful resource sites that can assist in learning more about mentoring
96. Demonstrate increasing speed and accuracy on the computer keyboard, medical transcription, and acceptable progress through the identified text(s).
97. Demonstrate knowledge and skill in medical terminology and anatomy & physiology by utilizing software to enhance learning and assist in research material for essay assignments.
98. Demonstrate progressive skill acquisition related to word processing, computerized medical office application, and processing of insurance claim forms with acceptable progress through the identified text(s).

TOPIC OUTLINE

I. Terminology associated with the Skeletal, Reproductive, and Endocrine System
  A. Three types of word parts
    1. Prefixes
    2. Suffixes
    3. Root terms
  B. Prefixes
    1. Numbers
    2. Colors
    3. Opposites
    4. Negative
    5. Size/Comparison
    6. Position
  C. Suffixes
    1. Condition
    2. Surgical
    3. Diagnostic
    4. Clinical
    5. Miscellaneous
  D. Root Terms
  E. Anatomical Terms
  F. Medical Abbreviations
  G. The Medical Record
  H. Prescription and Delivery
  I. Using the Medical Dictionary
  J. Anatomy & Physiology Overview, Skeletal System, Reproductive System, Endocrine System
II. Anatomy & Physiology of the Organization of the Human Body
  A. Anatomy
  B. Physiology
  C. Cytology
  D. Histology
  E. Pathology
  F. Anatomical Directional Terms
    1. Median (Sagittal) Plane
    2. Proximal and Distal
    3. Frontal (Coronal) Plane
    4. Transverse Plane
    5. Superficial
    6. Deep
    7. Anatomical position
  G. Body Cavities—divided into two main cavities
    1. Dorsal—located on posterior side of body
      a. Cranial
      b. Spinal
    2. Ventral—located on the anterior side of body
      a. Thoracid cavity (chest)
      b. Abdominopelvic cavity (3 parts)
    3. Cranial cavity protects the brain
    4. Orbital cavity contains the eyes
    5. Nasal cavity contains the structure of the nose
    6. Buccal cavity contains the mouth
  H. Abdominal Regions
    1. Quadrant method of division
      a. right upper quadrant (RUQ)

      b. left upper quadrant (LUQ)
      c. right lower quadrant (RLQ)
      d. left lower quadrant (LLQ)
   2. Nine region method
      a. Epigastric
      b. Umbilical
      c. Hypogastric
      d. Hypochondriac
      e. Lumbar regions
      f. Iliac or Inguinal regions

I. Cell—basic building block of life
   1. Functions
   2. Cells vary, body contains 75 trillion cells
   3. Parts of a cell:
      a. Cytoplasm
      b. Cell membrane
      c. Organelles
        • Nucleus
        • Chromosomes
        • Nucleolus
        • Centrioles
        • Endoplasmic reticulum
        • Mitochondria
        • Golgi apparatus
        • Lysosomes
        • Pinocytic vessicles
   4. Passing molecules through cell membranes
      a. Diffusion
      b. Osmosis
      c. Filtration
      d. Active Transport
      e. Phagocytosis
      f. Pinocytosis
   5. Cellular division
      a. Mitosis
      b. Meiosis
   6. Homeostasis
   7. Mutations and traits

J. Three patterns of inheritance
   1. Dominant
   2. Recessive
   3. Sex-linked

K. DNA Fingerprinting

L. Genetic Conditions
   1. Cleft Lip
   2. Cleft Palate
   3. Cystic Fibrosis
   4. Down Syndrome
   5. Galactosemia
   6. Hemophilia
   7. Kinefelter's Syndrome
   8. Phenylketonuria
   9. Spina Bifida
  10. Talipes
  11. Turner's Syndrome

M. Tissues—cells join together and form tissue
   1. Made up of 60-99% water
      a. Dehydration
      b. Edema
   2. Four main types of tissue classifications
      a. Epithelial tissue
      b. Connective tissue
      c. Nerve tissue
      d. Muscle tissue
N. Organs—two or more tissues working together to perform a specific function
   1. Systems—types:
      a. Digestive
      b. Integumentary
      c. Skeletal
      d. Muscular
      e. Respiratory
      f. Circulatory
      g. Urinary
      h. Nervous
      i. Endocrine
      j. Reproductive
      k. Immune
III. Anatomy and Physiology of the Skeletal System
   A. Skeletal System—Function:
      1. Support
      2. Protection
      3. Leverage
      4. Storage
      5. Blood Cell Production
      6. Form
   B. Bone Structure
      1. Composition
      2. Types of bone tissue
         a. compact
         b. spongy
         c. marrow
         d. periosteum
      3. Four general shapes
         a. long
         b. short
         c. flat
         d. irregular
   C. Growth and development
      1. bone formation
      2. continues growing through 18-25 years of age
      3. growth increases at puberty
      4. grows in diameter
      5. bones become thinner and weaker with age
      6. specific bone mass reduction
   D. Number of bones
      1. 270 at birth
      2. 206 at adulthood
      3. difference between the bones is due to bone fusion

E. Divisions of the skeletal system
    1. Axial skeleton
        a. spinal column
        b. skull
        c. ribcage
    2. Appendicular
        a. arms
        b. hands
        c. legs
        d. feet
        e. shoulders
        f. pelvis

F. Identification of bones
    1. Spinal column
    2. Skull
    3. Rib cage
    4. Upper extremities
    5. Pelvic girdle
    6. Lower extremities

G. Joints—two or more bony parts joins together (articulation)
    1. Held together by ligaments
    2. Joint classifications
        a. Diarthrosis
        b. Amphiarthrosis / cartilaginous
        c. Synarthrosis / fibrous
    3. Types of joints
        a. Gliding joints
        b. Hinge joints
        c. Pivot joints
        d. Ball and socket joints
    4. Types of movement
        a. Flexion
        b. Extension
        c. Abduction
        d. Adduction
        e. Rotation

IV. Diagnostic Examinations
    A. Arthroscopy
    B. Computer Tomography (CT scan)
    C. Magnetic Resonance Imaging (MRI)

V. Fractures—Types
    A. Greenstick
    B. Simple or closed
    C. Compound or open
    D. Impacted
    E. Comminuted
    F. Depressed
    G. Spiral
    H. Colles
    I. Treatments
    J. Healing Process
    K. Amputation

VI. Common Diseases and Disorders
   A. Arthritis
   B. Bursitis
   C. Dislocation
   D. Herniated Disk
   E. Lumbar Myositis
   F. Osteoporosis
   G. Spinal Curvatures
   H. Sprain
VII. Anatomy and Physiology of the Female Reproductive System
   A. General information about the reproductive system
   B. Meiosis and sex determination
   C. Differentiation of reproductive organs
   D. Female reproductive organs
      1. Ovaries
      2. Primary follicles
      3. Fallopian Tubes
      4. Uterus
      5. Vagina
      6. Cul-de-sac
   E. Internal female reproductive organs
      1. Vulva
      2. Clitoris
      3. Perineum
      4. Mammary glands (breasts)
      5. Areola
   F. Menstral Cycle—when ovum is not fertilized, uterine lining deteriorates and is discharged from the body.
      1. Menstruation begins at menarche (first cycle) and ends with menopause (last cycle)
      2. Complete cycle is 28 days
      3. Cycle is divided into four phases:
         a. Phase I—Follicular Phase
         b. Phase II—Ovulation
         c. Phase III—Luteal Phase
         d. Phase IV—Menstruation
   G. Fertilization
      1. Millions of sperm are deposited
      2. Sperm travels to outer third of fallopian tube
      3. Sperm meets ovum and penetrates—ovum must be fertilized within 24 hours
      4. Zygote is formed
      5. Zygote starts to travel to uterus and implants into uterus
      6. Hormones support zygote
      7. Embryo develops and placenta begins to secrete progesterone and estrogen
      8. Twins
         a. fraternal
         b. maternal (identical)
         c. siamese
   H. Pregnancy
      1. Gestation period 38 weeks
      2. Embryonic state
      3. Fetal state
      4. Growth process
         a. First Trimester—0-3 months
         b. Second Trimester—3-6 months
         c. Third Trimester—6-9 months

5. Extra embryonic Membranes
    a. Yolk Sak
    b. Amnion
    c. Allantois
    b. Chorion
6. Pdacealia
7. Placental Circulation
8. Signs of pregnancy
9. Nagel's Rule
10. Birth Process
11. Stages of labor
12. Cesarean Section

I. Infertility—inability to become pregnant
1. affects 1 in 7 couples in United States
2. Causes
3. Treatment

J. Contraception—birth control
1. Reasons to practice birth control
2. Methods of contraception

K. Diagnostic tests for female reproductive system
1. Alpha-fetoprotein screening
2. Colposcopy
3. Diaphanogram
4. Hysteroscopy
5. Interventional hysterosalpingography
6. Mammogram
7. Maturation index
8. Papanicolaou smear (PAP)
9. Pregnancy test
10. Ultrasonography

L. Diseases and disorders of the female reproductive system
1. Abortion (Miscarriage)
2. Cervical erosion
3. Cystic breast disease
4. Cystocele
5. Dysmenorrhea
6. Endometriosis
7. Fibroids
8. Hysterectomy
9. Malignancy of the breast
10. Other malignancy's
11. Ovarian cysts
12. Premenstrual Syndrome (PMS)
13. Polyps
14. Rectocele
15. Vaginitis

M. Sexually transmitted diseases
1. AIDS
2. Chlamydia
3. Gonorrhea
4. Herpes
5. Nongonococcal Urethritis
6. Pelvic Inflammatory Disease (PID)

       7. Pediculosis Pubis (lice)

       8. Syphilis

       9. Trichomoniasis

     10. Vaginitis

VIII. Anatomy and Physiology of the Male Reproductive System

    A. Male Reproductive Organs-develop in the fetal abdomen and descend to the scrotum during the 8th -9th month of fetal development.

       1. Testes (male gonads)

       2. Epididymis

       3. Vas deferens

       4. Seminal vesicles

       5. Prostate gland

       6. Bulbourethral glands (Cowper's glands)

       7. Urethra

       8. Penis

    B. Vasectomy—Surgical sterilization

       1. Procedure

       2. Does not interfere with the function of the testes or sexual ability

    C. Diseases and disorders of the male reproductive system

       1. Epididymitis—SX, cause, TX

       2. Hydrocele—SX, cause, TX

       3. Impotence (Erectile dysfunction)—SX, cause, TX

       4. Prostatic Hypertrophy—SX, cause, TX

IX. Pediatrics

    A. Understanding pediatrics

       1. Pediatrics

       2. Pediatrician

       3. Pediatric examination

    B. Important concepts to remember when working with children

       1. Always explain

       2. Demonstrate procedures

       3. Allow the child to participate

    C. Types of pediatric visits—Two types

       1. Well child visit—description, medical assistant's responsibilities, and skills performed

       2. Sick child visit—description, medical assistant's responsibilities, and skills performed

    D. Administering medications—description

       1. Routes of administration

          a. Oral

          b. Nose drops

          c. Eye drops

          d. Ear drops

          e. Rectal

          f. Intramuscular injections

    E. Holding infants—transporting infants

       1. Cradle

       2. Football

       3. Upright

    F. Restraining—procedures sometimes require a child to be restrained to be performed correctly

       1. Total restraint methods

          a. Papoose board

          b. Mummy restraint

    G. Pediatric Vital signs

       1. Heart rate

       2. Respiratory rate

      3. Blood Pressure

      4. Temperature

  H. Pediatric dental care

      1. Teeth formation begins in the utero

      2. First tooth appears approximately at six months

      3. By age 3, all 20 primary teeth are present

      4. Nutrition affects teeth

      5. Parents responsibilities

      6. When to see the dentist

      7. Pacifiers and thumb sucking

      8. Nursing decay syndrome

      9. Routine dental care

     10. American Academy of Pediatric Dentistry

  I. Safety—Injury is the most common form of death in children

      1. Motor vehicle

      2. Pedestrian

      3. Submersion / drowning

      4. Burns

      5. Firearms

      6. Falls

      7. Poisons

X. Informed consent, Immunizations and Documentation

  A. Immunizations—known as vaccines

      1. Series—more than one immunization is necessary

      2. Booster—additional immunizations to ensure effectiveness of 1st immunization

      3. Titer—test to determine if antibodies are present

      4. Incubation—interval between exposure to infection and first symptom.

  B. How the body produces immunity against disease

      1. Natural immunity

      2. Artificial immunity

  C. Diseases prevented from immunizations

      1. Influenza (Flu)

      2. Pneumonia

      3. Haemophilus Influenza Type B

      4. Measles, Mumps, and Rubella (MMR)

      5. Diphtheria

      6. Pertussis (Whooping cough)

      7. Rabies

      8. Tetanus

      9. Varicella Zoster (Chicken Pox)

     10. Hepatitis B

     11. Poliomyelitis

     12. Cholera and Typhoid

  D. Immunization Schedule

  E. Informed consent, medication and documentation

      1. Informed consent—follow proper guidelines

      2. Medication and documentation protocol

  F. Medical Assistant legal and ethical concerns regarding immunizations

XI. Understanding Human Growth and Development

  A. Major theories of development

      1. Sigmund Freud—Psychosexual Development

      2. Erik Erikson—Psychosocial Development

      3. Jean Piaget—Cognitive Development

      4. Lawrence Kohlberg—Theory of Moral Development

5. Albert Bandura—Social Learning Theory
6. John Watson—Behaviorism
7. Urie Bronfenbrenner—Ecologic Theory
B. Infant Development
1. Neonate
2. Needs of an infant in the first 12 months
   a. comfort
   b. love
   c. warmth
   d. security
   e. stimulation to learn
3. When an infant's needs are met, the infant can progress normally through stages:
   a. neuromuscular (motor)
   b. intellectual (perceptual and sensory)
   c. psychosocial (adaptive, social, and emotional)
   d. language development
4. Development from three to twelve months of age
   a. neuromuscular
   b. intellectual
   c. psychosocial / language development
   d. medical assistant's implications
5. Toddler Development (1-3 years of age)
   a. changes
   b. basic needs
      • love
      • security
      • trust
      • discipline
      • autonomy
      • play
   c. Development from 18 to 30 months
      • Neuromuscular
      • Intellectual
      • Psychosocial / language
      • Medical Assistant's implications
6. Preschool Development
   a. changes
   b. basic needs
      • love
      • security
      • self-esteem
      • praise
   c. Preschool development from three to five years of age
      • Neuromuscular
      • Intellectual
      • Psychosocial / language
      • Medical Assistant's implications
7. Elementary Development—child takes steps towards adulthood
   a. changes
   b. basic needs
      • independence
      • forming peer relationships
      • self-esteem
      • respect

      c. Development of early to late elementary, ages 6 to 12
- Neuromuscular
- Intellectual
- Psychosocial / language
- Medical Assistant's implications

     8. Pre-adolescent Development—period of rapid physical and personality growth
      a. changes
      b. basic needs
- achieving independence
- respect
- trust
- to be listened to

      c. Development of the Pre-adolescent
- Neuromuscular
- Intellectual
- Psychosocial / language
- Medical Assistant's implications

     9. Adolescent Development—transition between childhood and adulthood
      a. changes
      b. basic needs
- respect
- autonomy
- authority

      a. Development of the Adolescent
- Neuromuscular
- Intellectual
- Psychosocial / language
- Medical Assistant's implications

   10. Adulthood—changes
   11. Early Adulthood—changes
   12. Middle Age—changes
   13. The older adult—changes
   14. Body system changes associated with aging (diseases and disorders)
      a. Skin
      b. Hair
      c. Muscles and bones
      d. Heart and blood vessels
      e. Respiration
      f. Brain
      g. Digestive System
      h. Urinary Tract
      i. Hormones
      j. Vision and hearing
   15. Special health risks of the older adult

XIII. Anatomy and Physiology of the Endocrine System
   A. Hormones—Two types
     1. Amino acid based
     2. Lipid-based
   B. Actions of hormones
   C. Control of hormone secretion (homeostasis)
   D. Major endocrine glands
     1. Pituitary
     2. Thyroid gland
     3. Parathyroid glands

       4. Adrenal glands

       5. Pancreas

       6. Thymus

       7. Pineal body

       8. Gonads

    E. Other hormone sources

       1. Kidneys

       2. Heart

       3. Digestive system

       4. Adipose tissue

    F. Hormones and stress

       1. Stress—any condition that threatens homeostasis

       2. Causes

         a. physical

         b. emotional

         c. environmental

         d. metabolic

       3. Responses—immediate

    G. Diagnostic Examinations

       1. Blood sugar

       2. T3, TSH and T4

       3. HCG—pregnancy test

       4. GTT—Glucose tolerance test

       5. GHB Alc (Glucohemoglobin)

       6. Scanning tests

       7. Specific tests to measure hormone levels in the blood

    H. Diseases and disorders of the endocrine system

       1. Cretinism—description, SX, cause, TX

       2. Cushing's Syndrome—description, SX, cause, TX

       3. Diabetes Mellitus—description, SX, cause, TX

       4. Grave's Disease—description, SX, cause, TX

       5. Myxedema—description, SX, cause, TX

XIII. Career Development—Success with Mentoring

    A. Role and responsibilities of a mentor and how mentors achieve success

    B. Mentor

    C. Who can be a mentor

    D. How to find work with a mentor

    E. Selecting a mentor

    F. The mentor-mentee relationship

    G. How to become a mentor

    H. Mentoring guidelines

    I. Student resource web sites

XIV. Technical Communication and Professional Development

    A. Medical Terminology

    B. Anatomy & Physiology

    C. Keyboarding

    D. Word Processing

    E. Medical Operations Software

    F. Medical Insurance

    G. Medical Transcribing

    H. Disease short essays

Day and Evening Schedule

MEDICAL ASSISTING
MODULE F- Endocrinology / Reproduction
Lecture Calendar

One (1) Hour Per Day

Unit 1 Day 1	Day 2	Day 3	Day 4	Day 5
Module Overview - Syllabus **Lecture:** Introduction of and the organization of the Human Body Chapter 1 & 2	**Lecture:** A & P of the Skeletal System Chapter 3 & 4	**Lecture:** A & P of the Skeletal System Chapter 3 & 4 **Exam Review**		**Unit 1 Theory Exam** Organization of the Human Body and the Skeletal System Chapter 1 - 4

Unit 2 Day 6	Day 7	Day 8	Day 9	Day 10
Lecture: Male Reproductive System Chapter 5 & 6 **Lab Lecture:** Assisting with Medical Specialties Chapter 11	**Lecture:** Female Reproductive System Chapter 5 & 6 **Lab Lecture:** Assisting with Medical Specialties Chapter 11	**Lecture:** Male Reproductive System Chapter 6 & 7	**Lecture:** Career Development Success with Mentoring **Exam Review**	**Unit II Theory Exam** Female & Male Reproductive System Chapters 5 & 7

Unit 3 Day 11	Day 12	Day 13	Day 14	Day 15
Lecture: Pediatrics Chapter 12 **Lab Lecture:** Immunization & Vaccine Documentation	**Lecture:** Pediatrics Chapter 12 **Lab Lecture:** Immunization & Vaccine Documentation	**Lecture:** Understanding Human Growth and Development Chapter 12	**Lecture:** Understanding Human Growth and Development Chapter 12 **Exams Review**	**Unit III Theory Exam** Pediatrics & Human Growth & Development Chapter 12 **Unit II & III Lab Exam- Ch 10**

Unit 4 Day 16	Day 17	Day 18	Day 19	Day 20
Lecture: A & P of the Endocrine System Chapters 9 & 10	**Lecture:** A & P of the Endocrine System Chapters 9 & 10	**Lecture:** A & P of the Endocrine System Chapters 9 & 10	**Lecture:** Career Development Success with Mentoring 1-10 Female Reprosystem Pregnancy Development and Inheritance **Final Exam Review** **and collect all assignments**	**Unit IV Module Final Exam** Chapters 1 - 12

Revised 5-5-03

MEDICAL ASSISTING—MODULE F

Standard Lab / Clinical Calendar

Day and Evening Schedule   **Two (2) Hours Per Day**

Group 1

	Day 1	Day 2	Day 3	Day 4	Day 5
	Demo Vital Signs	Demo Injections	Demo Venipuncture	Demo Coding	Demo PDR
1	Practice Core Skills	Practice Core Skills	Practice Core Skills	Practice Core Skills	Practice Core Skills
2	Practice Core Skills	Practice Core skills	Practice Core Skills	Practice Core Skills	Practice Core Skills
3	Practice Core Skills	Practice Core skills	Practice Core Skills	Practice Core Skills	Practice Core Skills
4	Practice Core Skills	Practice Core skills	Practice Core Skills	Practice Core Skills	Practice Core Skills

Group 2

	Day 6	Day 7	Day 8	Day 9	Day 10
	Demo Rectal Tray Set-up	Demo Pap tray	Demo Pelvic exam	Demo Self-breast exam	Open Lab
1	Check-off Core	Practice Skills	Practice Skills	Practice Skills	Practice Skills
2	Practice Skills	Check-off Core	Practice Skills	Practice Skills	Practice Skills
3	Practice Skills	Practice Skills	Check-off Core	Practice Skills	Practice Skills
4	Practice Skills	Practice Skills	Practice Skills	Check-Offs	Check-Offs

Group 3

	Day 11	Day 12	Day 13	Day 14	Day 15
	Demo Peds Vital Signs	Demo Peds Restraining	Demo PKU	Demo Peds Measurement	Demo Immunization Doc
1	Practice vital signs	Practice Peds Restraining	Practice PKU	Practice Peds measurement	Practice Skills
2	Practice vital signs	Practice Peds Restraining	Check-offs	Practice Peds measurement	Practice Skills
3	Practice vital signs	Check-offs	Practice PKU	Practice Peds measurement	Practice Skills
4	Check-offs	Practice Peds Restraining	Practice PKU	Practice Peds measurement	Practice Skills

Group 4

	Day 16	Day 17	Day 18	Day 19	Day 20
	Lab	Lab	Lab	Lab	Open Lab
1	Practice Skills	Practice Skills	Practice Skills	Check-Offs	Check-Offs
2	Practice Skills	Practice Skills	Practice Skills	Check-Offs	Check-Offs
3	Check-offs	Practice Skills	Check-offs	Check-Offs	Check-Offs
4	Practice Skills	Practice Skills	Practice Skills	Check-Offs	Check-Offs

MODULE CHECK-OFFS:

Pediatric Vitals	PKU Test	CPT/ICD-9 Coding	Intradermal Injections	
Pelvic Exam	Immunization Documentation	PDR Exercises	Subcutaneous Injections	
Pediatric Restraining	Breast self-exam	Charting	Vital Signs I & II	Deltoid Injections
Pediatric Measurement	Rectal Exam	Professionalism	Venipuncture	Z-Track Injections

Appendix B

PROCEDURE COMPETENCY CHECKLISTS AND ASSIGNMENTS

_____   _____   _____
Student Name (Print)   **Instructor's Name (Print)**   **Date**

MODULE F
STUDENT ASSIGNMENTS AND PROCEDURE LOCATION LIST

It is recommended that students read the assigned chapters thoroughly every week. Be sure to include the items labeled in the chapters: Med Tips located *in* the chapter, and On The Job, Legal and Ethical Issues, and the Study Outline and Chapter Review that are located *at the end of* the chapters.

To assist you in preparing for the Certification Exam to become a Certified Medical Assistant when your program is complete, we have provided review questions to study at the end of each chapter and at the end of your textbook.

Your instructor will assign 25 vocabulary words from the chapters you are reading for the week to study for your weekly Spelling and Terminology Exam.

In addition to your regular assignments, every module you will be expected to complete PDR (Page 457), CPT Coding (Page 459), and ICD-9 (Page 461) exercises that you have in your text. It is recommended that you begin these exercises as soon as the module begins to ensure that they are complete by the end of the module. If you have never done these exercises before, your instructor will go over them with you.

WEEK 1 ASSIGNMENTS:

Read:

Chapter 1-4 – Medical Terminology and A & P of the Skeletal System and Introduction to the Organization of the Human Body.

Assignments:

Complete the following assignments that are due according to your instructor's direction:

Chapter 1, Pages 28 – 33

Chapter 2, Pages 47 – 50

Chapter 3, Pages 80 – 89

Chapter 4, Pages 119 – 125

WEEK 2 ASSIGNMENTS:

Read:

Chapter 5 – 7 & 11 – Medical Terminology and A & P of the Reproductive System (Male & Female) and Assisting with Medical Specialties

The Career Development reading assignment is located in the appendix of your student handbook. This reading assignment must be completed prior to your scheduled career development lecture that will be conducted this week.

Assignment:

Chapter 5, Pages 146 - 153

Chapter 6, Pages 180 - 190

Chapter 7, Pages 209 - 214

Chapter 10, Pages 309 - 315

WEEK 3 ASSIGNMENTS:

Read:

Chapter 8 & 12 – Development, and Inheritance and Pediatrics

Assignment:

Chapter 8 & 12, NO HOMEWORK for this week unless the instructor provides an assignment

WEEK 3 ASSIGNMENTS:

Read:

Chapter 9 & 10 – Medical Terminology and A & P of the Endocrine System

Assignment:

Chapter 9, Pages 261 - 269

Chapter 9, Pages 284 - 289

PROCEDURE LOCATION LIST

Pediatric Restraining	Pages 323 - 324
(Injections & Head Circumference)	
Pediatric Measurements	Pages 323 - 324
(Height / Weight & Head Circumference)	
Pediatric Vital Signs	In the appendix of the student handbook
(Pulse, Temp- rectal & tympanic)	
Pelvic Exam	Page 304 - 306
Breast Exam	Page 302 - 303
Immunization Documentation	Pages 334
Charting	In the appendix of the student handbook
Vital Signs	In the appendix of the student handbook
Venipuncture	In the appendix of the student handbook
Injections:	
Intradermal	In the appendix of the student handbook
Subcutaneous	Same as above
Intramuscular	Same as above
Z-track	Same as above

MEDICATION LEARNING EXERCISE

STUDENT _____

INSTRUCTOR _____

MOD & UNIT _____

DATE _____

1. Locate the Drug Name in PINK section (Alphabetical Index by Brand Name) Of the PDR (Physicians Desk Reference). This will give the page number of the WHITE section to complete the exercise.

2. Give indications. Some lists will be extensive, select a few uses.

3. Drug Classification will be given under indications or action (i.e., antibiotic, diuretic).

4. Contraindications: Conditions when the drug would not be used.

5. Dosage—Give the usual dose. Also list the forms of the drug (i.e., tablets, suppositories).

6. Side Effects or Adverse Reactions: Conditions that may arise as a result of taking the drug. (i.e., nausea, vomiting)

NAME OF DRUG CATEGORY (GENERIC/TRADE)	INDICATION (USE)	CONTRAINDICATIONS (PRECAUTIONS/WARNINGS)	FORM, DOSAGE AND INSTRUCTIONS	SIDE EFFECTS

NAME OF DRUG	INDICATION (USE)	CONTRAINDICATIONS (PRECAUTIONS/WARNINGS)	FORM, DOSAGE AND INSTRUCTIONS	SIDE EFFECTS

NAME OF DRUG	INDICATION (USE)	CONTRAINDICATIONS (PRECAUTIONS/WARNINGS)	FORM, DOSAGE AND INSTRUCTIONS	SIDE EFFECTS

Appendix C

REFERENCE TO COMMON ALLERGIES, INFECTIONS, DISORDERS, PROCEDURES, AND TESTS

TABLE 1   Common Types of Allergies

Allergy	Description
Allergic rhinitis	Inflammation of the nasal mucosa which results in nasal congestion, rhinorrhea (runny nose), sneezing and itching of the nose. Seasonal allergic rhinitis, such as seen in hay fever, occurs only during certain seasons of the year. Children suffering from this type of allergy may rub their nose in an upward movement, called the "allergic salute."
Asthma	A condition seen most frequently in early childhood in which wheezing, coughing, and dyspnea are the major symptoms. Asthmatic attacks may be caused by allergens inhaled from the air, food, and drugs. The patient's airway is affected by a constriction of the bronchial passages. Treatment is medication and control of the causative factors.
Contact dermatitis	Inflammation and irritation of the skin due to contact with an irritating substance, such as soap, perfume, cosmetics, plastic, dyes, and plants such as poison ivy. Symptoms include itching, redness, and skin lesions with blistering and oozing. Treatment consists of topical and systemic medications and removal of the causative item.
Eczema	A superficial dermatitis accompanied by papules, vesicles, and crusting. This condition can be acute or chronic.
Urticaria	A skin eruption of pale reddish wheals (circular elevations of the skin) with severe itching. It is usually associated with a food allergy, stress, or drug reactions. Also called hives.

TABLE 2   Common Skin Lesions

Type of Lesion	Description
Cyst	A fluid-filled sac or pouch under the skin.
Fissure	Crack-like lesion or groove in the skin.
Macule	Small, flat discolored area that is flush with the skin surface. An example would be a freckle and the flat rash of roseola.
Nodule	Solid, raised group of cells.
Papule	Small, solid, circular raised spot on the surface of the skin.
Polyp	Small tumor with a pedicle or stem attachment. They are commonly found in vascular organs such as the nose, uterus, and rectum.
Pustule	Raised spot on the skin containing pus.
Vesicle	Small, fluid-filled raised spot on the skin; blister.
Wheal	Small, round, raised area on the skin that may be accompanied by itching.

TABLE 3   Common Skin Infections

Infection	Description
Boil	Acute inflammation of the subcutaneous layer of skin, or hair follicle. Also called a furuncle. Treatment consists of the application of moist heat until the boil comes to a "head" or softens. An incision and drainage (I&D) may be performed to allow the purulent material to drain. Antibiotics may be prescribed.
Carbuncle	Inflammation and infection of the skin and hair follicle that may result from several untreated boils. They are most commonly found on the neck, upper back, or head. Treatment is similar to that for a single boil. Systemic antibiotics may be prescribed. A gauze bandage is applied when drainage is present.
Furuncle	Staphylococcal skin abscess with redness, pain and swelling. Also called a boil.
Herpes simplex	Infectious disease caused by the herpes simplex virus 1 and characterized by thin vesicles that tend to recur in the same area such as the lips or conjunctiva. Treatment consists of the drug acyclovir either locally or orally.
Herpes zoster	A painful, infectious viral disease which attacks the nerve endings. It is also called shingles and is caused by the same virus as chickenpox. Treatment consists of analgesics to relieve pain, and antiviral medications, such as acyclovir. In severe cases a nerve block may be necessary to relieve pain.
Impetigo	A highly contagious inflammatory skin disease with pustules that become crusted and rupture. Treatment consists of thorough cleansing using separate towels and wash cloths for the patient. These should be washed daily. Topical medications may be prescribed.
Scabies	Contagious skin disease caused by an egg-laying mite that causes intense itching. The lesions appear as small, red papules and vesicles between the fingers, toes, genitalia, and beneath the breasts. Treatment consists of a methrin cream from the neck down. All clothing and bedding need careful laundering.
Sebaceous cyst	Cyst filled with sebum (oil) from a sebaceous gland. This can grow to a large size and may need to be excised.

(continued)

TABLE 3   *(continued)*

Infection	Description
Tinea	A fungal skin disease resulting in itching, scaling lesions. Tinea pedis is also called athlete's foot. Diagnosis of tinea is made with the use of a Wood's light which are ultraviolet rays used to detect fluorescent materials in the skin and hair of patients with tinea. Topical treatment consists of fungicidal agents, such as griseofulvin.
Verruca	A benign neoplasm (tumor), which has a rough surface that is removed by chemicals and /or laser therapy, and is caused by a virus. Also called warts.

TABLE 4   Neoplasms

Benign (non-cancerous) Neoplasms	Description
Dermatofibroma	A fibrous tumor of the skin. It is painless, round, firm, red, and generally found on the extremities.
Hemangioma	Benign tumor of dilated vessels.
Keloid	The formation of a scar after an injury or surgery, which results in a raised, thickened, red area.
Keratosis	Overgrowth and thickening of cells in the epithelium located in the epidermis of the skin.
Leukoplakia	A change in the mucous membrane that results in thick, white patches on the mucous membrane of the tongue and cheek. It is considered precancerous and is associated with smoking.
Lipoma	Fatty tumor that generally does not metastasize (spread).
Nevus	A pigmented (colored) congenital skin blemish. It is usually benign but may become cancerous. Also called a birthmark or mole.

Malignant (cancerous) Neoplasms	Description
Basal cell carcinoma	An epithelial tumor of the basal cell layer of the epidermis. A frequent type of skin cancer that rarely metastasizes.
Kaposi's sarcoma	A form of skin cancer frequently seen in acquired immune deficiency syndrome (AIDS) patients. It consists of brownish-purple papules that spread from the skin and metastasize to internal organs.
Malignant melanoma	A dangerous form of skin cancer caused by an overgrowth of melanin in the skin. It may metastasize.
Squamous cell carcinoma	Epidermal cancer that may go into deeper tissue but does not generally metastasize.

TABLE 5   Diagnostic Procedures and Tests Relating to the Integumentary System

Procedure/Test	Description
Adipectomy	Surgical removal of fat.
Biopsy	Removal of a piece of tissue by syringe and needle, knife, punch, or brush to examine under a microscope as an aid in diagnosis.
Cauterization	The destruction of tissue with a caustic chemical, electric current, freezing, or hot iron.
Chemobrasion	Abrasion of the skin using chemicals. Also called a chemical peel.
Cryosurgery	The use of extreme cold to freeze and destroy tissue.
Curettage	The removal of superficial skin lesions with a curette or scraper.
Debridement	The removal of foreign material or dead tissue from a wound.
Dermabrasion	Abrasion or rubbing using wire brushes or sandpaper.
Dermatoplasty	The transplantation of skin. Also called skin grafting. May be used to treat large birthmarks (hemangiomas) and burns.
Electrocautery	To destroy tissue with an electric current.
Exfoliative cytology	Scraping cells from tissue and then examining them under a microscope.
Frozen section	Taking a thin piece of tissue from a frozen specimen for rapid examination under a microscope. This is often performed during a surgical procedure to detect the presence of cancer in a diseased organ.
Fungal scrapings (FS)	Scrapings taken with a curette or scraper of tissue from lesions are placed on a growth medium and examined under a microscope to identify fungal growth.
Incision and drainage (I & D)	Making an incision to create an opening for the drainage of material such as pus.
Laser therapy	Removal of skin lesions and birthmarks using a laser that emits intense heat and power at close range. The laser converts frequencies of light into one small beam.
Lipectomy	The surgical removal of fat.
Marsupialization	Creating a pouch to promote drainage by surgically opening a closed area, such as a cyst.
Needle biopsy	Using a sterile needle to remove tissue for examination under a microscope.
Plication	Taking tucks surgically in a structure to shorten it.
Rhytidectomy	Surgical removal of excess skin to eliminate wrinkles. Commonly referred to as a face lift.
Skin grafts	The transfer of skin from a normal area to cover another site. Used to treat burn victims and after some surgical procedures.
Sweat test	Test performed on sweat to see the level of chloride. There is an increase in skin chloride in some diseases, such as cystic fibrosis.

TABLE 6   Disorders of the Cardiovascular System

Disorder	Description
Anemia	A reduction in the number of circulating red blood cells per cubic millimeter of blood. It is not a disease but a symptom of disease.
Aneurysm	An abnormal dilation of a blood vessel, usually an artery, due to a congenital weakness or defect in the wall of the vessel.
Angina pectoris	Condition in which there is severe pain with a sensation of constriction around the heart. It is caused by a deficiency of oxygen to the heart muscle.
Angioma	Tumor, usually benign, consisting of blood vessels.
Angiospasm	Spasm or contraction of blood vessels.
Aortic aneurysm	Localized, abnormal dilation of the aorta, causing pressure on the trachea, esophagus, veins, or nerves. This is due to a weakness in the wall of the blood vessel.
Aortic insufficiency	A failure of the aortic valve to close completely which results in leaking and inefficient heart action.
Aortic stenosis	Condition caused by a narrowing of the aorta.
Arrhythmia	An irregularity in the heartbeat or action.
Arterial embolism	Blood clot moving within an artery. This can occur as a result of arteriosclerosis.
Arteriosclerosis	Thickening, hardening, and loss of elasticity of the walls of arteries.
Atherosclerosis	This is the most common form of arteriosclerosis. It is caused by the formation of yellowish plaques of cholesterol building up on the inner walls of the arteries.
Bradycardia	An abnormally slow heart rate (under 60 beats per minute).
Congenital heart disease	Heart defects that are present at birth, such as patent ductus arteriosus, in which the opening between the pulmonary artery and the aorta fails to close at birth. This condition requires surgery.
Congestive heart failure	Pathological condition of the heart in which there is a reduced outflow of blood from the left side of the heart. This results in weakness, breathlessness, and edema.
Coronary artery disease	A narrowing of the coronary arteries that is sufficient enough to prevent adequate blood supply to the myocardium.
Coronary thrombosis	Blood clot in a coronary vessel of the heart causing the vessel to close completely or partially.
Embolus	Obstruction of a blood vessel by a blood clot that moves from another area.
Endocarditis	Inflammation of the membrane lining the heart. May be due to microorganisms or to an abnormal immunological response.
Fibrillation	Abnormal quivering or contractions of heart fibers. When this occurs within the fibers of the ventricle of the heart, arrest and death can occur. Emergency equipment to defibrillate, or convert the heart to a normal beat, will be necessary.
Hypertensive heart disease	Heart disease as a result of persistently high blood pressure which damages the blood vessels and ultimately the heart.
Hypotension	A decrease in blood pressure. This can occur in shock, infection, anemia, cancer, or as death approaches.
Infarct	Area of tissue within an organ or part that undergoes necrosis (death) following the cessation of the blood supply.
Ischemia	A localized and temporary deficiency of blood supply due to an obstruction to the circulation.
Mitral stenosis	Narrowing of the opening (orifice) of the mitral valve which causes an obstruction in the flow of blood from the atrium to the ventricle on the left side of the heart.
Mitral valve prolapse (MVP)	Common and serious condition in which the cusp of the mitral valve drops back (prolapses) into the left atrium during systole.
Murmur	A soft blowing or rasping sound heard upon auscultation of the heart.
Myocardial infarction	Condition caused by the partial or complete occlusion or closing of one or more of the coronary arteries. Symptoms include a squeezing pain or heavy pressure in the middle of the chest. A delay in treatment could result in death. This is also referred to as MI or heart attack.
Myocarditis	An inflammation of the myocardial lining of the heart resulting in extremely weak and rapid beat, and irregular pulse.
Patent ductus arteriosus	Congenital presence of a connection between the pulmonary artery and the aorta that remains after birth. This condition is normal in the fetus.
Pericarditis	Inflammatory process or disease of the pericardium.
Phlebitis	Inflammation of a vein.
Reynaud's phenomenon	Intermittent attacks of pallor or cyanosis of the fingers and toes associated with the cold or emotional distress. There may also be numbness, pain, and burning during the attacks. It may be caused by decreased circulation due to smoking.
Rheumatic heart disease	Valvular heart disease as a result of having had rheumatic fever.
Tetralogy of Fallot	Combination of four symptoms (tetralogy), resulting in pulmonary stenosis, a septal defect, abnormal blood supply to the aorta, and the hypertrophy of the right ventricle. A congenital defect that is present at birth and needs immediate surgery to correct.
Thrombophlebitis	Inflammation and clotting of blood within a vein.
Thrombus	A blood clot.
Varicose veins	Swollen and distended veins, usually in the legs, resulting from pressure, such as occurs during a pregnancy.

TABLE 7   Diagnostic Procedures and Tests Relating to the Cardiovascular System

Procedure/Test	Description
Aneurysmectomy	The surgical removal of the sac of an aneurysm, which is an abnormal dilatation of a blood vessel.
Angiography	X-rays taken after the injection of an opaque material into a blood vessel. Can be performed on the aorta as an aortic angiogram, on the heart as an angiocardiogram, and on the brain as a cerebral angiogram.
Angioplasty	A surgical procedure of altering the structure of a vessel by dilating the vessel using a balloon inside the vessel.
Arterial blood gases	Measurement of the amount of oxygen (O_2), carbon dioxide (CO_2), and nitrogen in the blood. Also gives a pH reading of the blood. Blood gases are performed in emergency situations and provide valuable evaluation of cardiac failure, hemorrhage, and kidney failure.
Artery graft	A piece of blood vessel that is transplanted from a part of the body to the aorta to repair a defect.
Artificial pacemaker	Electrical device that substitutes for the natural pacemaker of the heart. It controls the beating of the heart by a series of rhythmic electrical impulses. An external pacemaker has the electrodes on the outside of the body. An internal pacemaker will have the electrodes surgically implanted within the chest wall.
Cardiac catheterization	Passage of a thin tube (catheter) through an arm vein and the blood vessels leading into the heart. It is done to detect abnormalities, to collect cardiac blood samples, and to determine the pressure within the cardiac area.
Cardiac enzymes	Complex proteins that are capable of inducing chemical changes within the body. Cardiac enzymes are taken by blood sample to determine the amount of heart disease or damage.
Cardiac magnetic resonance imaging (MRI)	A noninvasive procedure in which images of the heart and blood vessels are captured for examination to determine effects.
Cardiolysis	A surgical procedure to separate adhesions which involves a resection of the ribs and sternum over the pericardium.
Cardiorrhaphy	Surgical suturing of the heart.
Cardioversion	Converting a cardiac arrhythmia (irregular heart action) to a normal sinus rhythm using a cardioverter to give countershocks to the heart.
Commissurotomy	Surgical incision to change the size of an opening. For example in mitral commissurotomy, a stenosis or narrowing is corrected by cutting away at the adhesions around the mitral opening (orifice).
Coronary artery bypass surgery	Open-heart surgery in which a shunt is created to permit blood to travel around the constriction in coronary blood vessel(s).
Doppler ultrasonography	Measurement of sound-wave echoes as they bounce off tissues and organs to produce an image. Can assist in determining heart and blood vessel damage. Also called echocardiogram.
Electrocardiogram	Record of the electrical activity of the heart. Useful in the diagnosis of abnormal cardiac rhythm and heart muscle (myocardium) damage. This procedure is explained fully in Chapter 29.
Electrolytes	Measurement of blood sodium (Na), potassium (K), and chlorides (Cl).
Embolectomy	Surgical removal of an embolus or clot from a blood vessel.
Heart transplantation	Replacement of a diseased or malfunctioning heart with a donor's heart.
Holter monitor	Portable ECG monitor worn by the patient for a period of a few hours to a few days to assess the heart and pulse activity as the person goes through the activities of daily living. Used to assess a patient who experiences chest pain and unusual heart activity during exercise and normal activities when a cardiogram is inconclusive.
Lipoproteins	Measurement of blood to determine serum cholesterol and triglycerides.
Open-heart surgery	Surgery that involves the heart, coronary arteries, or the heart valves. The heart is actually entered by the surgeon.
Percutaneous balloon valvuloplasty	Insertion through the skin of a balloon catheter across a narrowed or stenotic heart valve. When the balloon is inflated, the narrowing or constriction is decreased.
Percutaneous transluminal coronary angioplasty (PTCA)	Method for treating localized coronary artery narrowing. A balloon catheter is inserted through the skin into the coronary artery and inflated to dilate the narrow blood vessel.
Phleborrhaphy	Suturing of a vein.
Prothrombin time	Measurement of the time it takes for a sample of blood to coagulate.
Stress testing	Method for evaluating cardiovascular fitness. The patient is placed on a treadmill or bicycle and then subjected to steadily increasing levels of work. An EKG and oxygen levels are taken while the patient exercises. The test is stopped if abnormalities occur on the EKG.
Treadmill test	Also called a stress test.
Valve replacement	Surgical procedure to excise a diseased heart valve and replace with an artificial valve.
Venography	X-ray of the veins by tracing the venous flow. Also called phlebography.

TABLE 8   Disorders of the Endocrine System

Disorder	Description
Acidosis	Excessive acidity of bodily fluids due to the accumulation of acids, as in diabetic acidosis.
Acromegaly	Chronic disease of middle-aged persons which results in an elongation and enlargement of the bones of the head and extremities. There can also be mood changes.
Addison's disease	A disease resulting from a deficiency in adrenocortical hormones. There may be an increased pigmentation of the skin, generalized weakness, and weight loss.
Adenoma	A neoplasm or tumor of a gland.
Cretinism	Congenital condition due to a lack of thyroid, which may result in arrested physical and mental development.
Cushing's syndrome	Set of symptoms which result from hypersecretion of the adrenal cortex. This may be the result of a tumor of the adrenal glands. The syndrome may present symptoms of weakness, edema, excess hair growth, skin discoloration, and osteoporosis.
Diabetes insipidus (DI)	Disorder caused by the inadequate secretion of the antidiuretic hormone ADH by the posterior lobe of the pituitary gland. There may be polyuria and polydipsia.
Diabetes mellitus (DM)	Chronic disorder of carbohydrate metabolism which results in hyperglycemia and glycosuria. Type I diabetes mellitus (IDDM) involves insulin dependency, which requires that the patient take daily injections of insulin. Type II (NIDDM) patients may not be insulin dependent.
Diabetic retinopathy	Secondary complication of diabetes mellitus (DM) which affects the blood vessels of the retina, resulting in visual changes and even blindness.
Dwarfism	Condition of being abnormally small. It may be the result of a hereditary condition or an endocrine dysfunction.
Gigantism	Excessive development of long bones of the body due to overproduction of the growth hormone by the pituitary gland.
Goiter	Enlargement of the thyroid gland.
Graves' disease	Disease that results from an over activity of the thyroid gland and can result in a crisis situation. Also called hyperthyroidism.
Hashimoto's disease	A chronic form of thyroiditis.
Hirsutism	Condition of having an excessive amount of hair on the body. This term is used to describe females who have the adult male pattern of hair growth. Can be the result of a hormonal imbalance.
Hypercalcemia	Condition of having an excessive amount of calcium in the blood.
Hyperglycemia	Having an excessive amount of glucose (sugar) in the blood.
Hyperkalemia	Condition of having an excessive amount of potassium in the blood.
Hyperthyroidism	Condition that results from over activity of the thyroid gland. Also called Graves' disease.
Hypothyroidism	Result of a deficiency in secretion by the thyroid gland. This results in a lowered basal metabolism rate with obesity, dry skin, slow pulse, low blood pressure, sluggishness, and goiter. Treatment is replacement with synthetic thyroid hormone.
Ketoacidosis	Acidosis due to an excess of ketone bodies (waste products) which can result in death for the diabetic patient if not reversed.
Myasthenia gravis	Condition in which there is great muscular weakness and progressive fatigue. There may be difficulty in chewing and swallowing and drooping eyelids. If a thymoma is causing the problem, it can be treated with removal of the thymus gland.
Myxedema	Condition resulting from a hypofunction of the thyroid gland. Symptoms can include anemia, slow speech, enlarged tongue and facial features, edematous skin, drowsiness, and mental apathy.
Thyrotoxicosis	Condition that results from overproduction of the thyroid gland. Symptoms include a rapid heart action, tremors, enlarged thyroid gland, exophthalmos, and weight loss.
von Rechlinghausen's disease	Excessive production of parathyroid hormone, which results in degeneration of the bones.

TABLE 9   Procedures and Tests Relating to the Endocrine System

Procedure/Test	Description
Basal metabolic rate (BMR)	Somewhat outdated test to measure the energy used when the body is in a state of rest.
Blood serum test	Blood test to measure the level of substances such as calcium, electrolytes, testosterone, insulin, and glucose. Used to assist in determining the function of various endocrine glands.
Fasting blood sugar	Blood test to measure the amount of sugar circulating throughout the body after a 12-hour fast.
Glucose tolerance test (GTT)	Test to determine the blood sugar level. A measured dose of glucose is given to a patient either orally or intravenously. Blood samples are then drawn at certain intervals to determine the ability of the patient to utilize glucose. Used for diabetic patients to determine their insulin response to glucose.
Parathyroidectomy	Excision of one or more of the parathyroid glands. This is performed to halt the progress of hyperparathyroidism.
Protein bound iodine (PBI) test	Blood test to measure the concentration of thyroxin (T4) circulating in the bloodstream. The iodine becomes bound to the protein in the blood and can be measured. This test is useful in establishing thyroid function.
Radioactive iodine uptake (RAIU) test	Test in which radioactive iodine is taken orally (PO) or intravenously (IV) and the amount that is eventually taken into the thyroid gland (the uptake) is measured to assist in determining thyroid function.
Radioimmunoassay (RIA) test	Test used to measure the levels of hormones in the plasma of the blood.
Serum glucose test	Blood test performed to assist in determining insulin levels and useful for adjusting medication dosage.
Thymectomy	Surgical removal of the thymus gland.
Thyroid echogram	Ultrasound examination of the thyroid which can assist in distinguishing a thyroid nodule from a cyst.
Thyroidectomy	Surgical removal of the thyroid gland. The patient is then placed on replacement hormone (thyroid) therapy.

(continued)

TABLE 9   *(continued)*

Procedure/Test	Description
Thyroid function tests	Blood tests used to measure the levels of T3, T4, and TSH in the bloodstream to assist in determining thyroid function.
Thyroparathyroidectomy	Surgical removal (excision) of the thyroid and parathyroid glands.
Thyroid scan	Test in which a radioactive element is administered which localizes in the thyroid gland. The gland can then be visualized with a scanning device to detect pathology such as tumors.
Total calcium	Blood test to measure the total amount of calcium to assist in detecting parathyroid and bone disorders.
Two-hour postprandial glucose tolerance test	Blood test to assist in evaluating glucose metabolism. The patient eats a high-carbohydrate diet and fasts overnight before the test. A blood sample is then taken two hours after a meal.

TABLE 10   Disorders and Pathology of the Digestive System

Disorder/Pathology	Description
Anorexia	Loss of appetite that can accompany other conditions such as a gastrointestinal (GI) upset.
Ascites	Collection or accumulation of fluid in the peritoneal cavity.
Bulimia	Eating disorder that is characterized by recurrent binge eating and then purging of the food with laxatives and vomiting.
Cholecystitis	Inflammation of the gallbladder.
Cholelithiasis	Formation or presence of stones or calculi in the gallbladder or common bile duct.
Cirrhosis	Chronic disease of the liver.
Cleft lip	Congenital condition in which the upper lip fails to come together. This is often seen along with cleft palate and is corrected with surgery.
Cleft palate	Congenital condition in which the roof of the mouth has a split or fissure. It is corrected with surgery.
Constipation	Experiencing difficulty in defecation or infrequent defecation.
Crohn's disease	Form of chronic inflammatory bowel disease affecting the ileum and/or colon. Also called regional ileitis.
Diverticulitis	Inflammation of a diverticulum or sac in the intestinal tract, especially in the colon.
Diarrhea	Passing of frequent, watery bowel movements. Usually accompanies gastrointestinal (GI) disorders.
Dyspepsia	Indigestion.
Emesis	Vomiting usually with some force.
Enteritis	Inflammation of only the small intestine.
Esophageal stricture	Narrowing of the esophagus which makes the flow of foods and fluids difficult.
Fissure	Cracklike split in the rectum or anal canal or roof of mouth.
Fistula	Abnormal tubelike passage from one body cavity to another.
Gastritis	Inflammation of the stomach which can result in pain, tenderness, nausea, and vomiting.
Gastroenteritis	Inflammation of the stomach and small intestine.
Halitosis	Bad or offensive breath, which is often a sign of disease.
Hepatitis	Inflammation of the liver.
Ileitis	Inflammation of the ileum of the small intestine.
Inflammatory bowel syndrome	Ulceration of the mucous membranes of the colon of unknown origin. Also known as ulcerative colitis.
Inguinal hernia	Hernia or outpouching of intestines into the inguinal region of the body. May require surgical correction.
Intussusception	Result of the intestine slipping or telescoping into another section of intestine just below it. More common in children.
Irritable bowel syndrome	Disturbance in the functions of the intestine from unknown causes. Symptoms generally include abdominal discomfort and an alteration in bowel activity.
Malabsorption syndrome	Inadequate absorption of nutrients from the intestinal tract. May be caused by a variety of diseases and disorders, such as infections and pancreatic deficiency.
Peptic ulcer	Ulcer occurring in the lower portion of the esophagus, stomach, and duodenum thought to be caused by the acid of gastric juices. Some peptic ulcers are now successfully treated with antibiotics.
Pilonidal cyst	Cyst in the sacrococcygeal region due to tissue being trapped below the skin.
Polyphagia	To eat excessively.
Polyps	Small tumors that contain a pedicle or footlike attachment in the mucous membranes of the large intestine (colon).
Reflux esophagitis	Acid from the stomach backs up into the esophagus causing inflammation and pain. Also called GERD (gastroesophageal reflux disease).
Regurgitation	Return of fluids and solids from the stomach into the mouth. Similar to emesis but without the force.
Ulcerative colitis	Ulceration of the mucous membranes of the colon of unknown source. Also known as inflammatory bowel disease.
Volvulus	Condition in which the bowel twists upon itself and causes an obstruction. Painful and requires immediate surgery.

TABLE 11   Procedures and Tests Relating to the Digestive System

Procedure/Test	Description
Abdominal ultrasonography	Using ultrasound equipment for producing sound waves to create an image of the abdominal organs.
Air contrast barium enema	Using both barium and air to visualize the colon on x-ray.
Anastomosis	Creating a passageway or opening between two organs or vessels.
Appendectomy	Surgical removal of the appendix.
Barium enema (Lower GI)	Radiographic examination of the small intestine, large intestine, or colon in which an enema containing barium is administered to the patient while the x-ray pictures are taken.
Barium swallow (Upper GI)	A barium mixture swallowed while x-ray pictures are taken of the esophagus, stomach, and duodenum used to visualize the upper gastrointestinal tract. Also called esophagram.
Colectomy	Surgical removal of the entire colon.
Cholecystectomy	Surgical excision of the gallbladder. Removal of the gallbladder through the laparoscope is a newer procedure with fewer complications than the more invasive abdominal surgery. The laparoscope requires a small incision into the abdominal cavity.
Cholecystogram	Dye given orally to the patient is absorbed and enters the gallbladder. An x-ray is then taken.
Choledocholithotomy	Removal of a gallstone through an incision into the bile duct.
Choledocholithotripsy	Crushing of a gallstone in the common bile duct. Commonly called lithotripsy.
Colonoscopy	A flexible fiberscope passed through the anus, rectum, and colon is used to examine the upper portion of the colon. Polyps and small growths can be removed during the procedure.
Colostomy	Surgical creation of an opening of some portion of the colon through the abdominal wall to the outside surface.
Diverticulectomy	Surgical removal of a diverticulum.
Endoscopic retrograde cholan giopancreatography (ERCP)	Using an endoscope to x-ray the bile and pancreatic ducts.
Esophagoscopy	The esophagus is visualized by passing an instrument down the esophagus. A tissue sample for biopsy may be taken.
Esophagram (barium swallow)	As barium is swallowed the solution is observed traveling from the mouth into the stomach over a television monitor.
Esophagogastrostomy	Surgical creation of an opening between the esophagus and the stomach. Also called Upper GI.
Esophagostomy	Surgical creation of an opening into the esophagus.
Exploratory laparotomy	Abdominal operation for the purpose of examining the abdominal organs and tissues for signs of disease or other abnormalities.
Fistulectomy	Excision of a fistula.
Gastrectomy	Surgical removal of a part of or whole stomach.
Gastrointestinal endoscopy	A flexible instrument or scope is passed either through the mouth or anus to facilitate visualization of the gastrointestinal (GI) tract.
Glossectomy	Complete or partial removal of the tongue.
Hemorrhoidectomy	Surgical excision of hemorrhoids from the anorectal area.
Hepatic lobectomy	Surgical removal of a lobe of the liver.
Ileostomy	Surgical creation of a passage through the abdominal wall into the ileum. The fecal material (stool) drains into a bag worn on the abdomen.
Intravenous cholangiogram	A dye is administered intravenously to the patient that allows for visualization of the bile vessels.
Intravenous cholecystography	A dye is administered intravenously to the patient that allows for visualization of the gallbladder.
Jejunostomy	Surgical creation of a permanent opening into the jejunum.
Lithotripsy	Crushing of a stone located within the gallbladder.
Liver biopsy	Excision of a small piece of liver tissue for microscopic examination. This is generally used to determine if cancer is present.
Liver scan	A radioactive substance is administered to the patient by an intravenous (IV) route. This substance enters the liver cells, and this organ can then be visualized. This is used to detect tumors, abscesses, and other hepatomegaly.

TABLE 12   Disorders and Pathology of the Lymphatic System

Disorder/Pathology	Description
Acquired immune deficiency syndrome (AIDS)	A disease that involves a defect in the cell-mediated immunity system. A syndrome of opportunistic infections occur in the final stages of infection with the human immunodeficiency virus (HIV). This virus attacks T4 lymphocytes and destroys them, which reduces the person's ability to fight infection.
AIDS-related complex (ARC)	A complex of symptoms which appears in the early stages of AIDS. This is a positive test for the virus but only mild symptoms of weight loss, fatigue, skin rash, and anorexia.
Elephantiasis	Inflammation, obstruction, and destruction of the lymph vessels which results in enlarged tissues due to edema.
Epstein-Barr virus	Virus which is believed to be the cause of infectious mononucleosis.
Hodgkin's disease	Lymphatic system disease that can result in solid tumors in any lymphoid tissue.
Lymphadenitis	Inflammation of the lymph glands. Referred to as swollen glands.
Lymphangioma	A benign mass of lymphatic vessels.
Lyphoma	Malignant tumor of the lymph nodes and tissue.
Lymphosarcoma	Malignant disease of the lymphatic tissue.
Mononucleosis	Acute infectious disease with a large number of atypical lymphocytes. Caused by the Epstein-Barr virus. There may be abnormal liver function and spleen enlargement.
Multiple sclerosis	Autoimmune disorder of the central nervous system in which the myelin sheath of nerves is attacked.
Non-Hodgkin's lymphoma	Malignant, solid tumors of lymphoid tissue.
Peritonsillar abscess	Infection of the tissues between the tonsils and the pharynx. Also called quinsy sore throat.
Sarcoidoisis	Inflammatory disease of the lymph system in which lesions may appear in the liver, skin, lungs, lymph nodes, spleen, eyes, and small bones of the hands and feet.
Splenomegaly	Enlargement of the spleen.
Systemic lupus erythematosis (SLE)	A chronic autoimmune disorder of connective tissue that causes injury to the skin, joints, kidneys, mucous membranes, and nervous system.
Thymoma	Malignant tumor of the thymus gland.

TABLE 13   Procedures and Tests Relating to the Lymphatic System

Procedure/Test	Description
Bone marrow aspiration	Removing a sample of bone marrow by syringe for microscopic examination. Useful for diagnosing such diseases as leukemia. For example, a proliferation (massive increase) of white blood cells could confirm the diagnosis of leukemia.
ELISA	Enzyme immunoassay test used to test blood for an antibody to the AIDS virus. A positive test means that the person has been exposed to the virus. There may be a false-positive reading and then the Western blot test would be used to verify the results.
Lymphadenectomy	Excision of a lymph node. This is usually done to test for a malignancy.
Lymphangiogram	X-ray taken of the lymph vessels after the injection of dye into the foot. The lymph flow through the chest is traced.
Splenopexy	The artificial fixation of a movable spleen.
Tonsillectomy	The surgical removable of the tonsils. Usually the adenoids are removed at the same time. This procedure is known as a T & A.
Western Blot	The test that is used as backup to the ELISA blood test to detect the presence of the antibody to HIV (AIDS virus) in the blood.

TABLE 14   Disorders of the Musculoskeletal System

Disorder	Description
Arthritis	Inflammation of the bone joints.
Bunion	Enlargement of the joint at the base of the great toe caused by inflammation of the bursa of the great toe.
Bursitis	Inflammation of the bursa, the connective tissue surrounding a joint.
Carpal tunnel syndrome	Pain caused by compression of the nerve as it passes between the bones and tendons of the wrist.
Fibromyalgia	Chronic widespread pain characterized by tender trigger points at specific body locations. Patients are diagnosed when eleven of eighteen points are painful.
Gout	Inflammation of the joints caused by excessive uric acid.
Kyphosis	Abnormal increase in the outward curvature of the thoracic spine. Also known as hunchback or humpback.
Lordosis	Abnormal increase in the forward curvature of the lumbar spine. Also known as swayback.
Muscular dystrophy	Inherited disease causing a progressive muscle weakness and atrophy.
Myasthenia gravis	An autoimmune disorder causing loss of muscle strength and paralysis.
Osteoarthritis	Noninflammatory type of arthritis resulting in degeneration of the bones and joints, especially those bearing weight.
Osteomalacia	Softening of the bones caused by a deficiency of phosphorus or calcium. It is thought that in children the cause is insufficient sunlight and vitamin D.
Osteomyelitis	Inflammation of the bone and bone marrow due to infection; can be difficult to treat.
Osteoporosis	Decrease in bone mass that results in a thinning and weakening of the bone with resulting fractures. The bones become more porous, especially in the spine and pelvis.
Paget's disease	A fairly common metabolic disease of the bone from unknown causes. It usually attacks middle-aged and elderly people and is characterized by bone destruction and deformity.
Polymyositis	A disease causing muscle inflammation and weakness from an unknown cause.
Rheumatoid arthritis	Chronic form of arthritis with inflammation of the joints, swelling, stiffness, pain, and changes in the cartilage that can result in crippling deformities.
Rickets	Deficiency in calcium and vitamin D in early childhood which results in bone deformities, especially bowed legs.
Ruptured intervertebral disk	Herniation or outpouching of a disk between two vertebrae—also called a slipped or herniated disk.
Scoliosis	Abnormal lateral curvature of the spine.
Spinal stenosis	Narrowing of the spinal canal causing pressure on the cord and nerves.
Sprain	Complete or incomplete tear of a ligament caused by severe twisting action of a joint.
Strain	Painful muscle caused by applying excessive stress during exercising or other physical activity.

TABLE 15   Procedures and Diagnostic Tests Relating to the Musculoskeletal System

Procedure/Test	Description
Amputation	Partial or complete removal of a limb for a variety of reasons, including tumors, gangrene, intractable pain, crushing injury, or uncontrollable infection.
Anterior cruciate ligament (ACL) reconstruction	Replacing a torn ACL with a graft by means of arthroscopy.
Arthrocentesis	Removal of synovial fluid with a needle from a joint space, such as in the knee, for examination.
Arthrodesis	Surgical reconstruction of a joint.
Arthrography	Visualization of a joint by a radiographic study after injection of a contrast medium into a joint space.
Arthroplasty	Surgical reconstruction of a joint.
Arthroscopic surgery	Use of an arthroscope, a lighted instrument with camera/video capabilities, to facilitate performing surgery on a joint.
Arthrotomy	Surgically cutting into a joint.
Bone graft	Piece of bone taken from the patient that is used to take the place of a removed bone or a bony defect at another site, or to be wedged between bones for fusion of a joint.
Bone scan	Use of scanning equipment to visualize bones. It is especially useful in observing progress of treatment for osteomyelitis and cancer metastases to the bone.
Bunionectomy	Removal of the bursa at the joint of the great toe.
Carpal tunnel release	Surgical cutting of the ligament in the wrist to relieve nerve pressure caused by repetitive motion, for example typing (carpal tunnel disease).
Computerized axial tomography (CAT)	Computer-assisted x-ray used to detect tumors and fractures. Also referred to as CT-scan.
Electromyography	Study and record of the strength of muscle contractions as a result of electrical stimulation. Used in the diagnosis of muscle disorders and to distinguish nerve disorders from muscle disorders,.
Fasciectomy	Surgical removal of the fascia, which is the fibrous membrane covering and supporting muscles.
Laminectomy	Removal of the vertebral posterior arch to correct severe back problems caused by compression of the lamina.
Magnetic resonance imaging (MRI)	Medical imaging that uses radio-frequency radiation as its source of energy. It does not require the injection of contrast medium or exposure to ionizing radiation. The technique is useful for visualizing large blood vessels, the heart, brain, and soft tissues.

(continued)

TABLE 15   *(continued)*

Procedure/Test	Description
Menisectomy	Removal of the knee cartilage (meniscus).
Muscle biopsy	Removal of muscle tissue for pathological examination.
Myelography	Study of the spinal column after injecting opaque contrast material.
Photon absorptiometry	Measurement of bone density using an instrument for the purpose of detecting osteoporosis.
Reduction	Correcting a fracture by realigning the bone fragments. A closed reduction of the fracture is the manipulation of the bone into alignment and the application of a cast or splint to immobilize the part during the healing process. Open reduction is the surgical incision at the site of the fracture to perform the bone re-alignment. This is necessary when there are bone fragments to be removed.
Spinal fusion	Surgical immobilization of adjacent vertebrae. This may be done for several reasons, including correction of a herniated disk.
Total hip replacement	Surgical reconstruction of a hip by implanting a prosthetic or artificial joint.

TABLE 16   Disorders and Diseases of the Nervous System

Disorder/Disease	Description
Amnesia	Loss of memory in which people forget their identity as a result of head injury or a disorder, such as epilepsy, senility, and alcoholism. This can be either temporary or permanent.
Amyotrophic lateral sclerosis (ALS)	Disease with muscular weakness and atrophy due to degeneration of motor neurons of the spinal cord. Also called Lou Gehrig's disease, after the New York Yankees' baseball player who died from the disease.
Aneurysm	Localized abnormal dilatation of a blood vessel, usually an artery; the result of a congenital defect or weakness in the wall of the vessel.
Anorexia nervosa	Loss of appetite, which generally occurs in females between the ages of 12 and 21, due to a fear of obesity. The patient believes that she is fat even when thin. Psychiatric treatment may be necessary if the patient refuses to eat, since death can occur.
Aphasia	Loss of ability to speak.
Asthenia	Lack or loss of strength, causing extreme weakness.
Astrocytoma	Tumor of the brain or spinal cord that is composed of astrocytes.
Ataxia	Lack of muscle coordination as a result of a disorder or disease.
Autism	Form of mental introversion in which the patient, usually a child, shows no interest in anything or anyone except himself or herself.
Bell's palsy	One-sided facial paralysis caused by herpes simplex virus. The person cannot control salivation, tearing of the eyes, or expression but will usually recover.
Brain tumor	Intracranial mass, either benign or malignant. A benign tumor of the brain can be fatal since it will grow and cause pressure on normal brain tissue. The most malignant form of brain tumor in children is the glioma.
Cerebral palsy	Nonprogressive paralysis resulting from a defect or trauma at the time of birth.
Cerebrovascular accident (CVA)	Hemorrhagic lesion in the brain which can result in paralysis and the inability to speak.
Chorea	Involuntary nervous disorder that results in muscular twitching of the limbs or facial muscles.
Coma	Abnormal deep sleep or stupor resulting from an illness or injury.
Concussion	Injury to the brain that results from an illness or injury.
Convulsion (seizure)	Sudden severe involuntary muscle contractions and relaxations. These have a variety of causes, such as head injury, epilepsy, fever, and toxic conditions.
Encephalitis	Inflammation of the brain due to disease factors, such as rabies, influenza, measles, or smallpox.
Embolism	Obstruction of a blood vessel by a blood clot or foreign substance, such as air and/or fat.
Epidural hematoma	Mass of blood in the space outside the dura mater of the brain and spinal cord.
Epilepsy	A recurrent disorder of the brain in which convulsive seizures and loss of consciousness occurs.
• Grand mal	Severe seizures in which loss of consciousness and muscular contractions occur.
• Petit mal	Form of epilepsy in which there is an alteration in the level of consciousness but an absence of seizures or convulsions.
• Jacksonian	A localized form of epilepsy with spasms confined to one part or one group of muscles.
Glioma	Sarcoma of neurological origin.
Hematoma	Swelling or mass of blood confined to a specific area, such as in the brain.
Herniated nucleus pulposa	Protrusion of the nucleus pulposa of the intervertebral disk into the spinal canal. This is also called a herniated disk.
Huntington's chorea	Disease of the central nervous system that results in progressive dementia with bizarre involuntary movements of parts of the body.
Hydrocephalus	Accumulation of cerebrospinal fluid within the ventricles of the brain, causing pressure on the brain and for the head to be enlarged. It is treated by creating an artificial shunt for the fluid to leave the brain.
Meningioma	Slow-growing tumor in the meninges of the brain.
Meningitis	Inflammation of the membranes of the spinal cord and brain that is caused by a microorganism.

(continued)

TABLE 16   *(continued)*

Disorder/Disease	Description
Meningocele	Congenital hernia in which the meninges, or membranes, protrude through an opening in the spinal column or brain.
Multiple sclerosis	Degenerative, demyelination, inflammatory disease of the central nervous system in which there is extreme weakness and numbness.
Narcolepsy	Chronic disorder in which there is an extreme uncontrollable desire to sleep.
Neuritis	Inflammation of a nerve or nerves, causing pain.
Neuroblastoma	Malignant metastatic hemorrhagic tumor that originates in the sympathetic nervous system, especially in the adrenal medulla. Occurs mainly in infants and children.
Palsy	Temporary or permanent loss of the ability to control movement.
Paralysis	A temporary or permanent loss of the ability to control movement.
• Paraplegia	Paralysis of the lower portion of the body and both legs.
• Hemiplegia	Paralysis of only one side of the body. This is the same as hemiparesis.
• Quadriplegia	Paralysis of all four limbs. This is the same as tetraplegia.
Parkinson's disease	Chronic progressive disorder of the nervous system with fine tremors, muscular weakness, rigidity, and a shuffling gait.
Pica	An eating disorder in which there is a craving for material that is not food, such as clay, grass, wood, dirt, paper, soap, and plaster.
Reye's syndrome	A combination of symptoms that generally occurs in children under 15 years of age one week after they have had viral infection. It begins with a rash, vomiting, and confusion and may lead to coma, seizures, or respiratory arrest.
Shingles	Eruption of vesicles on the trunk of the body along a nerve path. Can be painful and generally occurs on only one side of the body. It is caused by the herpes zoster.
Spina bifida	Congenital defect in the walls of the spinal canal in which the laminae of the vertebra do not meet or close. May cause membranes and/or the spinal cord to herniate through the opening. This condition can also result in other defects such as hydrocephalus (fluid on the brain).
Subdural hematoma	Mass of blood forming beneath the dura mater of the brain.
Syncope	Fainting.
Tic douloureaux	Painful condition in which the trigeminal nerve is affected by pressure or degeneration. The pain is of a severe stabbing nature and radiates from the jaw and along the face.
Transient ischemic attack (TIA)	Temporary interference with blood supply to the brain, causing neurological symptoms, such as dizziness, numbness, and hemiparesis. May lead eventually to a full-blown stroke (CVA).

TABLE 17   Procedures and Tests Relating to the Nervous System

Procedure/Test	Description
Babinski's sign	Reflex test developed by John Babinski, a French neurologist, to determine lesions and abnormalities in the nervous system. The Babinski reflex is present, for a positive Babinski, if the great toe extends instead of flexes when the lateral sole of the foot is stroked. The normal response to this stimulation would be a flexion, or upward movement of the toe.
Brain scan	Injection of radioactive isotopes into the circulation to determine the function and abnormality of the brain.
Carotid endarterectomy	A surgical procedure for removing an obstruction within the carotid artery. It was developed to prevent strokes but is found to be useful only in severe stenosis with TIA.
Cerebral angiogram	X-ray of the blood vessels of the brain after the injection of radiopaque dye.
Cerebrospinal fluid shunts	Surgical creation of an artificial opening to allow for the passage of fluid. Used in the treatment of hydrocephalus.
Cordectomy	Removal of part of the spinal cord.
Craniotomy	Surgical incision into the brain through the cranium.
Cryosurgery	Use of extreme cold to produce areas of destruction in the brain. Used to control bleeding and treat brain tumors.
Echoencephalogram	Recording of the ultrasonic echoes of the brain. Useful in determining abnormal patterns of shifting in the brain.
Electromyogram	Written recording of the contraction of muscles as a result of receiving electrical stimulation.
Laminectomy	Removal of a vertebral posterior arch.
Lumbar puncture	Puncture with a needle into the lumbar area (usually the fourth intervertebral space) to withdraw fluid for examination and for the injection of anesthesia.
Nerve block	A method of regional anesthetic to stop the passage of sensory stimulation along a nerve path.
Pneumoencephalography	X-ray examination of the brain following withdrawal of cerebrospinal fluid and injection of air or gas via spinal puncture.
Positron emission tomography (PET)	Use of positive radionuclides to reconstruct brain sections. Measurement can be taken of oxygen and glucose uptake, cerebral blood flow, and blood volume.
Romberg's sign	Test developed to establish neurological function in which the person is asked to close their eyes and place their feet together. This test for body balance is positive if the patient sways when the eyes are closed.
Spinal puncture	Puncture with a needle into the spinal cavity to withdraw spinal fluid for microscopic analysis. Anesthetic is also administered by this route. This is also called a spinal tap.
Sympathectomy	Excision of a portion of the sympathetic nervous system. Could include a nerve or ganglion.
Transcutaneous electrical nerve stimulation (TENS)	Application of a mild electrical stimulation to skin electrodes placed over a painful area, causing interference with the transmission of the painful stimuli. Can be used in pain management to interfere with the normal pain mechanism.
Trephination	Process of cutting out a piece of bone in the skull to gain entry into the brain to relieve pressure.
Vagotomy	Surgical incision into the vagus nerve. Medication can be administered into the nerve to prevent its function.

TABLE 18   Common Disorders of the Eye

Disorder	Description
Achromatopsia	The condition of color blindness. This is more common in males.
Astigmatism	An eye disorder in which light rays are focused unevenly on the retina, resulting in a distorted image due to the abnormal curvature of the cornea.
Blepharitis	Inflammatory condition of the eyelash follicles and glands of the eyelids which results in swelling, redness, and crusts of dried mucus on the lids. This can be the result of allergy or infection.
Blepharochalasis	In this condition, the upper eyelid increases in size due to loss of elasticity, which is followed by swelling and recurrent edema of the lids. The skin may droop over the edges of the eyes when the eyes are open.
Cataract	Diminished vision resulting from the lens of the eye becoming opaque or cloudy. Treatment is usually surgical removal of the cataract.
Chalazion	A small, hard tumor or mass, similar to a sebaceous cyst, developing on the eyelid. This may require incision and drainage (I & D).
Conjunctivitis	An inflammation of the conjunctiva which is also called pinkeye.
Diabetic retinopathy	Small hemorrhages and edema that develop as a result of diabetes mellitus. Laser surgery and vitrectomy may be necessary for treatment.
Ectropion	Refers to an enversion (outward turning) of the eyelid, exposing the conjunctiva.
Entropion	Inversion (inward turning) of the eyelid.
Esotropia	Inward turning of the eye. An example of strabismus (muscle weakness of the eye).
Exophthalmus	Abnormal protrusion of the eyeball. Can be due to hyperthyroidism.
Esotropia	Outward turning of the eye. Also an example of strabismus (muscle weakness of the eye).
Glaucoma	Increase in intraocular pressure, which, if untreated, may result in atrophy (wasting away) of the optic nerve and blindness. Glaucoma is treated with medication and surgery. There is an increased risk of developing glaucoma in persons over 60 years of age, in people of African ancestry, after sustaining a serious eye injury, and in anyone with a family history of diabetes or glaucoma. Figure 22-8 [ID23-19] illustrates a glaucoma test.
Hemianopia	Loss of vision in half of the visual field. A stroke patient may suffer from this condition.
Hordeolum	Refers to a sty which is a small purulent inflammatory infection of a sebaceous gland of the eye. This is treated with hot compresses and, if necessary, surgical incision.
Hyperopia	With this condition a person can see things in the distance but has trouble reading material at close vision. It is also known as farsightedness.
Keratitis	Inflammation of the cornea.
Macular degeneration	Degeneration or deterioration of the macular area of the retina of the eye. It may be treated with laser surgery to destroy the blood vessels beneath the macula.
Myopia	With this condition a person can see things close up but distance vision is blurred. It is also known as nearsightedness.
Nystagmus	Jerky-appearing involuntary eye movement.
Presbyopia	Visual change due to aging, resulting in difficulty in focusing for near vision (such as reading).
Retinal detachment	A disorder that occurs when the two layers of the retina become separated or detached. The treatment is surgery.
Retinitis pigmentosa	Progressive disease of the eye which results in the retina becoming hard (sclerosed), pigmented, and atrophying (wasting away). There is no known cure for this condition.
Strabismus	An eye muscle weakness resulting in the eyes looking in different directions at the same time. (The eyes may be divergent or convergent). May be corrected with glasses, and/or surgery. Also called lazy eye, crossed eyes, or squint.
Trachoma	A chronic infectious disease of the conjunctiva and cornea caused by bacteria. This occurs more commonly in people living in hot, dry climates. Untreated, it may lead to blindness when the scarring invades the cornea. Trachoma can be treated with antibiotics.

TABLE 19   Procedures and Diagnostic Tests Relating to the Eye

Disorder	Description
Fluorescein angiography	The process of injecting a dye (fluorescein) to observe the movement of blood for detecting lesions in the macular area of the retina. This is used to determine if there is a detachment of the retina.
Gonioscopy	Use of an instrument called a gonioscope to examine the anterior chamber of the eye to determine ocular motility and rotation.
Keratometry	Measurement of the cornea using an instrument called a keratometer.
Laser Surgery	Surgical procedure performed with a laser handpiece that transfers light into intense, small beams capable of destroying or fixing tissue in place.
Slit lamp microscope	The instrument used in ophthalmology for examining the posterior surface of the cornea.
Tonometry	Measurement of the intraocular pressure of the eye using a tonometer to check for the condition of glaucoma. After a topical anesthetic is applied, the physician places the tonometer lightly upon the eyeball and a pressure measurement is taken. An air-puff tonometer similarly records the cornea's resistance to pressure, but uses more expensive equipment. This is generally part of a normal eye examination for adults.
Visual acuity	Measurements of the sharpness of a patient's vision. Usually a Snellen chart is used for this test and the patient identifies letters from a distance of 20 feet.
Vitrectomy	A surgical procedure for replacing the contents of the vitreous chamber of the eye.

TABLE 20   Common Disorders of the Ear

Disorder	Description
Acoustic neuroma	Benign tumor of the eighth cranial nerve sheath which can cause symptoms from pressure being exerted on tissues.
Anacusis	Total loss of hearing. Also called deafness.
Cerumen block	Ear wax causing a blockage in the external canal of the ear.
Conductive hearing loss	Loss of hearing as a result of the blocking of sound transmission in the middle ear or outer ear.
Meniere's disease	An abnormal condition within the labyrinth of the inner ear that can lead to a progressive hearing loss. The symptoms are dizziness or vertigo, hearing loss, and tinnitus (ringing in the ears).
Otitis media	Commonly referred to as a middle ear infection. This is seen frequently in children and is often preceded by an upper respiratory infection.
Otosclerosis	Progressive hearing loss caused by immobility of the stapes bone.
Presbycusis	Loss of hearing that can accompany the aging process.

TABLE 21   Procedures and Diagnostic Tests Relating to the Ear

Procedure/Test	Description
Audiogram	A chart that shows the faintest sounds a patient can hear during audiometry testing.
Audiometric test	A test of hearing ability by determining the lowest and highest intensity and frequencies that a person can distinguish. The patient may sit in a soundproof booth and receive sounds through earphones as the technician decreases and changes the volume or tones.
Falling test	A test used to observe balance and equilibrium. The patient is observed on one foot, then with one foot in front of the other, and then walking forward with eyes open. The same test is conducted with the patient's eyes closed. Swaying and falling with the eyes closed can indicate an ear and equilibrium malfunction.
Mastoid antrotomy	Surgical opening made in the cavity within the mastoid process to alleviate pressure from infection and allow for drainage.
Mastoid x-ray	X-ray taken of the mastoid bone to determine the presence of an infection, which can be an extension of a middle ear infection.
Myringoplasty	Surgical reconstruction of the eardrum.
Myringotomy	Surgical puncture of the eardrum with removal of fluid and pus from the middle ear, to eliminate a persistent ear infection and excessive pressure on the tympanic membrane. A tube is placed in the tympanic membrane to allow for drainage of the middle ear cavity.
Otoplasty	Corrective surgery to change the size of the external ear or pinna. The surgery can either enlarge or decrease the size of the pinna.
Otoscopy	The use of a lighted instrument (otoscope) to examine the external auditory canal and the middle ear.
Rinne and Weber tuning-fork tests	The physician holds a tuning fork, an instrument that produces a constant pitch when it is struck, against or near the bones on the side of the head. These tests assess both nerve and bone conduction of sound.
Sensorineural hearing loss	A type of hearing loss in which the sound is conducted normally through the external and middle ear but there is a defect in the inner ear or with the auditory nerve (eighth cranial nerve), resulting in the inability to hear.
Stapedectomy	Removal of the stapes bone to treat otosclerosis (hardening of the bone). A prosthesis or artificial stapes is implanted.
Tympanometry	Measurement of the movement of the tympanic membrane. Can indicate the presence of pressure in the middle ear.
Tympanoplasty	Another term for the surgical reconstruction of the eardrum. Also called myringoplasty.

TABLE 22   Common Disorders and Pathology of the Reproductive System

Disorder/Pathology	Description
Abruptio placenta	An emergency condition in which the placenta tears away from the uterine wall before the 20th week of pregnancy. This requires immediate delivery of the baby.
Amenorrhea	An absence of menstruation, which can be the result of many factors, including pregnancy, menopause, and dieting.
Breech presentation	Position of the fetus within the uterus in which the buttocks or feet are presented first for delivery rather than the head.
Carcinoma in situ	Malignant tumor that has not extended beyond the original site.
Cervical cancer	A malignant growth in the cervix of the uterus. This is an especially difficult type of cancer to treat, and causes 5 percent of the cancer deaths in women. PAP tests have helped to detect early cervical cancer.
Cervical polyps	Fibrous or mucous tumor or growth found in the cervix of the uterus. These are removed surgically if there is a danger that they will become malignant.
Cervicitis	Inflammation of the cervix of the uterus.
Choriocarcinoma	A rare type of cancer of the uterus which may occur following a normal pregnancy or abortion.
Condyloma	A wartlike growth on the external genitalia.

(continued)

TABLE 22   *(continued)*

Disorder/Pathology	Description
Cystocele	Hernia or outpouching of the bladder that protrudes into the vagina. This may cause urinary frequency and urgency.
Dysmenorrhea	Painful cramping that is associated with menstruation.
Eclampsia	Convulsive seizures and coma occurring between the 20th week of pregnancy and the first week of postpartum.
Ectopic	A fetus that becomes abnormally implanted outside the uterine cavity. This is a condition requiring immediate surgery.
Endometrial cancer	Cancer of the endometrial lining of the uterus.
Fibroid tumor	Benign tumor or growth that contains fiberlike tissue. Uterine fibroid tumors are the most common tumors in women.
Mastitis	Inflammation of the breast, which is common during lactation but can occur at any age.
Menorrhagia	Excessive bleeding during the menstrual period. Can be either in the total number of days or the amount of blood or both.
Ovarian carcinoma	Cancer of the ovary.
Ovarian cyst	Sac that develops within the ovary.
Pelvic inflammatory disease (PID)	Any inflammation of the female reproductive organs, generally bacterial in nature.
Placenta previa	When the placenta has become attached to the lower portion of the uterus and, in turn, blocks the birth canal.
Preeclampsia	Toxemia of pregnancy which if untreated can result in true eclampsia. Symptoms include hypertension, headaches, albumin in the urine, and edema.
Premature birth	Delivery in which the infant (neonate) is born before the thirty-seventh week of gestation (pregnancy).
Premenstrual syndrome (PMS)	Symptoms that develop just prior to the onset of a menstrual period, which can include irritability, headache, tender breasts, and anxiety.
Prolapsed uterus	A fallen uterus that can cause the cervix to protrude through the vaginal opening. It is generally caused by weakened muscles from vaginal delivery or as a result of pelvic tumors pressing down.
Rh factor	A condition developing in the baby when the mother's blood type is Rh-negative and the father's is Rh-positive. The baby's red blood cells can be destroyed as a result of this condition. Treatment is early diagnosis and blood transfusion.
Salpingitis	Inflammation of the fallopian tube or tubes.
Spontaneous abortion	Loss of a fetus without any artificial aid. Also called a miscarriage.
Stillbirth	Birth in which the fetus dies before or at the time of delivery.
Toxic shock syndrome	Rare and sometimes fatal staphylococcus infection that generally occurs in menstruating women.
Tubal pregnancy	Implantation of a fetus within the fallopian tube instead of the uterus. This requires immediate surgery.
Vaginitis	Inflammation of the vagina, generally caused by a microorganism.

TABLE 23   Procedures and Diagnostic Tests Relating to the Female Reproductive System

Procedure/Test	Description
Abortion	The termination of a pregnancy before the fetus reaches a viable point in development.
Amniocentesis	Puncturing of the amniotic sac using a needle and syringe for the purpose of withdrawing amniotic fluid for testing. Can assist in determining fetal maturity, development, and genetic disorders.
Cauterization	The destruction of tissue using an electric current, a caustic product, a hot iron, or freezing.
Cervical biopsy	Taking a sample of tissue from the cervix to test for the presence of cancer cells.
Cesarean section (C-section)	Surgical delivery of a baby through an incision into the abdominal and uterine walls.
Colposcopy	Visual examination of the cervix and vagina.
Conization	Surgical removal of a core of cervical tissue or a partial removal of the cervix.
Cryosurgery	Exposing tissues to extreme cold in order to destroy tissues. This procedure is used in treating malignant tumors, to control pain and bleeding.
Culdoscopy	Examination of the female pelvic cavity using an endoscope.
Dilation and curettage (D&C)	Surgical procedure in which the opening of the cervix is dilated and the uterus is scraped or suctioned of its lining or tissue. A D & C is performed after a spontaneous abortion and to stop excessive bleeding from other causes.
Doppler ultrasound	Using an instrument placed externally over the uterus to detect the presence of fibroid tumors to outline the shape of the fetus.
Endometrial biopsy	Taking a sample of tissue from the lining of the uterus to test for abnormalities.
Episiotomy	Surgical incision of the perineum to facilitate the delivery process. Can prevent an irregular tearing of tissue during birth.
Fetal monitoring	Using electronic equipment placed on the mother's abdomen to monitor the baby's heart rate and strength of uterine contractions during labor.
Hymenectomy	Surgical removal of the hymen.
Hysterectomy	Surgical removal of the uterus.
Hysterosalpingography	Taking an x-ray after injecting radiopaque material into the uterus and oviducts.
Hysteroscopy	Inspection of the uterus using a special endoscope instrument.
Intrauterine device (IUD)	A device inserted into the uterus by a physician for the purpose of contraception.

(continued)

TABLE 23   *(continued)*

Procedure/Test	Description
Kegel exercises	Exercises named after A.H. Kegel, an American gynecologist, who developed them to strengthen female pelvic muscles. The exercises are useful in treating incontinence and as an aid in childbirth.
Laparoscopy	Examination of the peritoneal cavity using an instrument called a laparoscope. The instrument is passed through a small incision made by the surgeon into the peritoneal cavity.
Laparotomy	Making a surgical opening into the abdomen.
Oophorectomy	Surgical removal of an ovary.
Panhysterectomy	Excision of the entire uterus, including the cervix.
Panhysterosalpingo-oophorectomy	Surgical removal of the entire uterus, cervix, ovaries, and fallopian tubes. Also called a total hysterectomy.
PAP (Papanicolaou) smear	Test for the early detection of cancer of the cervix named after the developer of the test, George Papanicolaou, a Greek physician. A scraping of cells is removed from the cervix for examination under a microscope.
Pelvic examination	The physical examination of the vagina and adjacent organs performed by a physician by placing the fingers of one hand into the vagina. A visual examination is performed using a speculum.
Pelvimetry	Measurement of the pelvis to assist in determining if the birth canal will allow the passage of the fetus for a vaginal delivery.
Pelvic ultrasonography	The use of ultrasound waves to produce an image or photograph of organ or fetus.
Pregnancy test	A chemical test on urine that can determine pregnancy during the first few weeks. This can be performed in the physician's office or with an at-home test.
Salpingo-oophorectomy	Surgical removal of the fallopian tube and ovary.
Tubal ligation	Surgical tying off of the fallopian tube to prevent conception from taking place. This results in the sterilization of the female.

TABLE 24   Disorders of the Male Reproductive System

Disorder	Description
Anorchism	A congenital absence of one or both testes.
Aspermia	The lack of, or failure to, eject sperm.
Azoospermia	Absence of sperm in the semen.
Balanitis	Inflammation of the skin covering the glans penis.
Benign prostatic hypertrophy	Enlargement of the prostate gland commonly seen in males over 50.
Carcinoma of the testes	Cancer of one or both testes.
Cryptorchidism	Failure of the testes to descend into the scrotal sac before birth. Generally, the testes will descend permanently before the boy is one year old. A surgical procedure called an orchidopecy may be required to bring the testes down into the scrotum permanently and secure them permanently. Failure of the testes to descend could result in sterility in the male.
Epididymitis	Inflammation of the epididymis which causes pain and swelling in the inguinal area.
Epispadias	Congenital opening of the male urethra on the dorsal surface of the penis.
Hydrocele	Accumulation of fluid within the testes.
Hypospadias	Congenital opening of the male urethra on the underside of the penis.
Impotent	Inability to copulate due to inability to maintain an erection or to achieve orgasm.
Perineum	In the male, the external region between the scrotum and the anus.
Phimosis	Narrowing of the foreskin over the glans penis which results in difficulty with hygiene. The condition can lead to infection or difficulty with urination. The condition is treated with circumcision, the surgical removal of the foreskin.
Prostate cancer	A slow-growing cancer that affects a large number of males after 50. The PSA (prostate-specific antigen) test is used to assist in early detection of this disease.
Prostatic hyperplasia	Abnormal cell growth within the prostate.
Prostatitis	An inflamed condition of the prostate gland which may be the result of infection.
Varicocele	Enlargement of the veins of the spermatic cord which commonly occurs on the left side of adolescent males. This seldom needs treatment.

TABLE 25   Procedures and Diagnostic Tests Relating to the Male Reproductive System

Procedure/Test	Description
Castration	Excision of the testicles in the male or the ovaries in the female.
Cauterization	Destruction of tissue with an electric current, a caustic agent, hot iron, or by freezing.
Circumcision	Surgical removal of the end of the prepuce or foreskin of the penis. Generally performed on the newborn male at the request of the parents. The primary reason is for ease of hygiene. Circumcision is also a ritual practiced in some religions.
Orchidopexy	Surgical fixation to move undescended testes into the scrotum, and attaching them to prevent retraction.
Prostatectomy	Surgical removal of the prostate gland.
Sterilization	Process of rendering a male or female sterile or unable to conceive children.
Transurethral resection of the prostate (TUR)	Surgical removal of the prostate gland by inserting a device through the urethra and removing prostate tissue.
Vasectomy	Removal of a segment or all of the vas deferens to prevent sperm from leaving the male body. Used for contraception purposes. A bilateral vasectomy would render the male sterile.
Semen analysis	This procedure is used when performing a fertility workup to determine if the male is able to produce sperm. Sperm is collected by the patient after abstaining from sexual intercourse for a period of three to five days. Also used to determine if a vasectomy has been successful. After a period of six weeks, no further sperm should be present in a sample from the patient.

TABLE 26   Sexually Transmitted Diseases

Disease	Description
Acquired immune deficiency syndrome (AIDS)	The final stage of infection from the human immunodeficiency virus (HIV). At present there is no cure.
Candidiasis	A yeastlike infection of the skin and mucous membranes which can result in white plaques on the tongue and vagina.
Chancroid	Highly infectious nonsyphilitic ulcer.
Chlamydial infection	Parasitic microorganism causing genital infections in males and females. Can lead to pelvic inflammatory disease (PID) in females and eventual infertility.
Genital herpes	Growths and elevations of warts on the genitalia of both males and females which can lead to cancer of the cervix in females. These painful vesicles on the skin and mucosa erupt periodically and can be transmitted through the placenta or at birth.
Genital warts	Growths and elevations of warts on the genitalia of both males and females which can lead to cancer of the cervix in females. There is currently no cure.
Gonorrhea	Sexually transmitted inflammation of the mucous membranes of either sex. Can be passed on to an infant during the birth process.
Hepatitis	Infectious, inflammatory disease of the liver. Hepatitis B and C types are spread by contact with blood and bodily fluids of an infected person.
Syphilis	Infectious, chronic, venereal disease that can involve any organ. May exist for years without symptoms.
Trichomoniasis	Genitourinary infection that is usually without symptoms (asymptomatic) in both males and females. In women the disease can produce itching and/or burning, a foul-smelling discharge, and results in vaginitis.

TABLE 27   Genetic Disorders

Disorder/Disease	Description
Alopecia	Baldness in particular patterns, especially on the head.
Cleft lip	A structural defect of the upper lip caused by the failure of the soft tissue to unite during gestation.
Cleft palate	A structural defect in the roof of the mouth caused by the failure of the two sides of the palate to fuse together during gestation.
Cooley's anemia	A rare form of anemia or a reduction of red blood cells which is found in some people of Mediterranean origin.
Cystic fibrosis	A disorder of the exocrine glands which causes these glands to produce abnormally thick secretions of mucus. The disease affects many organs, including the pancreas and the respiratory system. One reliable diagnostic test in children is the sweat test, which will show elevated sodium and potassium levels. There is presently no known cure for the disease, which can shorten the life span.
Down syndrome	A disorder which produces moderate-to-severe mental retardation and multiple defects. The physical characteristics of a child with this disorder are a sloping forehead, flat nose or absent bridge to the nose, low-set eyes, and a general dwarfed physical growth. The disorder occurs more commonly when the mother is over 40. Also called Trisomy 21.

(continued)

TABLE 27   *(continued)*

Disorder/Disease	Description
Duchene muscular dystrophy	A muscular disorder in which there is progressive wasting away of various muscles, including leg, pelvic, and shoulder muscles. Children with this disorder have difficulty climbing stairs and running. They may eventually be confined to a wheelchair. Other complications relating to the heart and respiratory system can be present. It is caused by a recessive gene and is more common in males. This disorder often results in a shortened life-span.
Hemophilia	A bleeding disorder in which there is a deficiency in one of the factors necessary for blood to clot. There is an abnormal tendency to bleed, and victims of this disorder may require frequent blood transfusions. The female (mother) carries this recessive gene and it is passed on to males. Therefore, it is found almost exclusively in boys.
Huntington's chorea	A rare condition characterized by bizarre involuntary movements called chorea. The patient may have progressive mental and physical disturbances, which generally begin around 40.
Phenylketonuria	A metabolic disease causing brain damage due to the inability of the newborn's body to act upon an amino acid called phenylalanine.
Retinitis pigmentosa	Chronic progressive disease that begins in early childhood and is characterized by degeneration of the retina. This can lead to blindness by middle age.
Sickle cell anemia	Severe, chronic, incurable disorder that results in anemia and causes joint pain, chronic weakness, and infections. Occurs more commonly in people of Mediterranean and African heritage. The blood cell in this disease is sickle shaped.
Spina bifida	A congenital disorder that results in a defect in the walls of the spinal column, causing the membranes of the spinal cord to push through to the outside. It may be associated with other defects, such as hydrocephalus, which is an enlarged head as a result of the accumulation of fluid on the brain.
Talipes	A structural malformation of the foot, commonly called club foot, caused by a deformed foot bone and shortened Achilles tendon.
Tay-Sachs disease	A disorder caused by a deficiency of an enzyme, which can result in mental and physical retardation and blindness. It is transferred by a recessive trait and is most commonly found in families of Eastern European Jewish decent. Death generally occurs before the age of 4.

TABLE 28   Respiratory Disorders and Pathology

Disorder/Pathology	Description
Asthma	Disease caused by various conditions, such as allergens, and resulting in constriction of the bronchial airways and labored respirations. It can cause violent spasms of the bronchi (bronchospasms) but is not generally life-threatening. Medication can be very effective.
Atelectasis	A condition in which the lung tissue collapses, which prevents the respiratory exchange of oxygen and carbon dioxide. It can be caused by a variety of conditions, including pressure upon the lung from a tumor or other object.
Bronchiectasis	An abnormal stretching of the bronchi which results from a dilation of a bronchus or the bronchi that can be the result of an infection. The major symptom is a large amount of purulent (pus-filled) sputum. Rales (bubbling chest sounds) and hemoptysis (spitting up blood) may be present. This can be irreversible and may result in destruction of the bronchial walls.
Bronchitis	Inflammation of the mucous membranes of the bronchial tubes which results in a typical barking cough, fever, and **malaise** or discomfort.
Bronchogenic carcinoma	Malignant lung tumor that originates in the bronchi. It is usually associated with a history of cigarette smoking.
Chronic obstructive pulmonary disease (COPD)	Progressive, chronic, and usually irreversible condition in which the lungs have a diminished capacity for inspiration (inhalation) and expiration (exhalation). The patient may have difficulty breathing upon exertion (dyspnea) and a cough. Also called chronic obstructive lung disease.
Croup	An acute respiratory condition found in infants and children which is characterized by a barking type of cough or stridor.
Emphysema	Pulmonary condition that can occur as a result of long-term heavy smoking. Air pollution also worsens this disease. The patient may not be able to breath except in a sitting or standing position.
Empyema	Pus within the pleural space, usually the result of infection.
Epistaxis	Nosebleed.
Histoplasmosis	A pulmonary disease from dust in the droppings of pigeons and chickens.
Hyaline membrane disease	Condition seen in premature infants whose lungs have not had time to develop properly. The lungs are not able to expand fully and a membrane (hyaline membrane) actually forms which causes extreme difficulty in breathing and may result in death. It is also known as infant respiratory distress syndrome (IRDS).
Laryngitis	Inflammation of the larynx (voicebox) causing difficulty in speaking.
Legionnaires' disease	Severe, often fatal disease characterized by pneumonia and gastrointestinal symptoms. It is caused by a gram-negative bacillus and named after people who came down with it at an American Legion Convention in 1976.
Paroxysmal nocturnal dyspnea	Attacks of shortness of breath (SOB) which occur only at night and awaken the patient.
Pertussis	Commonly called whooping cough, due to the "whoop" sound made when coughing. It is an infectious disease which children receive immunization against as part of their DPT shots.
Pleural effusion	The abnormal presence of fluid or gas in the pleural cavity. Physicians can detect the presence of fluid by tapping the chest (percussion) or listening with a stethoscope (auscultation).
Pleurisy	Inflammation of the pleura surrounding the lungs. The patient will experience pain upon inspiration due to friction caused by a rubbing of the pleural lining.

(continued)

TABLE 28 *(continued)*

Disorder/Pathology	Description
Pneumonia	Inflammatory condition of the lung which can be caused by bacterial and viral infections, diseases, and chemicals.
Pneumoconiosis	A condition that occurs as a result of inhaling environmental particles that become toxic. Can be the result of inhaling coal dust (anthracosis), or asbestos (asbestosis).
Pneumonomycosis	A disease of the lungs caused by a fungus.
Pneumothorax	Collection of air or gas in the pleural cavity which may result in collapse of the lung.
Pulmonary edema	Condition in which lung tissue retains an excessive amount of fluid. This results in labored breathing.
Pulmonary embolism	Blood clot or air bubble that moves to the pulmonary artery or one of its branches.
Respiratory distress syndrome (RDS)	Impairment of the respiratory function in premature infants due to immaturity.
Silicosis	A form of respiratory disease resulting from the inhalation of silica (quartz) dust. It is considered an occupational disease. Unexpected and unexplained death of an apparently well infant.
Sudden infant death syndrome (SIDS)	A narrowing and stenosis of the lumen or opening into the trachea.
Tracheostenosis	An infectious disease caused by the tubercle bacillus, Mycobacterium tuberculosis. It most commonly affects the respiratory system and causes inflammation and calcification of the system. Tuberculosis is again on the uprise and is seen in many patients who have an impaired immune system, such as in AIDS.
Tuberculosis	

TABLE 29   Procedures and Tests Relating to the Respiratory System

Procedure/Test	Description
Arterial blood gases	Testing for the gases present in the blood. This test is generally used to assist in determining the levels of oxygen (O_2) and carbon dioxide (CO_2) in the blood.
Bronchography	X-ray of the lung after a radiopaque substance has been inserted into the trachea or bronchial tube.
Bronchoplasty	The surgical repair of a bronchial defect.
Bronchoscopy	Using an instrument, the bronchoscope, to visualize the bronchi. During this procedure, tissue can be obtained for biopsy and foreign bodies can be removed.
Bronchotomy	A surgical incision of a bronchus, larynx, or trachea.
Cardiopulmonary resuscitation (CPR)	Emergency treatment provided by persons trained in CPR given to patients when their respirations and heart stop. CPR provides oxygen to the brain, heart, and other vital organs until medical treatment can restore a normal heart and pulmonary function. See an illustration of adult and infant CPR in Chapter 35.
Chest x-ray	Taking a radiographic picture of the lungs and heart from the back and front of the patient.
Endotracheal intubation	Placing a tube through the mouth to create an airway.
Heimlich maneuver	A technique for removing a foreign body from the trachea or pharynx by exerting diaphragmatic pressure.
Hyperbaric oxygen therapy	The use of oxygen under greater than normal pressure to treat cases of smoke inhalation, carbon monoxide poisoning, and other conditions. In some cases, the patient is placed in a hyperbaric oxygen chamber for this treatment.
Intermittent positive pressure breathing (IPPB)	A method for assisting the breathing of patients with a mask that is connected to a machine that produces an increased pressure.
Laryngectomy	The surgical removal of the larynx. This procedure is most frequently performed for excision of cancer.
Laryngoplasty	Surgical repair of the larynx.
Laryngoscopy	Examination of the interior of the larynx with a lighted instrument.
Lobectomy	Surgical removal of a lobe of the lung. Often the treatment of choice for lung cancer.
Pneumonectomy	The surgical removal of lung tissue.
Postural drainage	Drainage of secretions from the bronchi by placing the patient in a position that uses gravity to promote drainage. It is used for the treatment of cystic fibrosis, bronchiectasis, and before lobectomy surgery. May be combined with clapping and vibrating maneuvers to dislodge secretions.
Pulmonary angiography	Injecting dye into a blood vessel for the purpose of taking an x-ray of the arteries and veins of the lungs.
Pulmonary function test (PFT)	Breathing equipment used to determine respiratory function and measure lung volumes and gas exchange. Also called spirometry.
Rhinoplasty	Plastic surgery of the nose performed for cosmetic reasons and to facilitate breathing.
Sinus x-ray	An x-ray view of the sinus cavities from the front of the head.
Spirometry	Using a device to measure the breathing capacity of the lungs.
Sputum culture and sensitivity (CS)	Testing sputum by placing it on a culture medium and observing any bacterial growth. The specimen is then tested to determine antibiotic effectiveness.
Sputum cytology	Testing for malignant cells in sputum.
Throat culture	Removing a small sample of tissue or material from the pharynx and placing it upon a culture medium to determine bacterial growth.
Thoracentesis	The surgical puncture of the chest wall for the removal of fluids.
Thoracostomy	An insertion of a tube into the chest for the purpose of draining off fluid or air.
Tracheotomy	Surgical incision into the trachea to provide an airway. This is generally performed as an emergency procedure to provide oxygen.
Tuberculin skin tests (TB test)	Applying a chemical agent (Tine or Mantoux tests) under the surface of the skin to determine if the patient has been exposed to tuberculosis.

TABLE 30   Disorders and Diseases of the Urinary System

Disorder/Disease	Description
Anuria	No urine formed by the kidneys and a complete lack of urine excretion.
Bladder neck obstruction	Blockage of the bladder outlet.
Dysuria	Abnormal secretion of large amounts of urine.
Enuresis	Involuntary discharge of urine after the age by which bladder control should have been established. This usually occurs by the age of 5. Also called bed-wetting at night.
Glomerulonephritis	Inflammation of the kidney (primarily of the glomerulus). Since the glomerular membrane is inflamed, it becomes more permeable and this results in protein (proteinuria) and blood (hematuria) in the urine.
Hematuria	A condition of blood in the urine. This is a symptom of disease process.
Hypospadius	A congenital opening of the male urethra on the underside of the penis.
Interstitial cystitis	Disease of an unknown cause in which there is inflammation and irritation of the bladder. It is most commonly seen in middle-aged women.
Lithotomy	Surgical incision to remove kidney stones.
Meatotomy	A surgical enlargement of the urinary opening (meatus).
Nocturia	Excessive urination during the night. This may or may not be abnormal.
Pyelitis	Inflammation of the renal pelvis.
Pyelonephritis	Inflammation of the renal pelvis and the kidney. This is one of the most common types of kidney disease. It may be the result of a lower urinary tract infection that moved up to the kidney via the ureters. There may be large quantities of white blood cells and bacteria in the urine. Hematuria may also be present. This condition can occur whenever there is an untreated or persistent case of cystitis.
Pyuria	Presence of pus in the urine.
Renal colic	Pain caused by a kidney stone. This type of pain can be excruciating and generally requires medical treatment.

TABLE 31   Procedures and Tests Relating to the Urinary System

Procedure/Test	Description
Catheterization	The insertion of a sterile tube through the urethra and into the urinary bladder for the purpose of withdrawing urine. This procedure is used to obtain a sterile urine specimen and also to relieve distension when the patient is unable to void on their own. See Chapter 26 for procedure.
Cystography	The process of instilling a contrast material or dye into the bladder by catheter to visualize the urinary bladder.
Cystoscopy	Visual examination of the urinary bladder using an instrument called a cystoscope. The patient may receive a general anesthetic for this procedure.
Dialysis	The artificial filtration of waste material from the blood. It is used when the kidneys fail to function.
Excretory urography	Injection of dye into the bloodstream followed by taking an x-ray to trace the action of the kidney as it excretes the dye.
Hemodialysis	Use of an artificial kidney that filters the blood of a person to remove waste products. Use of this technique in patients who have defective kidneys is lifesaving.
Intravenous pyelogram (IVP)	An x-ray examination of the kidneys, ureters, and bladder by injecting a radiopaque dye into the circulatory system and tracing its route as it is excreted.
Lithotripsy	Destroying or crushing kidney stones in the bladder or urethra with a device called a lithotriptor.
Peritoneal dialysis	The removal of toxic waste substances from the body by placing warm chemically balanced solutions into the peritoneal cavity. This is used in treating renal failure and in certain types of poisonings.
Renal transplant	Surgical placement of a donor kidney.
Urinalysis	A laboratory test that consists of the physical, chemical, and microscopic examination of urine.
Urography	The use of a contrast medium to provide an x-ray of the urinary tract.

INDEX